GREEN'S
RESPIRATORY THERAPY

A Practical and Essential Tutorial
on the Core Concepts of Respiratory Care

GREEN'S
RESPIRATORY THERAPY

A Practical and Essential Tutorial
on the Core Concepts of Respiratory Care

Robert J. Green Jr., ND, RRT

Published by Aventine Press
55 E Emerson Street
Chula Vista, CA 91911

ISBN: 978-1-59330-934-3

Library of Congress Control Number: 2017912828

Printed in the United States of America

Cover Design by Mira Parker

For John, Zarah, & Joseph

Table of Contents

2. Selected Topics in Physiologic Ventilation 55

3. Selected Topics in Gas Exchange   119

4. Selected Topics in Physical Assessment 165

5. Selected Topics in Acid/Base Chemistry and the Arterial Blood Gas 193

6. Selected Topics in Hemodynamics 213

7. Selected Topics in Oxygen Therapy (and Other Medical Gases)   231

8. Selected Topics in Mechanical Ventilation   261

10. Respiratory Pharmacology   417

Drug list to include drug class, generic names, mechanism of action, side effects, delivery routes, and recommended dosages of the drugs most often encountered in the practice of respiratory therapy.

Note to the Reader

Every attempt has been made to ensure accuracy and clarity in the writing and editorial process of creating this book. Students and/or clinicians must always rely on their own experience and knowledge in evaluating and using any of the information and methods described in this book. With regards to the drugs discussed in the pharmacology chapter, readers are advised to always check the most current information that is available to verify dosage information, methods and duration of administration, and contraindications. It is the responsibility of every clinician to rely on their own experience and knowledge of their patients to make diagnoses, to determine appropriate dosages, and to select the best treatment for each individual patient. It is incumbent upon the individual clinician to always make patient safety the highest priority. The author and the publisher of this work assume no legal liability for any injury or damage to persons or property from the use, operation, or application of any methods, instructions, or ideas contained in the material herein.

Formatting Note

Due to formatting limitations, $\dot{V}_E$ will often appear simply as V_E (without the dot above the V). Know that when you see it without the dot that it is implied that you know the dot should be there. The same thing goes for V_A, V/Q, VCO_2, VO_2, Q, V, etc.

Introduction

This book is essentially a thorough compilation and revision of selected lecture and clinical notes that I had formulated during my time as a respiratory therapy student and tutor. Prior to studying respiratory therapy, I received my bachelor's degree from San Diego State University where I had studied cellular and molecular biology. After obtaining my BA from San Diego State I attended medical school, however, during the course of my medical studies I developed a particular interest in the application of complimentary and integrative medicine to the area of chronic lung disease. This interest led me to pursue research in this area, and I ultimately completed an academic ND (doctor of natural health/naturopathy) where my dissertation research involved gaining an understanding of how the methods of nutrition and natural medicine could be employed as a means to provide scientifically grounded options in the treatment of chronic obstructive pulmonary disease (COPD). My dissertation evolved into my first full length text on the subject which then underwent revision into a second edition that was published in 2007, and eventually a Spanish edition that was published in 2016.

After several years of working in natural medicine I decided to return to school to study respiratory therapy in order to expand upon my previous education and training. Respiratory therapy was a perfect fit in that it was a natural extension of what I had already been doing for almost a decade. I want to mention here that despite my academic background prior to attending respiratory therapy school, I still had to study diligently. Even though I was a Sputum Bowl finalist and graduated first in my class, and passed both parts of the boards on the first attempt to earn my RRT credential, it was not without very hard work and persistent effort that any of that came to pass. As the majority of respiratory therapy programs are still associate degree programs, most students do not enter with an extensive academic background, nor do most students realize what they are getting themselves into regarding the intensity of a respiratory therapy program.

This brings us to the point of why I decided to write this

book. Given the background that I had acquired prior to attending respiratory therapy school, I was hired by my department chairman to be the departmental tutor for the respiratory therapy program. So not only was I a student in the program, but from the beginning of the second semester until graduation I also served as the tutor for the program and held regular office hours where I met with dozens of students several times a week for the next 4 semesters. It was through my interaction with these students and helping them to understand the material that I became acutely aware of the areas in which they struggled. Students struggle with material for a variety of reasons, but one of the main reasons I found was because they enter into the program without being sufficiently prepared in the basic sciences. This is due in part because in an associate degree program you take your basic science courses along with your respiratory therapy courses at the same time, yet the material you are covering in your respiratory therapy courses assumes that you already have the appropriate basic science background. In a bachelor's degree program, this is less of an issue because a student spends their first two years studying basic science and doesn't begin respiratory therapy courses until they are a junior. Associate degree program students do not have such a luxury and must study basic science along with respiratory therapy simultaneously and therein lies the significant challenge for many as it can get very overwhelming. It becomes overwhelming not only because of the sheer volume of material being presented at a quick pace, but also because they often find themselves struggling to be able to understand both their lectures and their primary textbook. The other main issue I found to be true was that most students were not experienced with knowing how to study properly or how to prioritize their time. It is important to know how to study – to know how to organize and prioritize material, and to know how to be disciplined and allocate the time needed to cover said material until it is mastered. The respiratory therapy curriculum is difficult and challenging - I can't put it any other way.

Being organized and knowing how to prioritize your time in becoming an effective student is something that each individual student will have to master in order to not only be a successful student, but to also be a good respiratory therapist. Having a solid base of knowledge in your head is only part of what is necessary to be a good practitioner. Proper management of your patients not only requires you to be knowledgeable, but also that you are able to prioritize tasks and effectively manage your time. These are things that you will hopefully learn as you progress through your clinical rotations as a student. Having said that, the aim of this text is to help you achieve mastery of the core concepts of respiratory care – the basics and the nuts and bolts of what you absolutely must have in your everyday working memory. When it comes to studying material (and especially preparing for an exam), I can't tell you the number of times that I heard students ask their professors "what do I need to know"? And the standard response at my school was "everything" - you need to know everything. This does not mean that you have to memorize every last word of your textbook, but it does mean that you must have a fluent grasp of core concepts and be well versed in the material such that you can competently think on your feet and solve the myriad problems that constantly arise in the clinical management of a patient. Very few of the questions you are going to be asked on an exam are going to be what we refer to as straightforward recall questions. Most of the questions you are going to be asked are going to be application and analysis questions that test your ability to take the factual knowledge you have learned and apply it to a clinical situation. The entire clinical simulation exam that you will take as the second part of your boards is going to question you exactly in this manner. It is incumbent upon you to understand this right now and begin to prepare yourself properly so that as you progress through your program you are learning how to not only master the facts that you need to know, but to then know how to apply that knowledge in the practice of clinical respiratory care.

This book is not intended to be a complete and comprehensive treatment of the entire subject of respiratory therapy. It is therefore never meant to replace your primary textbook. The purpose of this book is to serve as a tutorial – a supplement to your lectures and primary textbook that gives specific coverage to those areas that are often difficult for many students. Hopefully my explanations will help you understand the material. Before you get to the point where you can start thinking like a clinician and be able to analyze the complexities of clinical situations, you must first have a firm mastery of the material. The chief aim of this book is to present the material to you as succinctly as possible so as to enable you to not only grasp and understand the material, but to permanently retain it in your working memory. You will not find a table of formulas at the end of the book. Rather, you will find formulas and equations presented throughout the text in the sections where they are relevant so that you can understand them in context. Throughout my time as the departmental tutor in the respiratory therapy program I was always being asked by students if I would let them copy my notes. I very rarely obliged that request – not because I didn't want to share my notes, but mainly because the organization of them would not have been easy to follow. What follows in the pages of this book is a well-organized revision of all those notes along with the appropriate prose needed to explain the concepts in a manner that hopefully enables you to grasp and retain the material. In its own unique way, this text serves as my way of being able to act as your tutor. To obtain its maximum value, this book has to be read thoroughly and digested completely. As I said earlier – although this book covers a great deal of material, it is not wholly comprehensive as its primary mission is to address *only* those areas that are problematic for most students. It will present things in a very clear and well-organized manner so that you will have confidence in your understanding. I have made every attempt to write in such a way so that it seems as though if I was just talking to you. There is obviously much more material that you need to know besides just that which is in this book, but if you develop an attitude of wanting to know as much as you possibly can, you will have served yourself well. So – to ask the question again - "what do I need to know"? Know as much as you possibly can! I want to wish you all the very best in your studies and your pursuit of this most excellent profession.

Robert J. Green Jr.
August 2017

Chapter 1

Selected Topics in Physics

Having a solid understanding of certain basic fundamentals of physics is essential to just about everything that you will encounter in respiratory care. Normal physiologic ventilation, gas exchange, medical gas therapy, and mechanical ventilation are but just a few of the areas of respiratory care that involve concepts from physics that must be thoroughly understood. This chapter will highlight and explain some of the most important and fundamental concepts of physics that are necessary for you to have in your working memory. Many of these concepts and ideas will reappear in later chapters of this text, and they will be reinforced as they are applied to the material that is being discussed at that time.

A. The Gas Laws

This section is going to discuss and explain the gas laws, and show how and when they are applied in different situations.

Things to keep in mind when dealing with the gas laws

1.   All temperatures must be in K (Kelvin) when working a gas law problem. Depending upon how the data is presented in a problem, you may have to do some conversions first to get the temperature in Kelvin.

Temperature   1. $°F = (9/5 \times °C) + 32$ **or** $(1.8 \times °C) + 32$

Conversion   2. $°C = 5/9 (°F - 32)$ **or** $(°F - 32) / 1.8$

Equations   3. $K = °C + 273$

- Fahrenheit and Celsius expressions of temperature are based upon the freezing & boiling points of water, whereas Kelvin is based upon thermal motion.

- Temperature is a measure of the average kinetic energy of the molecules of a substance.

2. *Remember* that if water vapor is present in a mixture of gases, it must be accounted for because it lowers the partial pressures of the other gases in the mixture.

3. *Therefore - Remember* to correct P for water vapor when necessary - (P_{H20} = 47mmHg @ 37° C). This means for example that if you're doing a Boyle's law problem or a combined gas law problem, and you have to account for the presence of water vapor, then you must subtract the water vapor pressure from the pressure given in the problem before proceeding with solving the problem.

4. *Remember* that for a constant temperature and pressure, a saturated gas will always have a larger volume than that same gas would if it was dry.

5. *Remember* the following abbreviations as you will encounter them at times when dealing with combined gas law problems. There will be times when you will be given information in one form, but yet will be asked to give your result in another form. An example of this would be if you were given information about a gas at BTPS, but the question was asking for the answer in terms of STPD. An actual example of this will be illustrated when the combined gas law is discussed in a few pages.

ATPS – ambient temperature and pressure saturated
ATPD – ambient temperature and pressure dry
BTPS – body temperature and pressure saturated
STPD – standard temperature and pressure dry, which is
        0° C, 760 mmHg, dry

BOYLE'S LAW, CHARLE'S LAW, and GAY-LUSSAC'S LAW

* Note that mass is constant in all 3 of these laws.

* Note also that with problems involving these laws you have 4 variables – 3 of which you will already know - they will be given to you in the problem. It is just a matter of you utilizing basic algebra to solve for your unknown variable.

BOYLE'S LAW

$$P_1V_1 = P_2V_2$$

Volume varies <u>inversely</u> with pressure at *constant temperature*. This law applies in matters of *ventilation*. Boyle's law explains how changing the size (volume) of the thorax during spontaneous ventilation produces the pressure gradients necessary for normal breathing.

CHARLE'S LAW

$$\frac{V_1}{T_1} = \frac{V_2}{T_2}$$

Volume varies <u>directly</u> with temperature at *constant pressure*. This law is most often applied when doing *ATPS / BTPS corrections*. Note that you can change this formula from being expressed in terms of a division problem to that of a multiplication problem via cross multiplying and it will still mean the same thing.

$$V_1T_2 = V_2T_1$$

Just remember that if you do this – make sure you keep

track of your variables and ensure their proper placement in the equation.

GAY-LUSSAC'S LAW

$$\frac{P_1}{T_1} = \frac{P_2}{T_2}$$

Pressure varies <u>directly</u> with temperature at *constant volume*. This law is most often applied when doing problems involving *cylinder pressures*. Note that you can also change this formula from being expressed in terms of a division problem to that of a multiplication problem via cross multiplying and it will still mean the same thing.

$$P_1T_2 = P_2T_1$$

Again – make sure you keep track of your variables and ensure their proper placement in the equation.

I want to take a moment to clarify what is meant in the aforementioned gas laws when it is stated that one thing varies either *directly* or *inversely* with another thing. When it is said that something "varies directly" (another way of putting it is to say that it is "directly related to") with something else - this means that as one variable gets bigger, the other variable also gets correspondingly bigger. By the same token, it also means that if one variable gets smaller, the other variable also gets correspondingly smaller. Take Charles Law for example: It states that volume varies directly with temperature at constant pressure. This means that as the temperature increases, the volume will correspondingly increase. It also means that if the temperature decreases, the volume will decrease. *As temperature goes up, volume goes up – as temperature goes down, volume goes down.* The formula of Charles Law enables you to calculate by how much.   The same concept applies to Gay-Lussac's Law except in this case you are dealing with pressure and temperature rather than volume and temperature. In Gay-Lussac's Law, it states that pressure varies directly with temperature at constant volume. This means that as the temperature increases, the pressure will correspondingly increase.   It also means that if the temperature decreases, the pressure will decrease. *As temperature goes up, pressure goes up – As temperature goes down, pressure goes down.* The formula of Gay-Lussac's Law enables you to calculate by how much.

With Boyle's Law, however, the variables are not related to one another *directly*, but rather they are *inversely* related. This means that as one variable gets bigger, the other variable gets smaller. By the same token, it also means that if one variable gets smaller, the other variable gets bigger. Boyle's Law states that volume varies inversely (or is inversely related) with pressure at constant temperature. This means that as the volume increases, the pressure will correspondingly decrease. It also means that if the volume decreases, the pressure will correspondingly increase. *As volume goes up, pressure goes down – as volume goes down, pressure goes up.* The formula of Boyle's Law enables you to calculate by how much.

When used correctly, these formulas will always enable you to solve for your unknown variable. They are straightforward and simple enough formulas to use, however, it is important to take a moment to visualize them – especially Boyle's law as it is central to the dynamics of spontaneous ventilation. You will gain a fuller appreciation for Boyle's law in the next chapter on ventilation.

THE COMBINED GAS LAW

$$\frac{P_1 V_1}{T_1} = \frac{P_2 V_2}{T_2}$$

This law is a combination of all three gas laws. There are no constants except for mass. It involves slightly more complex interactions between the variables, but so long as you keep track of your variables you will be fine when solving problems of this type. Remember that despite there being six variables in a problem of this type, you will always be given five of them in the problem. *One of the more common ways* you will see this problem is when you will be given an initial volume (V_1), pressure (P_1), and temperature (T_1). You'll also be given a final pressure (P_2) and temperature (T_2), and will be asked to determine what the final volume (V_2) would be.

$$V_2 = \frac{P_1 V_1 T_2}{P_2 T_1}$$

At the end of the day your task is to be able to read the problem and determine what information you have been given (which 5 of the 6 variables have you been given) such that you then know the unknown variable you are solving for. The rest is simply a matter of very carefully rearranging the equation in order that you may solve it for your unknown. In the immediate example above the equation was rearranged in order to be able to solve for V_2. If the problem asks you to solve for a different variable other than a final volume, just make sure you properly rearrange the equation in order to solve for the unknown variable that you are looking for.

Example 1: $V_1 = 3500$ml $V_2 = ?$
               $P_1 = 720$ mmHg $P_2 = 750$ mmHg
               $T_1 = 35°C$ $T_2 = 30°C$

$$V_2 = \frac{P_1 V_1 T_2}{P_2 T_1} \qquad V_2 = \frac{(720)(3500)(303)}{(750)(308)}$$

don't forget to change temp. to K

(°C + 273)

$$V_2 = \frac{763{,}560{,}000}{231{,}000} = 3305\text{ml}$$

Let us now consider a problem where it involves converting from BTPS to STPD, or ATPS to BTPS, or whatever – it doesn't matter. These types of problems are handled exactly the same way as any other combined gas law problem would be handled – you just have to remember the values for the various parameters. That means that you need to remember that with STPD the temperature is 0°C, pressure is 760 mmHg, and it's dry – so there's no subtracting water vapor. With BTPS the temperature is 37°C, pressure is 760 mmHg, and it's saturated – so you'll need to subtract the water vapor pressure (47 mmHg) from the 760 mmHg.

Example 2: A volume of gas is 5000ml at BTPS. What is its volume at STPD?

BTPS is body temperature and pressure *saturated*
STPD is standard temperature and pressure *dry*

BTPS   STPD

V_1 = 5000ml V_2 = ?
P_1 = 760 mmHg P_2 = 760 mmHg
T_1 = 37°C ⟶ 310K T_2 = 0°C ⟶ 273K
P_{H2O} = 47 mmHg P_{H2O} = 0
  – this is an example where you   - there is no water vapor to
   have to account for water vapor   to account for because it is
   because BTPS means the gas is   STPD – it's dry.
   saturated.

$$V_2 = \frac{P_1 V_1 T_2}{P_2 T_1}$$

$$V_2 = \frac{(760 - 47)(5000)(273)}{(760)(310)}$$

$$V_2 = \frac{(713)(5000)(273)}{(760)(310)} = \frac{973,245,000}{235,600} = 4130.9 \text{ or } 4131\text{ml.}$$

Note – water vapor pressure (P_{H2O}) is only 47 mmHg at 37°C (body temperature) – that's good for BTPS. But remember that water vapor pressure varies with temperature – so if the problem is dealing with ATPS – then the P_{H2O} for the particular ambient temperature in the problem *must be given to you.*

B. Other Important Laws

GRAHAM'S LAW

Graham's law is used to compare the rates of diffusion of two gases at a *constant temperature and pressure.* The formula has two forms depending upon whether you are considering gas diffusion simply in the air or across the alveolar-capillary (A/C) membrane in the lung.

The following formula is the first form of Graham's Law. It is to be used when comparing the rates of diffusion of two gases that are simply diffusing in the air.

$$\frac{R_1}{R_2} = \frac{\sqrt{gmw_2}}{\sqrt{gmw_1}}$$

where R refers to the rates and gmw refers to the gram molecular weights of the gases.

- At constant pressure and temperature, the rates are *inversely related* to the square root of their molecular weights.
- Light gases diffuse at a rapid rate.
- Heavier gases diffuse at a slower rate.
- Increased heat and/or mechanical agitation accelerates the rate of diffusion.

This is the second form of Graham's law. It is to be used when comparing the rates of diffusion of two gases across the alveolar-capillary (A/C) membrane in the lung.

$$\frac{R_1}{R_2} = \frac{SC_1 \sqrt{gmw_2}}{SC_2 \sqrt{gmw_1}}$$

- Remember that the A/C membrane consists of the alveolar epithelium, the interstitial fluid, and the capillary endothelium.
- Therefore, when comparing the rates of diffusion of two gases across the A/C membrane, you must include the **solubility coefficient (SC)** in the Graham's Law formula because fluid is involved.
  - SC for oxygen is 0.023ml at 37°C & 760 mmHg.
  - SC for carbon dioxide is 0.510ml at 37°C & 760 mmHg.
  - *Carbon dioxide is 22 times more soluble in plasma than oxygen.*
- At constant temperature and pressure, the rates are *directly related* to the solubility coefficients and *inversely related* to the square root of their molecular weights.

A Word About the Solubility Coefficient

- The solubility coefficient (SC) of a gas in a liquid is the number of milliliters of the gas that will dissolve in 1ml of the liquid at a temperature of 37°C and 760 mmHg. *Note that 37°C is used in this definition because the fluid in this case is plasma at normal body temperature.*
- Note however that the SC varies inversely with temperature.
- As temperature increases, solubility coefficient decreases.

  A generic example of this is the illustration of carbonated soda pop. Soda pop will retain its carbonation better when kept refrigerated. If left out and it warms up, the solubility of the gas in the soda is lessened and thus the gas escapes quicker and the soda pop becomes flat. Hence gases in general are more soluble in liquids that are colder.

An example of utilizing Graham's Law (the second form) to compare the rates of diffusion of carbon dioxide and oxygen across the A/C membrane.

$$\frac{R_1}{R_2} = \frac{SC_1 \sqrt{gmw_2}}{SC_2 \sqrt{gmw_1}}$$

$$\frac{R_{CO2}}{R_{O2}} = \frac{.510 \sqrt{32}}{.023 \sqrt{44}}$$ (32 is the molecular wt. of O_2)

(44 is the molecular wt. of CO_2)

$$\frac{R_{CO2}}{R_{O2}} = \frac{.510}{.023} \quad \frac{5.65}{6.63}$$

$$\frac{R_{CO2}}{R_{O2}} = \frac{2.88}{.152}$$

$$\frac{R_{CO2}}{R_{O2}} \approx 19$$

Therefore, carbon dioxide diffuses across the A/C membrane about 19 times faster than oxygen – which is consistent with what we would expect due to carbon dioxide being so much more soluble than oxygen to begin with.

Don't let the solubility coefficient (SC) confuse you. When you are comparing two gases that are just diffusing in the air, you use the first form of Graham's Law without the solubility coefficient. When comparing two gases that are diffusing across the A/C membrane, you have to use the second form of Graham's Law which includes the solubility coefficient because remember that there is fluid (liquid) associated with the parts of the A/C membrane – the alveolar epithelium (which are cells), the interstitial fluid (very similar to/essentially plasma), and the capillary endothelium (which are cells).

HENRY'S LAW

Henry's Law addresses the question of *how much* of a gas will dissolve in a liquid (plasma again in our case). Specifically, the law states that the amount of gas that will dissolve in a liquid (plasma) is equal to the product of the partial pressure of the gas and its solubility coefficient. Consider oxygen as an example:

Amount of gas dissolved = PaO_2 x   SC

- Note here that we are talking about a gas *dissolving* in a liquid – we're not talking about gas diffusion as was the case in the aforementioned Graham's Law. Even though the SC was involved with the second form of Graham's Law due to fluid being involved, Graham's Law was still addressing gas diffusion whereas Henry's law is specifically talking about a gas dissolving, not a gas diffusing – remember to keep that straight.

Recall that the solubility coefficient (SC) given for oxygen in the previous section on Graham's law was 0.023ml at 37°C & 760 mmHg. Remember also from the previous section that the solubility coefficient was defined in terms of the number of milliliters of gas that would dissolve in **1ml** of plasma. In the case of Henry's Law, we are now dealing with **100 ml** of plasma – not just 1ml - and therefore the solubility coefficient (SC) to be used for oxygen is 0.003ml and *here is why*. The simplest and most practical way to explain this is to use the example of when Henry's Law is applied after obtaining the PaO_2 from an arterial blood gas (ABG). Arterial blood gases (ABG's) are determined as per 100ml of plasma, not 1ml. Hence the solubility coefficient number has to be converted to reflect per 100ml. It is also necessary to express the SC in terms of 1 mmHg rather than 760 mmHg. In Henry's Law, you're multiplying the PaO_2 by the SC, and the PaO_2 is expressed in terms of mmHg, therefore you need to have the SC expressed in terms of mmHg – not 760 mmHg.

Consider the following:

Previously in the Graham's Law section it was stated that the SC of oxygen was 0.023ml per 1ml of plasma at 37°C and 760 mmHg.

But remember that when it comes to analyzing an ABG that it is calculated in terms of 100ml – not 1ml.

Therefore, follow the math to understand how the SC gets converted in order to be able to be used with Henry's Law.

$$\frac{0.023ml}{1ml} = \frac{X}{100\ ml}$$

cross multiply and you get:

$$(X)\ ml\ =\ 2.3ml$$

therefore X = 2.3ml per 100ml of plasma @ 760 mmHg

Don't worry about reconciling the units in these equations as they are not going to cancel as you would expect. I've taken liberty to simplify things. Just know that this is how it is done and that this is the right way to determine the solubility coefficient for oxygen when being used with Henry's Law.

But remember also that you want to know the SC for 1 mmHg rather than 760 mmHg.

$$\frac{2.3\text{ml}}{760\text{ mmHg}} = \frac{X}{\textbf{1 mmHg}}$$

cross multiply and you get:

(X) 760 mmHg = 2.3ml

solve for X

therefore X = 0.003ml per 100ml of plasma @ 1 mmHg

The SC that was previously expressed as 0.023ml per 1ml of plasma at 760 mmHg is now expressed as 0.003ml per 100ml of plasma at 1 mmHg. It can also be noted that the temperature in both instances is 37°C (body temperature).

With this now being understood, it can be shown how this is used with Henry's Law. Say for example that you draw an ABG and it reveals that the patient has a PaO_2 of 100 mmHg. By using the properly converted form of the SC as just demonstrated, you can now determine the amount of oxygen dissolved per 100ml of plasma.

Henry's Law: Amount of gas dissolved = PaO_2 x SC

Amount of gas dissolved = 100 mmHg x 0.003ml

Amount of gas dissolved = 0.3ml

or 0.3ml O_2 per 100ml of plasma

DALTON'S LAW

Dalton's Law (or Dalton's Law of Partial Pressures) deals with the relationship between the partial pressures of the individual gases in a mixture and the total gas pressure of the mixture. Another way of stating this is to say that the whole (the total pressure of the gas mixture) is equal to the sum of its parts (the various partial pressures of the gases in the mixture).

Consider the atmosphere as an example for a general understanding of this idea. Generally speaking, the atmosphere *primarily* consists of:

O_2	.2095 or 21%	*These fractional*
N_2	.7808 or 78%	*percentages do*
CO_2	.0004 or .04%	*not change*

Dalton's Law states that the sum of the partial pressures of these constituent atmospheric gases must equal the total pressure. The total pressure in this case is what you know as the barometric pressure – and barometric pressure is expressed as P_B. Now P_B at sea level is 760 mmHg, and that consists of all three of the aforementioned gases. Since we know what the fractional percentages are for each of the gases in the atmosphere, we can readily determine their respective partial pressures.

The formula to calculate the particular partial pressure of a given gas in a mixture is as follows:

$$P_B \times F = P$$

where P_B is the barometric pressure (total pressure of all the atmospheric gases), F is the fractional percentage of whichever particular gas we are considering, and P is the partial pressure of that particular gas.

For oxygen it is: 760 mmHg x (.21)   =   160 mmHg

For nitrogen it is: 760 mmHg x (.78)   =   593 mmHg

For carbon dioxide it is: 760 mmHg x (.0004) =   .30 mmHg
                                                   _____

                                                   753.3 mmHg

Now Dalton's Law expressed as a formula is as follows:

$$P_{total} = P_1 + P_2 + P_3 + P_n$$

Applying this formula to the gases in the atmosphere gives:

$$P_B = P_{O2} + P_{N2} + P_{CO2}$$

where P_B is the total pressure (barometric pressure), and P_{O2}, P_{N2}, and P_{CO2} are the partial pressures of the constituent gases.

Therefore:

$$P_B \quad = \quad P_{O2} \quad + \quad P_{N2} \quad + \quad P_{CO2}$$
$$760 \text{ mmHg} \quad = \quad 160 \text{ mmHg} + 593 \text{ mmHg} + .30 \text{ mmHg}$$

$$760 \text{ mmHg} \quad \approx \quad 753.3 \text{ mmHg}$$

Dalton's Law thus demonstrates that the sum of the partial pressures of the gases in the atmosphere does indeed equal the total gas pressure in the atmosphere – which is 760 mmHg (barometric pressure). You may say how does 760 = 753.3? The other 6 – 7 mmHg (< 1%) is accounted for by the other trace gases in the atmosphere that were not included in this example for the sake of simplicity.

Thus far Dalton's Law has been discussed in terms of gases in the air (the atmosphere). Dalton's Law also applies to gases inside the lung, and although the basic conceptual idea is the same insofar as the total gas pressure inside the lung must be equal to the sum of the partial pressures of the constituent gases in the lung, the method of calculating the partial pressures in the lung is a bit different. Remember that the upper airway adds water vapor to inspired air – and that water vapor exerts a pressure (P_{H2O}) of 47 mmHg at 37°C that must be accounted for. At different temperatures the P_{H2O} will vary. And in general, there is also a *direct* relationship between gas partial pressures and the patient's temperature.

The modified version of the partial pressure formula when determining the partial pressures of *inspired* gases is as follows: (oxygen is being used as an example)

$$(P_B - P_{H2O}) \times FiO_2 = PIO_2$$

It's not all that different from $P_B \times F = P$. Just note that rather than just having P_B, you have to remember to subtract the water vapor (P_{H2O}) which is 47 mmHg. And rather than just having (F) you have (FiO_2) because the patient may not be breathing room air where oxygen is 21%. What if the patient is on oxygen therapy or is intubated and is being given a percentage of oxygen that is higher than 21%? You have to account for this because it will affect the partial pressure of oxygen (PIO_2). And "PIO_2" simply means partial pressure of *inspired* oxygen.

It is important to realize that PIO_2 is only talking about the partial pressure of inspired oxygen to about the level of the bronchi. At an FiO_2 of 21% (room air), the PIO_2 would be about 150 mmHg – and that is 10 mmHg less than what the partial pressure of oxygen was in the atmosphere due to the upper airway having added water vapor to the mixture of inspired gases.

$$(P_B - P_{H2O}) \times FiO_2 = PIO_2$$

$$(760 \text{ mmHg} - 47 \text{ mmHg}) \times (.21) \approx 150 \text{ mmHg}$$

PAO$_2$, however, is the partial pressure of oxygen in the *alveoli* – and that is what we are really interested in when we refer to the partial pressure of oxygen in the lung – and it is even lower than PIO$_2$ because at the level of the alveoli the presence of carbon dioxide becomes significant and must be accounted for when determining partial pressures. In the atmosphere and at the level of the bronchi, carbon dioxide has virtually no effect on the partial pressures of the other *inspired* gases because it's fractional percentage in those places is so small as to be insignificant. In the alveoli, however, the amount of carbon dioxide *is* significant, and therefore has a direct effect on the partial pressures of the other gases in the alveoli. This is why the modified equation just given is incomplete and not sufficient enough to determine a proper PAO$_2$ - because it doesn't account for carbon dioxide. Although the normal partial pressure of carbon dioxide in the alveoli is relatively stable at 40 mmHg, it can fluctuate due to metabolic and/or pathological reasons – and this must be accounted for because it will affect the PAO$_2$. Furthermore, the uptake per minute of oxygen from the alveoli into the blood is not equal to the excretion per minute of carbon dioxide from the blood into the alveoli – and this must also be accounted for. Proper determination of the partial pressure of oxygen in the alveoli (PAO$_2$) therefore requires using what is known as the alveolar air equation. The good news is that the modified formula just presented on the last page is about 90% of the alveolar air equation anyway. There are a few more concepts that you must learn first in order to have the full picture, and those concepts along with the alveolar air equation will be covered in chapter 3.

Finally - always remember that the fractional percentage of oxygen is constant at all points in the atmosphere - (.2095) or 21%. Therefore, as you go up in elevation and the P$_B$ drops, the partial pressure of O$_2$ in the atmosphere will be less according to Dalton's Law. This is why supplemental O$_2$ is needed at high elevations. By increasing the fractional percentage artificially by giving supplemental oxygen you will effectively maintain a proper partial pressure of oxygen in the blood.

C. Gas Behavior at Extreme Temperatures and Pressure

Changes in gas behavior at extreme temperatures and/or pressures are due to the involvement of forces known as Van der Waals forces. Under normal conditions most gases will display ideal behavior, but at extreme temperatures and/or pressures this can change due to the effect that Van der Waals forces can have on gas molecules under these extreme conditions. Van der Waals forces are encountered primarily in the area of physical chemistry; therefore, a thorough discussion of this matter is beyond the scope of this text or your curriculum. What is necessary for you to understand is that *they are mainly weak attractive forces that can oppose the motion of gas molecules*, and that extreme temperature and/or pressure can affect these forces.

Therefore - deviations in the ideal behavior of a gas can occur at:

1. Extremely low temperatures

   At extremely low temperatures, the movement of gas molecules is greatly reduced. With the gas molecules moving less, the Van der Waals forces of weak attraction between gas molecules are thus more pronounced, and are therefore able to exert a greater effect in being able to oppose gas motion since the gas molecules have significantly less kinetic energy at extremely low temperatures.

2. Extremely high pressures

   At extremely high pressure, the gas molecules are much closer to one another. With the gas molecules being so much closer together, the Van der Waals forces of weak attraction between gas molecules are thus more pronounced, and are therefore able to exert a greater effect in being able to oppose gas motion.

D. Critical Temperature & Critical Pressure

CRITICAL TEMPERATURE

Every substance has what is known as a critical temperature. The critical temperature of a substance is the temperature above which the gaseous state of the substance cannot be liquefied - no matter how much pressure is applied. This temperature therefore indicates the maximum temperature at which something is able to exist in the liquid state - beyond this temperature no amount of pressure will be able to maintain equilibrium between the liquid and gas phases of the molecules. Once you exceed the critical temperature, there is no amount of pressure that can liquefy the gas.

CRITICAL PRESSURE

The critical pressure therefore is the pressure required to maintain the liquid – gas equilibrium *at the critical temperature.*

* Furthermore – the cooler a gas is below its critical temperature, the less pressure it takes to liquefy it.

Consider the example of oxygen to illustrate these concepts:

Oxygen has a critical temperature of -181.5 °F and a critical pressure of 49.7 Atmospheres. *(1 atm = 760 mmHg)*

What this means from the explanations above is that -181.5 °F is the highest temperature at which oxygen can exist as a liquid (hence liquid oxygen is extremely cold), and above that temperature there is no amount of pressure that will keep oxygen in the liquid state. The critical pressure of 49.7 Atmospheres is the pressure required to maintain the liquid - gas equilibrium when oxygen is at its critical temperature of -181.5 °F.

When you are at both the critical temperature and the critical pressure – this is known as the *Critical Point*.

Now look at carbon dioxide:

Carbon dioxide has a critical temperature of 87.8 °F and a critical pressure of 73 Atmospheres. This means that 87.8 °F is the highest temperature at which carbon dioxide can exist as a liquid and that it will take a pressure of 73 Atmospheres to maintain the liquid – gas equilibrium at this temperature. Beyond this temperature there is no amount of pressure that will be able to maintain the equilibrium, therefore the carbon dioxide will be entirely in the gaseous phase.

So, when it comes to liquefying a gas you either **a)** lower the temperature to below its boiling point, or **b)** lower the temperature to below the critical temperature and apply pressure. Take note though in the case of carbon dioxide at room temperature - since its critical temperature is above ambient you can liquefy it with just pressure – there isn't the need to have to lower the temperature because at ambient (room) temperature you are already below the critical temperature for carbon dioxide.

Note - the difference between a true gas and a vapor

A true gas is a state of matter - a vapor is not. A vapor is a substance in its gas *phase* at a temperature lower than its critical temperature.

The fundamental difference between a gas and a vapor is that a gas has a single defined thermodynamic state at room temperature whereas a vapor is in equilibrium with a liquid because it is able to undergo phase changes. A gas only exists in the gaseous state at room temperature – the critical temperature is too low to allow otherwise. A vapor, however, is the gaseous phase of a substance that is below its critical temperature, and can therefore be liquefied by pressure alone. A vapor therefore is able to co-exist with its liquid phase at room temperature.

E. Flow   *to follow the presentation of this section, your algebra prowess needs to be solidly intact*

The concept of flow is a very important concept in respiratory care and it is also one of the concepts that is often misunderstood by students when they encounter it formally for the first time. In the most basic sense, flow is simply the movement of fluid per unit of time. This is true not only for liquids, but always remember that gases are classified as fluids as well, and much of what will be discussed about flow needs to be understood in the context of gas flow. Since flow by definition is the movement of fluid per unit time, it is useful to think of flow in terms of *flow rate*.

Flow rate and the Law of Continuity

$$\text{flow rate } (\dot{V}) = \frac{\text{volume (in ml or L)}}{\text{time (minutes or seconds)}}$$

This gives a flow rate ($\dot{V}$ – called "v dot") that is usually expressed in terms of LPM (liters per minute) or occasionally LPS (liters per second), but the most common way you will see flow rate expressed is LPM (liters per minute).

Consider now the following ideas:

Flow rate is expressed in terms of volume and time as just shown above, however, the *Law of Continuity* enables us to also know that for a given constant flow rate, the velocity of a fluid through a tube is inversely related to the cross-sectional area of the tube. And note here that the word "tube" not only applies to what one would think of as a normal tube like a hose for example, but also the airways of the respiratory tract – always remember that gases are fluids that flow thru tubes (the airways). When the inverse relationship between velocity and cross-sectional area (at a constant flow) is represented mathematically, it can then be shown how flow is also equal to the product of cross sectional area and velocity.

Follow this:

Given that:

$$\text{velocity} = \frac{\text{flow}}{\text{cross-sectional area}}$$

Then via
simple algebra: flow = cross sectional area x velocity

These equations show the inverse relationship between
velocity and cross-sectional area (at constant flow)
according to the Law of Continuity.

Therefore, if the cross-sectional area decreases, then the velocity must increase in order to maintain the same flow. **This is the key factor that relates velocity to flow.** And it will do this proportionally – meaning that cutting the cross-sectional area in half requires doubling the velocity in order to maintain the same flow rate.

Flow is generally discussed in terms of *type of flow* and/or the *pattern of flow*. Let us first address the two types of flow.

1. Bulk Flow – bulk flow is when all the molecules move together in response to a pressure gradient. **This is the type of flow seen in the large and medium airways.**

2. Diffusional Flow – diffusional flow is when *individual* molecules move from an area of higher partial pressure to an area of lower partial pressure – flow is down the concentration/diffusion gradient. **This is the type of flow in the smallest airways and across the A/C (alveolar-capillary) membrane.**

Resistance to flow

Before moving on to the three patterns of flow, it is necessary to have a discussion about resistance, and more specifically - flow resistance (or resistance to flow). In general, resistance will always be encountered when a fluid moves through a tube – and gas moving through the airway is analogous to fluid moving through a tube.

The *basic* equation for flow resistance is given by:

$$R = \frac{\Delta P}{\dot{V}}$$

Resistance is the ratio of pressure and flow

$\dot{V}$ = flow (volume/unit time – or LPM)
R = resistance
ΔP = difference in pressure ($P_1 - P_2$) – *the pressure gradient*

A simple rearrangement of the equation just given leads to:

$$\dot{V} = \frac{\Delta P}{R}$$

Flow is the ratio of pressure and resistance

ΔP (delta P) means "the change in P". ΔP is simply the shorthand way of expressing ($P_1 - P_2$). The first equation relates resistance to pressure and flow. The second equation shows how flow relates to pressure and resistance. But if you look closely at both equations, you will notice in each case that resistance and flow are inversely related to one another because either equation leads to $\Delta P = R \times V$. *For a given pressure that is constant, an increase in resistance will always result in a decrease in flow – and vice versa.*

Resistance can be caused by a variety of factors. In the case of fluid moving through a tube, what is often encountered is frictional resistance that is caused by the viscosity of the fluid and the friction that occurs between the fluid and the wall of the tube. More particularly as it pertains to the airways you will find resistance being created by the various pathologies that cause narrowing of the airways as well as occluding the airways. Consider the following which will illustrate the ramifications of resistance.

The equation that relates resistance to the radius of a tube is given by the following:

$$R = \frac{1}{r^4}$$

Where R = resistance
and r = radius of tube.

By way of example – take two tubes, one with a radius of 1mm and the other with a radius of 2mm. By substituting 1 into the equation for r, the first tube will have a resistance of 1. By substituting 2 into the equation for r, the second tube has a resistance of 1/16. This means that the first tube has a resistance that is 16 times greater than that of the second tube. That is a significant change in resistance for just a 1mm change in radius. This means that for a given pressure that is driving the flow through the 2mm tube – if the radius is reduced to 1mm, you will now have to increase the pressure by a factor of 16 in order to maintain the same flow as before. This should clearly illustrate why the various pathologies that cause narrowing of the airways (thus reducing the radius of the tube) have profound implications on respiratory health. Let us continue our discussion of flow by now considering the three patterns of flow.

3 PATTERNS OF FLOW

1. LAMINAR FLOW

- Laminar flow is characterized by the motion of fluid through discreet cylindrical layers called streamlines.
- Δv (the change in velocity) between these different layers is defined as the shear rate.
- The shear rate (Δv between the layers) is determined by:

  * Shear stress – the pressure behind the fluid
  * The fluid's viscosity

& if $\text{Viscosity} = \dfrac{\text{Shear Stress}}{\text{Shear Rate}}$ then $\text{Shear Rate} = \dfrac{\text{Shear Stress}}{\text{Viscosity}}$

Therefore: * Shear rate is directly related to shear stress
            * Shear rate is inversely related to the fluid's viscosity

Laminar flow is when you have concentric layers (streamlines) of fluid flowing parallel to the wall of a tube, and the velocities of those layers successively increases as the center of the fluid is approached.

Laminar Flow - cross-sectional view of fluid flowing through a tube

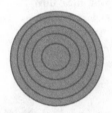

* Each of the concentric circles defines the border of one of the streamlines of flow – these are the "layers" of flowing fluid.

* As you go from the edge (the wall of the tube) to the center of the fluid, the velocity of the flow in each layer successively increases.

- The fluid in the outermost layer has the lowest velocity.
- The fluid in the innermost layer has the highest velocity.

In the case of laminar (smooth) flow, *Poisseuille's Law* is applied in order to understand the relationship between driving pressure and flow. Poisseuille's Law also explains the relationship between the diameter (although expressed as the radius in the equation, it is still speaking to the lumen) of a tube and the resistance to flow through the tube.

The form of **Poisseuille's Law** to consider is:

$$\Delta P = \frac{8\mu l V}{\pi\, r^4}$$

The equation here for Poisseuille's Law is just a more elaborate and more sophisticated expression of the ideas expressed in the resistance equations a couple pages back. If you were to combine those previous 3 equations, you would see that $\Delta P = V/r^4$ This should enable you to see the similarity of Poisseuille's equation.

V is flow
ΔP is the pressure gradient

8 and π are constants
μ is the fluid's viscosity
l is the length of the tube, and r is the radius of the tube

ΔP varies directly with μ, l, and V.
ΔP varies inversely with r.

Depending upon the emphasis of your professor, you may be tested on using the actual Poisseuille's Law equation. Or you may be tested on just your conceptual understanding. In either case, it is very important for you to understand the relationships that

Poisseuille's Law describes. *Fundamentally what it is showing is that when it comes to laminar flow – the relationship between pressure and flow is linear – it's an expression of the form f(x) = x.*

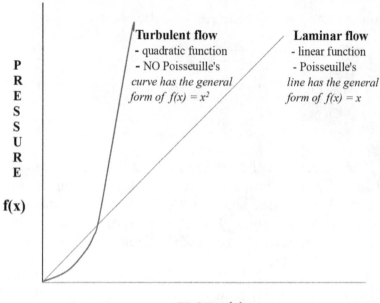

P
R
E
S
S
U
R
E

f(x)

Turbulent flow
- quadratic function
- NO Poisseuille's
curve has the general
form of f(x) = x^2

Laminar flow
- linear function
- Poisseuille's
line has the general
form of f(x) = x

FLOW (x)

The graph above is the correct graphical representation of how pressure relates to flow for both laminar flow and turbulent flow. Turbulent flow will be discussed next; however, it is presented in this graph along with laminar flow so that you can see the difference between the two. *The main point with laminar flow is that the relationship between pressure (ΔP) and flow (V) is linear - it's an expression of the form f(x) = x, the implication of which means that in order to double the flow you double the pressure.*

Note also that although Poisseuille's Law has been discussed to show the relationship between driving pressure and flow, if you look closely you will see that the radius term of the Poisseuille's Law equation is in the denominator. Recall the equation that related resistance to tube radius given a couple of pages back and note that in that equation the radius is also in the denominator. Both cases (both equations) are illustrating that there is an inverse relationship between the radius of a tube and either resistance or driving pressure. What does this mean or why is it important to point out this subtlety?   It's important because if you appreciate this nuance you will have grasped a fundamentally crucial concept that is central to understanding the flow of gas through the airways as it relates to the work of breathing. With the equation that expresses the inverse relationship between resistance and the radius of the tube you realize that as the tube (airway) gets smaller (or constricted) that resistance to flow becomes much greater. When you look at the inverse relationship between driving pressure and the radius of the tube as shown with Poisseuille's equation you realize that as the radius of the tube (airway) gets smaller (or constricted) that it causes the driving pressure (the ΔP term) to increase for a given constant flow. All of this translates directly to what is known as the work of breathing (WOB) – being done either by the patient spontaneously or by the ventilator mechanically. In either case, what both of these equations illustrate is that when the radius of the tube (airways) becomes smaller (constricted) that the resistance to flow becomes greater and that means that it will require much more effort (pressure) to maintain the same flow of gas. This will result in either the patient having to work a whole lot harder to maintain adequate flow (which is increased work of breathing) - or if they are intubated and receiving mechanical ventilation it means that increased pressures will be required to maintain adequate flow.

2. TURBULENT FLOW

- Turbulent flow is characterized by the loss of regular streamlines of flow.
- Turbulent flow is characterized by irregular currents, and these irregular currents create back flow (resistance).
- Turbulent flow is not linear like laminar flow, but rather it is expressed by a quadratic function – see the previous graph.
- The transition from laminar flow to turbulent flow involves the following four variables:

1) fluid density ρ *Density is more of an influence than viscosity.*
2) viscosity μ
3) linear velocity v *Sharp increases in velocity cause turbulence.*
4) tube diameter D

These four variables, when arranged in the form of the equation below, give what is known as *Reynold's Number* – a dimensionless number designated as R_e. In the academic sense of it, the calculation of Reynold's Number enables you to predict whether flow will be laminar or turbulent.

$$R_e = \frac{v \rho D}{\mu}$$

When $R_e < 2000$, flow is laminar. When $2000 < R_e < 4000$, flow is transitional, and when $R_e > 4000$, flow is turbulent. Physiologically it can indicate that turbulence and back pressure are more likely at high flow rates, and it may help clinicians to manage inspiratory flow rates during mechanical ventilation in order to optimize distribution of ventilation.

What is most important to understand about turbulent flow is that the relationship between pressure and flow is no longer linear, but rather it is expressed by a quadratic function – it is of the form of f(x) = x² - and therefore Poisseuille's Law can no longer be used.

The equation to describe turbulent flow is as follows:

$$\Delta P = \frac{f_D \, l \, \dot{V}^2}{4 \pi^2 r^5}$$

$\dot{V}$ is flow l is the tube length
ΔP is the pressure gradient r is the tube radius
π is constant f_D is the friction factor

One of the first things you should notice is that unlike Poisseuille's equation, this equation has a squared variable (the flow term) in the numerator. Mathematically this tells you right away that this can't possibly be expressing a linear relationship. Rather it is a quadratic function and this is illustrated by the curve that represents turbulent flow on the graph a couple of pages back.

The point to remember is that with turbulent flow the relationship between pressure (ΔP) and flow (V) is expressed by a quadratic function - it's an expression of the form f(x)= x^2, the implication of which means that in order to double the flow you need to increase the pressure by a factor of 4. Review the graph from a couple pages back.

3. TRANSITIONAL FLOW

Transitional flow is simply a combination of laminar flow and turbulent flow. Not much more needs to be said as both laminar flow and turbulent flow have been covered. *The main take home point for transitional flow is to remember that* FLOW IN THE AIRWAYS IS PREDOMINANTLY TRANSITIONAL.

F. Bernoulli & Fluid Entrainment

The Bernoulli Principle and fluid (to include gases) entrainment are concepts that are actually much easier to comprehend than they may appear to be at first glance. Bernoulli's Principle in essence is a derivation of the Law of Continuity that is also consistent with the law of conservation of energy whereby energy must always be conserved. In the case of steady fluid flow, this means that the sum of all forms of energy in a fluid that is flowing in a streamline is the same at all points along the streamline – in other words the sum of the various forms of energy has to remain constant. And when speaking of fluids, this includes not only kinetic and potential energy, but also the lateral pressure exerted by the fluid against the wall of the tube through which it is flowing. Also, keep in mind that a gas is a fluid – so these concepts pertain to a gas flowing through a tube.

Previously in the section on flow, the Law of Continuity was introduced and that law stated that for a given constant flow rate, the velocity (kinetic energy) of a fluid through a tube varies inversely with the cross-sectional area of the tube. Bernoulli's Principle simply extends this concept by now including pressure (specifically lateral pressure). Bernoulli's Principle tells us that an increase in the velocity of a fluid occurs simultaneously with a decrease in pressure. Whereas the Law of Continuity tells us that the velocity of a fluid flowing through a tube will increase if the cross-sectional area of the tube decreases, Bernoulli's Principle now tells us that when this happens – when the velocity of the fluid increases – the lateral pressure of the fluid will decrease. Energy is conserved (the Law of Conservation of Energy is upheld) because the sum of the energy *after* the tube got smaller is the same as the sum of the energy *before* the tube got smaller. The increase in velocity is offset by the decrease in lateral pressure such that the sum of the energy *after* the tube got smaller is the same as the sum of the energy *before* the tube got smaller.

Remember to envision these concepts with respect to gas flow because the next idea to be discussed will bring the concept of the Bernoulli Principle full circle and show how it relates to fluid (and thus gas) entrainment. These are important ideas because they explain how certain pieces of respiratory therapy equipment work-particularly the air entrainment mask.

Consider the drawing below as a generic illustration to convey the idea of air entrainment (air which of course is by definition a mixture of gases and thus a fluid).

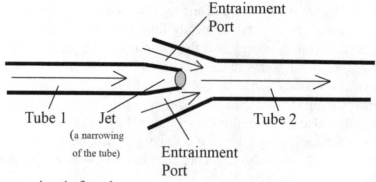

The arrows show the flow of gas

Tube 1 represents the tube that is coming from the gas source (either the wall source or a tank). Tube 2 represents the portion that is part of the apparatus of the air entrainment mask. Keep in mind though that this diagram is a schematic to illustrate a concept – it's not what the actual set up looks like. In real life, and you'll learn this when you get to medical gas therapy, what you have is usually one of two things – either a variety of color coded adapters for various FiO_2's, or a single adapter that has a dial on it where you can set a desired FiO_2. What this means is as follows: Oxygen coming out of the wall source or a tank is always 100% O_2. But you're not always going to want to give a patient 100% O_2 - so you therefore need to have a way to be able to reduce that 100% O_2 down to the percentage of oxygen (FiO_2) you desire to give to the patient. FiO_2 simply means the fractional percentage of inspired oxygen. Say for example that the MD wants the patient to be getting 60% O_2 (an FiO_2 of 60%). When you set up the air entrainment mask you are going to either use the colored adapter that is for 60%, or you are going to use the adapter with a dial and set it at 60%. But how does the adapter accomplish reducing the 100% O_2 from the source down to 60%?

The adapter itself is the part that actually contains the jet. In reality, the tube coming from the wall gets connected to the adapter, and within the structure of the adapter itself is the jet. If you refer back to the diagram on the previous page - the middle portion of the diagram where you see the jet and the entrainment port – that's actually the adapter. Tube 2 is the connecting tube from the adapter to the mask. In addition to housing the jet itself, the adapter also has an opening on the side - that is the entrainment port. Now how does this all work? When a fluid (gas flowing from the wall through tube 1) encounters a very narrow passageway (the jet), the velocity of the gas increases and the lateral pressure decreases (Bernoulli's Principle). Note the inverse relationship between velocity and lateral pressure because this is in essence what Bernoulli's Principle is ultimately illustrating. *The increase in velocity can be so great that it will cause the lateral pressure to drop below ambient.* Remember that the lateral pressure is the pressure that the gas is exerting inside the tube. Remember also that there is not only gas flowing through the tube that is feeding into the adapter, but there is also gas (air) in the room surrounding the adapter. If the gas that is flowing through tube 1 is forced into a jet of much smaller diameter such that its velocity increases to the point where that causes the lateral pressure to drop below ambient (and thus become negative with respect to the pressure in the room), then the air in the room surrounding the adapter is going to flow into the opening on the adapter (the entrainment port) and thus be *entrained* into the overall flow of gas going to the patient. This happens because gases will naturally flow from areas of higher pressure to lower pressure. If the pressure has dropped to below ambient within the adapter, then the air in the room which is at higher pressure is going to flow into the entrainment port on the adapter. Thus, you have room air at 21% O_2 flowing into the entrainment port that is now being combined with the 100% O_2 that is coming from the wall – and that mixing will result in the 100% O_2 from the wall being reduced down to the FiO_2 desired.

The air entrainment device then serves 2 overall purposes:

1) You already have flow coming from the wall according to however many LPM you have the flow meter set at. Now that you are also entraining room air as well, you have effectively increased the total flow of gas to the patient. This is important as you always want to be able to deliver enough flow to meet a patient's inspiratory flow demand.

2) As already discussed, it is a way to be able to deliver a specific percentage of gas (FiO_2). To reiterate – Oxygen comes out of the wall at 100%. If you only want 60%, then you attach an adapter that has an entrainment port of appropriate size so as to mix enough room air with the 100% oxygen coming from the wall in order to bring the percentage of oxygen down to 60%.

The amount of entrained air depends on 2 things.

1) The size of the jet
   - Making the jet smaller increases the amount of air entrained and thus increases total flow.

2) The size of the air entrainment ports
   - For a fixed jet size – increasing the size of the air entrainment ports will increase the volume of air that is entrained and thus increase total flow.

G. States of Matter & Heat

When discussing the states of matter, it is important to remember that the physical state of any substance is determined by the relationship between its kinetic energy (KE) and the potential energy (PE) stored within its intermolecular bonds. Without going into the mathematics of kinetic and potential energy, it is sufficient to say that kinetic energy is the energy of motion whereas potential energy is the energy that is stored. This will become clearer as the following states of matter are discussed.

SOLIDS
- Fixed volume & shape – usually crystalline (lattice) or amorphous (less rigid structure)
- High degree of internal structural order
- Incompressible
- Solids have the lowest KE and high PE

LIQUIDS
- Fixed volume
- Have adaptable shape – liquids can "flow"
- Liquids are somewhat dense and not easily compressible (they are essentially incompressible except under extreme pressure)
- Have higher KE than solids and a somewhat high PE

GASES

- No defined volume or shape
- Much weaker intermolecular attraction than liquids/solids
- Much less dense than liquids or solids
- Velocity of gas is directly proportional to temperature.
- Have the highest KE and low PE

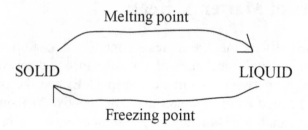

The temperature at which a solid transforms into a liquid is called the melting point. Conversely, the temperature at which a liquid transforms into a solid is called the freezing point. *Note that the melting point and the freezing point are the same temperature – it's just a matter of which direction you are going.* If you are going from solid to liquid you're melting – if you're going from liquid to solid you're freezing, but in either case they're both happening at the same temperature.

$$\text{LIQUID} \xrightarrow{\text{Boiling point}} \text{GAS}$$

The transition from liquid to gas is known as vaporization. It is a process that requires heat from the surroundings. The temperature at which a liquid will transform into a gas is called the boiling point. "Boiling" is the rapid vaporization that occurs at this temperature. This temperature is the temperature at which the vapor pressure of the liquid is equal to the atmospheric pressure. Reducing the atmospheric pressure above a liquid lowers its boiling point. This is why a liquid at high altitude will boil at a temperature that is lower than what would be needed for it to boil at sea level. The second type of vaporization – which you already know as evaporation - is when a liquid transitions into a gas at a temperature lower than its boiling point.

The transition from a gas into a liquid is called condensation. This process gives heat back to the environment. A common example of this would be the condensation that is seen along the side of a glass that is full of cold liquid. Water vapor in the room that is in contact with the side of the cold glass will yield some of its heat to the cold glass – by giving up some of its heat (energy), the water vapor becomes a liquid and forms the condensation that is seen along the side of the glass.

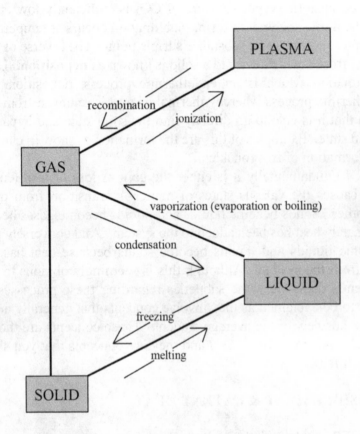

The diagram above shows a schematic of the states of matter and the processes they undergo in changing from one form to another. Plasma is indicated however it wasn't discussed in this section as it is not relevant to respiratory therapy. Plasma is a very complicated electrically neutral medium of unbound positive and negative particles, the subject of which is well beyond the scope of a respiratory therapy curriculum. Notice the vertical line that directly connects solid and gas. There are no arrows indicating anything between those two as that is going to be discussed now. Going from the solid phase directly to the gas phase and bypassing the liquid phase is known as **sublimation.** An example of this is dry ice where you have solid CO_2 going directly to gaseous CO_2. The solid CO_2 doesn't melt into liquid CO_2 and then vaporize into gaseous CO_2. Rather it goes from solid CO_2 directly to gaseous CO_2. It does this because the vapor pressure of CO_2 is sufficiently low enough for the liquid state not to form. Sublimation occurs at temperatures and pressures below a substance's triple point. The reverse of this – going from a gas directly to a solid is known as **deposition.** Unlike sublimation which is an endothermic process, deposition is an exothermic process whereby thermal energy is removed from a gas such that it is able to go directly into the solid state and bypass the liquid state. Examples of this are the formation of snow in clouds or the formation of frost on a leaf.

Fundamentally it is either the gain or loss of heat (energy) that causes the various states of matter to transition from one to the other. Solids become liquids and liquids become gases because ultimately heat has been added to the system. And conversely gases become liquids and liquids become solids because heat has been lost from the system. Although this is seemingly obvious to most students, there are some subtleties regarding these processes that need to be explained as they involve concepts that generally are not in the purview of the average student. These concepts are those of *sensible heat* and *latent heat* and they are concepts that you should be well familiar with.

SENSIBLE HEAT & LATENT HEAT

Sensible heat is the heat (energy) required to change the temperature, but not a change of state. Consider the following example of water. When water is below 0°C it is in the form of ice (solid water). Let's say you have a piece of ice and the temperature of that piece of ice is -10°C. As that piece of ice absorbs heat (energy) the temperature is going to start to rise. The heat (energy) that the ice cube is absorbing during this time is called sensible heat. The ice cube is gaining heat and the temperature is rising, but it is not yet transforming into liquid water. It won't start transforming into liquid water until the temperature gets to 0° C. Now when the temperature does reach 0° C the ice cube will start to melt and begin its transition into the liquid state of water. But notice – it is at this point that as additional heat continues to be added to the ice – the ice undergoes complete transformation into liquid water, but during the time that this transition is occurring the temperature does not rise. This extra heat (energy) that is absorbed during the time of the actual change of state is what is called *latent heat*. Another way of thinking of latent heat is to think of it as the additional amount of heat needed to cause a complete change of state. In going from a solid to a liquid it is referred to as the latent heat of fusion (or melting) and when going from a liquid to a gas it is referred to as the latent heat of vaporization.

Once the ice has been completely transformed into liquid water, if heat continues to be added to the system - then at this point the temperature is going to start to rise again. And if sufficient heat (sensible heat) is applied, the temperature is going to continue to rise until you get to the boiling point of water which is 100°C. At the point of reaching 100°C the same process is going to happen as before. At the point of 100°C the liquid water is going to start transitioning into steam, but in order to convert all of the liquid water into steam requires the additional latent heat to finish completing the change of state from liquid to gas. Remember that during this time period when the change of state is occurring (or being completed) that heat (latent heat) is being absorbed in order to complete the transition, but the temperature is not increasing. If you think about this, you will then understand why steam is so much more dangerous than boiling water. Being burned by boiling water which is at 100°C is bad enough, but being burned by steam is much worse because of all the additional latent heat that is contained in the steam. Boiling water and steam may both have the same temperature, but never forget that it is the addition of latent heat that causes the complete change of state into steam, and although there may not have been a rise in temperature during the completion of the change of state, that latent heat is still present and that additional energy in the form of latent heat will make for a very serious burn.

Let it be said that although the aforementioned discussion regarding sensible and latent heat was presented from the perspective of going from a solid to a liquid to a gas, the same concepts apply when going from a gas to a liquid to a solid – it's just the reverse process where you have heat being lost to the environment when going from a gas to a liquid to a solid.

Let us now turn our attention to a brief and generic

discussion of just how heat is transferred. The previous section discussed how heat is involved when a substance undergoes a change of state, but here the discussion will just speak about how heat itself is transferred without necessarily involving a substance changing its state.

HEAT TRANSFER

1. **Conduction** – conduction is one of the ways in which heat is transferred that involves direct physical contact between hot (molecules with higher energy) and cold (molecules with lower energy) objects. This is what is seen when you have two solid objects in contact with one another. Heat moves from hot to cold so the heat will move from the hot object to the cold object until equilibrium is reached.

2. **Convection** – convection is the mixing of fluid molecules (gases or liquids) from areas that are warmer (higher energy) to areas that are cooler (lower energy). The principle is similar to conduction in the sense that heat (energy) moves from hot to cold – except that in this case it involves gases or liquids rather than solids. An example of convection is when a radiator warms the air in a room. The air closest to the radiator is warmed first, but then that warm air circulates throughout the room and eventually all the cool air becomes warm. Note that convection, like conduction, also involves direct contact – the gas molecules in the air that are being warmed by the radiator are in contact with the cooler gas molecules – and by virtue of their contact with each other all the gas molecules circulating in the room will eventually be moving about with more energy which you perceive as the room becoming warmer.

3. **Radiation** – radiation is heat energy carried by electromagnetic waves and/or photons of light. An example of this is the way in which the Sun heats the Earth. When you do your NICU rotation you will see a heating unit that is positioned above the newborn infant. This unit functions by delivering radiant heat energy.

H. Thermodynamics

The laws of thermodynamics address **A)** the relationship between thermal energy (heat) and other forms of energy, **B)** how energy affects matter, and **C)** entropy. Thermodynamics will be covered in much more detail in your physics courses, however, the basic laws of thermodynamics are worth mentioning here as they are some of the most important laws in physics and you should have a basic understanding of these concepts. There are four basic laws of thermodynamics and they are as follows:

Zeroth Law of Thermodynamics

If two thermodynamic systems are each in thermal equilibrium with a third system, then they are in thermal equilibrium with each other.

First Law of Thermodynamics *(addresses the quantity of energy)*

The first law of thermodynamics is an expression of the *law of conservation of energy* to a thermodynamic system. It states that energy can neither be created nor destroyed – it can only change forms. For any process, the total energy of the universe remains constant. The total amount of energy in a particular thermodynamic system is the amount of heat supplied to the system minus the net work done by the system.

Second Law of Thermodynamics *(addresses the quality of energy)*

The second law of thermodynamics states that the entropy of an isolated system not in equilibrium will tend to increase over time, approaching a maximum value at equilibrium. This is based on the universal principle of decay that is seen in nature – it is an observable fact that over time systems move towards having greater disorder and randomness. Entropy is simply a measure of how far this has progressed. It is also indicating the amount of energy that is unavailable for work. *Given time, all systems will seek to achieve the lowest possible energy state – and thus the highest amount of entropy.*

All processes result in an increase in entropy. By way of example, consider the crystals that are formed through the evaporation of a solution of salt water. The crystals themselves are obviously more orderly than the salt ions were in the solution, however, vaporized (evaporated) water is much more disorderly than liquid water. The crystal formation and the evaporation of water are both occurring within the same system, and the mathematical analysis of the thermodynamics of these events will always indicate an overall net increase in disorder (entropy).

Why doesn't heat spontaneously flow from cold to hot? Because that would violate the very idea of a system naturally seeking to achieve the lowest possible energy state - and this is what the second law of thermodynamics illustrates. The consistent observation in nature is that energy (heat) moves from high to low (or hot to cold) and this behavior is indicative of the underlying idea that systems seek to achieve the lowest energy state possible.

Third Law of Thermodynamics

The third law of thermodynamics simply states that as temperature approaches absolute zero (0 K), the entropy of the system approaches a constant minimum. Although this may appear contradictory to what is stated in the second law with regard to the relationship between entropy and energy, there are quantum considerations that come into play at this point that are well beyond the scope of this text. In practice it is not possible to achieve absolute zero because at absolute zero all processes would cease.

I. Humidity

Humidity refers to the amount of moisture (water vapor) in the atmosphere. It is necessary to discuss humidity not only in terms of general concepts, but to also apply those general concepts to the respiratory system as water vapor is also present in the respiratory system. The first two concepts that need to be understood are *content* and *capacity*.

Content – Content, or **absolute humidity (AH),** is the actual amount of water molecules. It is simply the total mass of water vapor present for a given volume of air and it is expressed in mg/L (milligrams per liter).

Capacity – Capacity is the maximum amount of water vapor that the air *could* hold at a given temperature. It is also expressed in mg/L.

- As temperature increases, the capacity for air to hold water vapor increases.
- As temperature decreases, the capacity for air to hold water vapor decreases.

Therefore, content is telling you how much water vapor you actually have, and capacity is telling you the maximum amount you *could have* at a given temperature. At higher temperatures the air is able to hold more water vapor, and at lower temperatures the air is less able to hold water vapor – and this is because capacity is directly related to temperature.

Now – the **relative humidity (RH)**, or the % RH, is given by the following equation:

$$\% \, RH \;=\; \frac{Content \, (AH)}{Capacity} \; X \; 100$$

Since content is the amount of water vapor you actually have – if you divide that by the capacity (the maximum amount you could have for a given temperature) – then the resulting quotient tells you the percentage that you have. If the content you actually have is equal to the capacity for the temperature you are currently at, then you are going to end up with a quotient of 1, and 1 X 100 = 100%. So, remember that when content and capacity are the same, RH is 100% and that means that the air (gas) is fully saturated with water vapor. You can then see that if they are not equal – if the content is actually less than the capacity at the given temperature, then you are going to end up having a quotient that is less than 1, and thus a percentage that is less than 100% - hence the notion of it being called *relative humidity.*

Humidity Facts - Fully saturated air at 37°C (body temperature) and 760 mmHg has a vapor pressure of 47 mmHg and a content (absolute humidity) of 43.8 mg/L. And since it was just stated that the air is fully saturated, you should have then realized that the capacity at 37°C is also 43.8 mg/L. This 43.8 mg/L is also referred to as the alveolar gas vapor density. Don't let the word density confuse you – remember that density is expressed as mass/volume and this is what you have here with humidity being expressed in terms of mg/L. The 47 mmHg vapor pressure is the partial pressure that is being exerted by the water vapor. This was mentioned earlier in the section on the gas laws and Dalton's Law, and this 47 mmHg will be an important number later on when working with the alveolar air equation because the water vapor in the lungs needs to be accounted for when doing calculations.

% BH (body humidity) – when talking about the body humidity percentage, realize that conceptually it is the same as relative humidity with the exception that capacity is always 43.8 mg/L at 37°C (body temperature). Remember that capacity is the amount of water vapor that can be held at a particular temperature. Normal body temperature is 37°C, and at this temperature 43.8 mg/L of water vapor can be held so that is why the capacity term of this equation will always be 43.8 mg/L. Obviously if the patient has a fever, or for some reason has a body temperature lower than normal that this would change the scenario because remember that capacity is directly related to temperature. For the purposes of your understanding, however, this is being presented under the conditions of normal body temperature.

Hence:

$$\% \ BH \ = \ \frac{Content \ (AH)}{43.8 \ mg/L} \ X \ 100$$

Humidity Deficit

- The humidity deficit is what must be considered when the % RH or the % BH is less than 100%.
- The body humidity deficit represents the amount of water vapor the body needs to add to inspired gas in order to achieve saturation at body temperature.

There are two humidity deficits to be considered, and if you keep that in mind they won't be confusing. Your first concern is to determine the humidity deficit in the air – that is the 1° deficit. Then you can determine the humidity deficit in the body (lungs) – that is the 2° deficit.

1° deficit – The primary deficit tells you the humidity deficit that is occurring in the air. It means that the inspired air is not fully saturated at the air's current temperature. In this case you are looking at the (% RH) and seeing how far that is from 100%. In other words – the 1° deficit is the difference between the humidity you actually have (% RH) and being fully saturated at 100%.

1) Use the % RH formula to determine the % RH

2) Then subtract your answer from 100%

3) 100% - % RH = **% primary deficit**

<u>Example 1:</u> If you have a capacity of 25mg/L at a given temperature and your content for example is 11.25 mg/L, then according to the % RH formula, your % RH is going to be 45%. The percentage of primary deficit would therefore be 55%, *but more than likely you are going to be asked to express that deficit in terms of actual mg/L rather than a percentage.* Remember that when content equals capacity, humidity is 100% (fully saturated). Therefore, if you are asked to calculate the actual 1° humidity deficit in actual mg/L, all you need to do is subtract the content you have from the capacity given and that will tell you the additional amount of humidity in mg/L that you need to be at 100% full saturation with respect to the air. Referring back to the example above – if you have a content of 11.25 mg/L and your capacity is 25 mg/L, then you are going to need an additional 13.75 mg/L of content in order to be fully saturated - and that 13.75 mg/L is your 1° deficit.

Therefore:

Capacity (for the temperature you're at) – Content = **1° deficit in mg/L**.

<u>2° deficit</u> – Now that you have determined the primary deficit (which remember is the humidity deficit in the air), you can now determine the secondary deficit (which is the body humidity deficit). The body humidity deficit represents the additional amount of water vapor the upper airway needs to add to inspired gas in order to achieve saturation in the lungs at body temperature. You have either already learned, or will soon learn, that gas traveling through the airway must be completely humidified. Dry gas is damaging to the airway and therefore the upper airway has mechanisms in place to ensure the proper humidification of inspired air. There is always supposed to be 100% humidification of the airway. The 2° deficit tells you how far off from that you are. In determining the 2° deficit you are looking at the (% BH) and seeing how far that is from 100%. In other words – the 2° deficit is the difference between the humidity you actually have (% BH) and being fully saturated at 100%.

1) Use the % BH formula to determine the % BH

2) Then subtract your answer from 100%

3) 100% - % BH = % secondary deficit

Consider again the information given in example 1 where you have a content of 11.25mg/L (this is the absolute humidity of the room air that is being inspired). If that was the only amount of water molecules to reach the lung without any further humidity being added, then according to the % BH formula you would end up having a % BH of only 25.6%. That means that there would be a secondary humidity deficit of 74.4%. It was already previously mentioned that the lungs need inspired gas to be humidified to the point of full saturation at body temperature. This means that the % BH needs to be 100%, and this is accomplished one of two ways – either the body itself (the mucosa of the upper airway) adds the additional humidity needed to achieve full saturation or the additional humidity needed to achieve full saturation needs to be provided to the patient by the respiratory therapist (e.g.: when the patient is receiving oxygen therapy or is intubated).

Example 2: On an exam you will rarely be given a % BH in a humidity problem that asks you to solve for the 2° deficit. That would make the problem too easy for you. And more than likely, just like it was for the primary deficit, you're going to be asked to give the secondary deficit in terms of mg/L rather than a percentage. Often you will see the problem presented in the form of a clinical scenario that will give you the % RH and the capacity, and then ask you to solve for the 1°, 2°, and total humidity deficits in terms of mg/L. Say for example that you are given a problem in the form of a clinical scenario that tells you a patient is being given oxygen via a nasal cannula where they are getting 45% RH and the capacity is 25 mg/L (and remember that this is with respect to the air), and then the problem asks you to figure out the 1°, 2°, and total humidity deficits. Note that the numbers used for this made up clinical scenario are consistent with those used in example 1 in order that you may follow the train of thought here. Refer back to example 1 that was just given to illustrate the 1° deficit. The capacity was given as 25mg/L, the content was given as 11.25 mg/L, and thus the % RH was calculated to be 45%. This resulted in a 55% primary deficit, and it was also shown how this amounted to being a deficit of 13.75mg/L. And remember that this 1° deficit of 13.75 mg/L indicates the additional amount of humidity that would be needed in order to reach saturation for the capacity that was given.

Realize that example 1 gave the content and capacity because it was being used to illustrate how to solve for % RH. On an exam they may give you the % RH and capacity (like I did in the clinical scenario I just gave you as part of this example) – and you have to determine the content. This is how they will twist things around to try to make it more difficult for you. Now look again at the clinical scenario problem I just gave you - you're given a % RH of 45% and a capacity of 25mg/L as part of the problem - if you plug those numbers into the % RH formula you will then be able to figure out that the content is 11.25 mg/L. You have to be able to apply the formula. You have to be able to discern the information you've been given in a problem in order to determine what you need to know.

Your task in determining the 2° deficit is to determine the additional amount of humidity that is needed in order to be fully saturated inside the lung. The 1° deficit was determined to be 13.75 mg/L – but this was based on the capacity being 25 mg/L. Remember that capacity inside the lung is different – it is 43.8 mg/L - so you have to figure out how much additional humidity is needed (the 2° deficit) in order to be fully saturated at 100% inside the lung.

The following calculations will show you how to calculate the 2° deficit as well the total humidity deficit. The numbers are based upon the clinical scenario I just presented - a patient on a nasal cannula that is providing a % RH of 45% and the capacity is 25 mg/L. You've already determined the content to be 11.25 mg/L and the 1° deficit to be 13.75 mg/L. Knowing that the capacity in the lung is 43.8 mg/L, the following calculations will show you how to determine the additional amount of humidity needed (the 2° deficit) in order to achieve 100% saturation in the lung.

Therefore:

43.80 mg/L —   capacity for the lung
— 11.25 mg/L —   the amount of absolute humidity (content) you already have
_____   from the information given in the clinical scenario problem - see
                           also example 1

32.55 mg/L —   this is the **total humidity deficit** with respect to inside the lung.

32.55 mg/L
— 13.75 mg/L   1° deficit – determined in example 1
_____   (the additional humidity needed to reach
                             saturation with respect to the air)

18.8 mg/L   2° deficit
                 (the additional humidity needed to reach
                 saturation with respect inside the lungs)

If you round the 43.8 mg/L to 44 mg/L it will look like this:

44.00 mg/L -   capacity for the lung
— 11.25 mg/L -   the amount of absolute humidity (content) you already have
_____   from the information given in the clinical scenario problem – see
                           also example 1

32.75 mg/L —   this is the **total humidity deficit** with respect to inside the lung.

32.75 mg/L
— 13.75 mg/L   1° deficit – determined in example 1
_____   (the additional humidity needed to reach
                             saturation with respect to the air)

19 mg/L   2° deficit
                 (the additional humidity needed to reach
                 saturation with respect inside the lungs)

Realize that in some respects we are splitting hairs with regards to primary or secondary humidity deficits. Indeed, the primary deficit speaks to the additional amount of humidity that is needed to have 100% saturation with respect to the air at whatever the particular temperature happens to be, and the secondary deficit speaks to the additional humidity needed to be provided by the upper airway to achieve saturation at body temperature, but realize the following: In the clinical scenario previously given, the patient was on a nasal cannula that was giving them 45% RH. With the capacity being given as 25mg/L, it was determined that the content (AH) was 11.25mg/L. This 11.25mg/L is the only humidity the patient is receiving. We know they need 43.8mg/L in order to be fully saturated inside the lungs, but since they are only getting 11.25mg/L coming from the humidification of the nasal cannula, there is a total humidity deficit of 32.55mg/L. Whether 13.75mg/L of the 32.55mg/L is called the primary deficit because that happens to be the deficit with respect to the air – or the other 18.8mg/L of the 32.55mg/L is called the secondary deficit because that happens to be the deficit with respect to the lungs – *the bottom line is that a total of 32.55mg/L of additional humidity is needed in order to achieve full saturation inside the lungs at body temperature.* And that additional humidity is going to be provided by either the mucosa of the upper airway or by increasing the % RH coming through a humidification device, or a combination of both. Everything else is academic. In clinical practice you are never going to do humidity calculations at the bedside. If a patient is intubated, you may have a heat/moisture exchanger (HME) attached to the endotracheal tube that is going to provide the necessary humidification. If they are receiving oxygen therapy at a flow rate high enough to cause irritation to the airway there will be a bubble humidifier attached to the oxygen delivery device that will deliver a high enough % RH to ensure sufficient humidification. Providing adequate humidity to the patient is always part of the standard of care. It is however still important that you understand the concepts presented in this section and be able to do the calculations as they are part of your foundational knowledge base and you will be tested on them in your exams.

Chapter 2

Selected Topics in Physiologic Ventilation

One of my professors often joked that it's just air moving in and out - "air goes in, air goes out". Quintessentially that is what is happening, but unfortunately it isn't quite that simple. However, it doesn't need to be all that complicated either – it's just a matter of staying focused and following a train of thought so as to see the total picture of this process that we call breathing. The aim of this chapter will be to highlight and explain the fundamental concepts that are most essential to understanding the process of normal physiologic ventilation – the movement of air in and out of the lungs.

I am going to begin this chapter by discussing the various pressure gradients that exist within the respiratory system. This particular topic is problematic for most students because of the ambiguity that is typically associated with the presentation of this material. This ambiguity is furthered by the fact that there is quite a bit of variety in the way these gradients are described amongst all the different respiratory therapy textbooks - and this occurs because there is still no real professional consensus concerning this particular topic. Confusion arises from the fact that the terminology used to label and describe these gradients tends to vary from one author to the next depending upon who you are reading. Further confusion is created by inconsistencies in the formulation and application of the equations used to represent the various gradients. Fortunately, you will not *usually* be required to utilize any of the pressure gradient equations on an exam. What is important is that you *conceptually* understand what is going on with these gradients with respect to how they affect the flow of gas. Regardless of the issues that cause confusion, *just realize that ultimately these pressure gradients between the different areas of the respiratory system are simply a way to describe the differences in pressure that drive the flow of air in and out of the lungs.* In light of the ambiguity associated with this particular topic, I hope I am able to help alleviate some of the confusion by explaining these gradients as best as I can with the goal that it gives some clarity to the role they play in the mechanics of normal physiologic ventilation.

Pressure gradients have to exist in order for normal spontaneous ventilation to occur - otherwise there would be no means by which to cause gas to flow. Before discussing the gradients themselves, let us first consider the various pressures associated with the different areas of the respiratory system that enable these gradients to be established.

A. Pressures Associated with the Different Areas of the Respiratory System

1. **P_{AO}** – This is the pressure at the **airway opening** (the inside of the mouth). At the end of expiration during normal spontaneous breathing this pressure is equal to the ambient pressure – usually 760 mmHg (or 0 PSIG).

2. **P_{PL} – (intrapleural pressure)** This is the pressure within the plural space. This pressure is produced by the opposition of the elastic forces between the lungs and the chest wall. Under normal conditions, the elastic forces of the lung cause it to want to contract whereas the elastic forces of the chest wall cause it to want to expand. *At rest,* the net effect of these opposing forces causes the pressure in the plural space to vary around -3 to -6 cmH$_2$O. Note that this is sub-ambient. *You may also see P_{PL} (intrapleural pressure) referred to as the intrathoracic pressure.*

   Note: P_{PL} cannot be directly measured. An accurate estimation however, may be obtained by measuring the pressure in the esophagus (P_{ES}) via a catheter that has been placed into the lower third of the esophagus so as to be positioned between the lungs.

3. **P_A – (alveolar pressure)** <u>This is the pressure in the alveoli at the end of expiration.</u> Remember that at the end of expiration gas flow has ceased and the glottis is open. The pressure throughout the airway from the mouth to the alveoli is equal to ambient pressure – usually 760 mmHg (or 0 PSIG). Think – if it was higher or lower, then air would still be flowing. Note however that during the rest of the breathing cycle when air is flowing, P_A varies. More will be said about this during the discussion to follow on the transrespiratory gradient. *You may also see P_A (alveolar pressure) referred to as the intrapulmonary pressure.*

4. **P_{BS} – (body surface pressure)** <u>This is the pressure at the body surface.</u> It is always the atmospheric or ambient pressure, and at sea level that is 760 mmHg (or 0 PSIG).

B. Respiratory System Pressure Gradients

The important pressure gradients for you to understand are as follows:

1. TRANSRESPIRATORY GRADIENT: $P_{TR} = P_{AO} - P_{BS}$

This is the "mother" gradient that is ultimately responsible for moving air in and out of the lungs. It is the gradient across the entirety of the lungs and thorax. All the other gradients that will be discussed subsequently are just sub divisions of this one.

As just mentioned in the discussion on P_{PL} – when a breath begins with the expansion of the rib cage pulling the parietal pleura outward while the elastic recoil of the lung is simultaneously pulling the visceral pleura inward – the net result is that the pressure in the pleural space (P_{PL}) becomes even more sub-ambient (negative with respect to the atmosphere). Here is your illustration of Boyle's law; you expanded the thorax thus making the volume bigger and therefore the pressure dropped. This sub-ambient pressure (around -8 cmH$_2$O) in the pleural space is reflected across the AC (alveolar-capillary) membrane and thus the P_A (alveolar pressure) begins to become sub-ambient as well. The sub-ambient P_{PL} that has been reflected into the alveoli and thus making the P_A sub-ambient is actually reflected all the way up to the inside of the mouth (P_{AO}). The net result of this is that the entire airway is now sub-ambient with respect to the atmosphere. *This is the gradient* (atmospheric pressure is greater than the pressure in the airway), and air will thus flow down this gradient into the lungs because gas will always flow from an area of higher pressure (the atmosphere) to an area of lower pressure (the airway).

Therefore: At the end of expiration, P_{AO} and P_{BS} are equal and there is no flow of air. During inspiration, P_{AO} (the inside of the mouth) becomes less than P_{BS} as just explained and thus air flows from the atmosphere into the lungs. Remember that P_{BS} is just atmospheric pressure.

Realize also that the sub-ambient pressure (-3 to -6 cmH$_2$O) in the pleural space at rest (the end of expiration) is what serves to keep the lung at FRC. FRC is the normal lung volume at rest after expiration. That -3 to -6 cmH$_2$O pressure in the pleural space (P_{PL}) is sufficient enough only to keep the lung at FRC – it is not enough to cause the P_A to become sub-ambient such that gas starts to flow into the airway. In order for gas to flow into the airway there needs to be chest wall expansion so as to cause the P_{PL} to become even more sub-ambient (-8 cmH$_2$O) such that THEN the P_A will become sub-ambient and thus the P_{AO} will then be sub-ambient, and then gas will flow from the atmosphere into the airway.

2. TRANSPULMONARY GRADIENT: $P_{TP} = P_A - P_{PL}$

This is the gradient between the alveoli and the pleural space. At rest (the end of expiration) the pressure in the pleural space (P_{PL}) is -3 to -6 cmH$_2$O (average is -5 cmH$_2$O), and the pressure in the alveoli (P_A) is ambient (760 mmHg or 0 PSIG). Remember that the pleural pressure (P_{PL}) of -5 cmH$_2$O is caused by the opposing forces of the chest wall and the lungs while at rest. Remember that at the moment expiration ends and gas flow stops - even though P_A is ambient at this moment and P_{PL} is -5 cmH$_2$O at this moment – the pressure gradient (difference in pressure) that exists between the alveoli and the pleural space at this moment is only sufficient enough to keep the lung at FRC – which is what it is supposed to be doing. It is only a moment later when chest wall expansion begins the next breath cycle that the gradient becomes sufficient enough (P_{PL} becomes even more negative) such that P_A then becomes sub-ambient and thus P_{AO} becomes sub-ambient and then gas flows into the airway again.

Perhaps by now you have realized that even through the previously discussed transrespiratory gradient was referred to as the "mother" gradient (the overall gradient responsible for moving air in and out of the lungs), it is actually the transpulmonary gradient that initiates all of this. A gradient by definition is simply a difference in pressure between two areas – and yes – the ultimate gradient that is moving air in and out of the lungs is the gradient between the atmosphere (P_{BS}) and the inside of the mouth (P_{AO}). When the pressure inside the mouth becomes sub-ambient with respect to the atmosphere, then obviously air is going to flow into the airway – hence the transrespiratory gradient being called the "mother" gradient. BUT REALIZE that the P_{AO} could have never become sub-ambient in the first place if it weren't for the fact that P_A became sub-ambient as a result of the P_{PL} reaching a sub-ambience of at least -8 cmH$_2$O due to chest wall expansion. So, if you think about it, it's the transpulmonary gradient that actually makes it possible for air to ultimately move in and out of the lungs. Without the -8 cmH$_2$O P_{PL} being reflected across the A/C membrane so as to make P_A sub-ambient, P_{AO} would never become sub-ambient with respect to the atmosphere (P_{BS}). Depending on what books you read, you may see the transpulmonary gradient written as $P_{TP} = P_{AO} - P_{PL}$. From everything that has just been explained it should not bother you to see it this way – remember that the sub-ambient P_{PL} that has been reflected across the A/C membrane that makes the P_A sub-ambient is also reflected all the way up to the inside of the mouth to also make P_{AO} sub-ambient. Gas flows into the airway because the sub-ambient pressure at the level of the alveoli is reflected up to the inside of the mouth. That means that whatever P_A is, P_{AO} is the same thing - it therefore makes no difference whether you use P_A or P_{AO} in the equation.

A word regarding expiration

Insofar as discussions on the pressure gradients of the respiratory system tend to focus on inspiration, I want to take a moment to clarify the role of the pressure gradients in expiration. The principle of Boyle's Law is still applied to understand how gas is exhaled from the lungs. All you have to realize is that the process is just the opposite of inspiration. Unlike inspiration which is an active process involving muscle contraction, expiration is a passive process that does not involve any muscle contraction (except under conditions of forceful breathing or exercise). Expiration occurs because of the elastic recoil of the lungs and the chest wall. Once inspiration ends, the respiratory muscles (mainly the diaphragm) relax. When the diaphragm and the intercostals relax, the previously expanded (during inspiration) thoracic cavity begins to decrease its volume because of its inherent property of elastic recoil. This decrease in lung volume due to elastic recoil causes the pressure of the gas in the alveoli to increase. This is just Boyle's law in the reverse. With inspiration – the pressure in the lungs decreases because chest expansion via muscle contraction has increased the volume of the thoracic cavity. With expiration – the pressure in the lungs increases because the elastic recoil of the lungs causes the volume to decrease. When elastic recoil reduces the volume of the lungs, it causes P_A to become greater than P_{BS}. And remember that P_A is reflected up to P_{AO}. If the pressure in the alveoli (P_A) becomes greater than ambient (P_{BS}), then gas is going to flow out of the lungs. When the reduction of lung volume occurs due to elastic recoil, and thus the pressure in the alveoli becomes greater than ambient, gas flows from the area of higher pressure in the alveoli to the area of lower pressure in the atmosphere. It is just the reverse of inspiration. *With expiration, it is the recoil of the lungs that creates the pressure gradient by causing the pressure in the alveoli (P_A) to become greater than the ambient pressure (P_{BS}) in the atmosphere.*

RESPIRATORY SYSTEM PRESSURE GRADIENTS

The following diagram will help you
conceptualize the pressure gradients

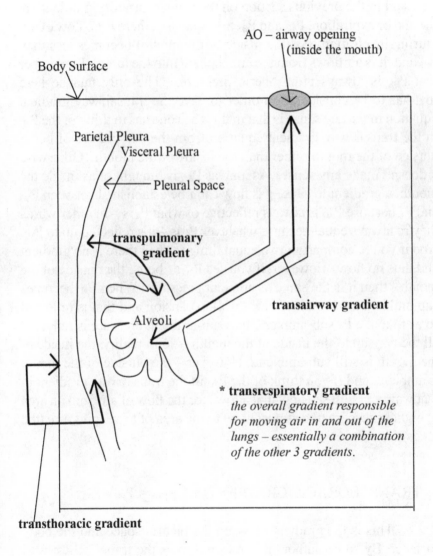

3. TRANSAIRWAY GRADIENT: $P_{TAW} = P_{AO} - P_A$

This is the gradient between the airway opening and the alveoli. *In practical terms*, this gradient is essentially the same thing as the transrespiratory gradient ($P_{TR} = P_{AO} - P_{BS}$). Remember what was said in the previous section on the transrespiratory gradient - at the end of expiration, P_{AO} and P_{BS} are equal and there is no flow of air. During inspiration, P_{AO} (the inside of the mouth) becomes less than P_{BS} and thus air flows from the atmosphere into the lungs. Remember that P_{BS} is always atmospheric pressure. The only nuance here that has to be considered in order to have the transairway gradient equation make any sense is that in this case one has to think of the P_{AO} in the transairway gradient equation from the perspective of being outside of the mouth rather than the inside of the mouth. Otherwise it doesn't make any sense. As long as P_{AO} is thought of as inside the mouth, a gradient to cause gas flow can't be established between P_{AO} and P_A because P_{AO} is always reflective of what P_A is – in other words they're always equal because whatever P_A is – it's reflected up to P_{AO}. And if you're comparing two equal things – then there is no gradient and thus no flow. However, if you see P_{AO} as being the outside of the mouth - then it is the same as ambient pressure. When P_{PL} becomes sub-ambient as a result of chest wall expansion and that is reflected so as to make P_A sub-ambient, that sub-ambient pressure is reflected all the way up to the inside of the mouth – so in reality, the inside of the mouth is still sub-ambient. However – the outside of the mouth is ambient, and if you think of the P_{AO} in the transairway gradient in that way, you will see how that allows for the flow of air from an area of higher pressure (the atmosphere) to the area of lower pressure (the lungs).

4. TRANSTHORACIC GRADIENT: $P_{TT} = P_{PL} - P_{BS}$

This is the gradient between the pleural space and the body surface. By some authors it is referred to as the trans – chest wall gradient. At rest it is representing the amount of force that is keeping the alveoli distended at FRC. During breathing it represents the total pressure required to expand or contract the lungs and chest wall.

C. Tidal Volume, IBW, and Respiratory Rate

Tidal Volume

- Tidal volume (V_T) is simply the volume of gas that is inhaled and exhaled with each normal breath.

- The average V_T for a normal adult at rest is between 5 – 8 ml/kg IBW.

- Average V_T is thus around 500ml.

IBW (Ideal Body Weight)

Tidal volume as just mentioned is in the context of the tidal volume that is breathed by a spontaneously breathing individual. Tidal volume does fluctuate somewhat from breath to breath, but as just stated – it averages around 500ml per breath for a normal adult. When a patient is being mechanically ventilated however, there are certain modes of mechanical ventilation where it is you the respiratory therapist that determines the V_T that the patient is going to get for each breath. The V_T that you have the ventilator deliver to the patient has to be determined according to their ideal body weight (IBW). I am jumping ahead here – IBW will be discussed in section I of chapter 8 – but since I just used the term in the second bullet point under tidal volume that was just discussed, I will also explain it to you now.

Formula for determining IBW in kg:

Males   50 + 2.3(height in inches – 60)

Females   45.5 + 2.3(height in inches – 60)

Example: you have a male patient that is 6'2" that weighs 230 lbs.

50 + 2.3(74 inches - 60 inches)
50 + 2.3(14)
50 + 32.2
82.2 kg is their IBW

If V_T is 5 – 8 ml/kg IBW, then 5 x 82.2 = 411, and 8 x 82.2 = 657.6
Therefore, you can set their V_T between $\approx$ 410 – 650 ml.

Note: Their IBW of 82.2 kg is the same as 181 lbs. (82.2 kg x 2.2 lbs./kg = 181 lbs.), which is 49 lbs. less than their actual weight of 230 lbs. But it is the IBW of 82.2 kg – not their actual weight that you must use when determining the range for tidal volume. IBW always has to be used because larger or heavier patients may have bigger bodies, but they don't have bigger lungs just because their bodies are bigger. Always be aware of this.

Respiratory Rate

The respiratory rate is the number of breaths a person takes per minute. The average respiratory rate for a normal, healthy individual is between 12 – 20 breaths per minute.

D. Breath Cycle Time (BCT), I:E Ratios, and T_I & T_E

Breath Cycle Time (BCT)

Every breath is a cycle of two distinct events – inspiration followed by expiration. Every breath cycle takes a certain amount of time – and that time is known as the breath cycle time. You may also hear it referred to as the total cycle time (TCT).

Calculation of the BCT

$$BCT = \frac{60}{RR}$$ gives you the number of seconds per breath (this includes inspiration & expiration)

60 is always a constant – it's the number of seconds in a minute. *Therefore it is the respiratory rate (frequency) that determines BCT.*

Example 1: RR is 12 breaths per minute.

$$BCT = \frac{60}{12} = 5 \text{ seconds per breath}$$

Example 2: RR is 14 breaths per minute.

$$BCT = \frac{60}{14} = 4.29 \text{ seconds per breath}$$

I:E Ratios and T_I & T_E

The BCT gives you the total amount of time for a breath, but the BCT consists of an inspiratory time (T_I) and an expiratory time (T_E) because a breath cycle consists of both inspiration and expiration. If the BCT is the total time for a breath, then obviously there is the portion of that total time that is accounted for by inspiration (T_I) and a portion of that total time that is accounted for by expiration (T_E).

The I:E ratio expresses the relationship between T_I and T_E. It is simply the ratio between inspiration and expiration. A ratio is a relationship between two numbers that compares values. A ratio tells you how much of one thing there is compared to another thing.

In this case we are comparing the amount of time for inspiration with the amount of time for expiration. We know from our understanding of human physiology that normal I:E ratios during normal tidal breathing are around 1:2 to 1:3. With a 1:2 ratio, that means that expiration is twice as long as inspiration. Realize that the amount of time spent on inspiration compared to the amount of time spent on expiration in a spontaneously breathing normal individual occurs naturally – that 1:2 ratio of inspiration to expiration just happens naturally on its own as part of the normal ventilatory process.

   If the BCT and the I:E ratio are known (and they will be known because BCT is determined by the simple calculation just shown, and the I:E for a normal person is 1:2), then you can determine the respective times for inspiration (T_I) and expiration (T_E) by using the following formula:

$$T_I = \frac{BCT \times I}{I + E}$$

This formula enables you to solve for T_I. Once you figure out T_I, you can then get T_E by subtracting T_I from BCT because

$$BCT = T_I + T_E$$

Therefore: $T_E = BCT - T_I$

Example:

Given that:

BCT = 5 seconds per breath
You determined this because we are using a RR of 12 for the hypothetical patient in this example, and $60/12 = 5$.

I:E ratio is 1:2
This is because you are dealing with a normal spontaneously breathing individual.

Therefore calculate T_I and T_E

$$T_I = \frac{BCT \times I}{I + E}$$

$$T_I = \frac{5 \times 1}{1 + 2} = \frac{5}{3} = 1.66 \text{ seconds}$$

And $T_E = BCT - T_I$ Therefore, $T_E = 5 - 1.66 = 3.34$ seconds

And to prove that this is correct:

The calculations just showed the T_I to be 1.66 seconds and the T_E to be 3.34 seconds – giving an I:E ratio of 1.66:3.34. But you know that when you express a ratio it has to be in terms of whole numbers – so you divide each of those terms by 1.66.

$$\frac{1.66 \; : \; 3.34}{1.66 \; : \; 1.66}$$ Gives you the ratio expressed as 1:2

and proves the correctness of the T_I and the T_E that you calculated because you solved that problem on the basis of an I:E ratio of 1:2.

There are various disease states that will alter the I:E ratio. You will become much more familiar with those conditions as you progress through your studies, but for now it would behoove you to understand the following:

- Obstructive lung disease generally causes T_E to INCREASE.

  - This is because in obstructive lung disease there is either a reduction in the elastic recoil ability of the lungs or an increase in resistance in the airway. It is often due to both.

- Restrictive lung disease generally causes T_E to DECREASE.

  - This is because in restrictive lung disease there is either an increase in the elastic recoil of the lungs or a decrease in alveolar filling. It is often due to both.

The End Expiratory Pause (EEP)

At the end of expiration, just before inspiration begins, there is a short period where there is no flow. That short period is known as the end expiratory pause (EEP).

- The EEP accounts for about 25% of the T_E. Therefore, EEP can be estimated as follows: $EEP = T_E \times 0.25$

E.   Resistance to Lung Inflation

It must be understood that in the normal process of breathing there are forces that naturally act to resist the inflation of the lung. In the last chapter resistance was introduced as it pertained to the resistance to flow (particularly the flow of gas), and from that discussion you should be able to appreciate that resistance is a force that opposes movement. In this section, the concept of resistance will now be extended to illustrate the forces involved that oppose (or resist) the inflation of the lung. There are two general categories of respiratory system resistances, and they are 1) elastic resistance and 2) frictional resistance.

1. Elastic Resistance

A. Elastance

There are millions of fibers (primarily elastic and collagen fibers) that are part of the anatomy of the airways and surround the alveoli. These fibers are what give the lungs their characteristic of *elasticity*. Think of elasticity as stretchiness + the ability to recoil – it is the propensity of a substance to return to its initial form after being stretched. This is why normal exhalation is passive (no muscle work is involved) – the natural elastic properties of the lung are sufficient to bring about exhalation without needing any additional muscle work. If the natural tendency of those fibers is to facilitate recoil, then they will also naturally tend to resist inflation. This natural tendency to resist inflation, which can be thought of as elastic resistance, must be overcome in order to get the lung inflated. Elastic resistance, or *elastance,* is the tendency of the lungs to resist a stretching force (inflation) and thus recoil or return to their original size and form after expansion. The greater the elastance of the lungs, the more work it is going to take to inflate the lunges. Lungs with really high elastance are stiff lungs – they resist inflation and are thus difficult to inflate. Let's backtrack for a moment and relate elastic resistance to the previous discussion on pressure gradients. When the diaphragm and intercostals contract during inspiration in order to expand the thoracic cavity and thus increase the volume of the thoracic cavity so as to cause the pressure in the alveoli to become sub-ambient so that gas can flow into the lungs – those muscles are having to exert enough force in order to overcome the elastic resistance of the lungs. When inspiration has ended and the muscles relax, the elastic recoil is then what causes the lung volume to go back down to what it was – and when the volume of the lungs decreases due to the elastic recoil – that's when the pressure in the alveoli becomes greater than atmospheric pressure such that gas then flows out of the lungs.

Mathematically, elastance is represented by the following:

$$\text{Elastance} \ = \ \frac{\Delta P}{\Delta V}$$

This equation is an interpretation of Hooke's Law. Hooke's Law explains how the elastic properties of the lungs and chest wall affect resistance during spontaneous inspiration and provide most of the energy for alveolar emptying during expiration. Hooke's Law essentially tells us that the tension that arises when an elastic structure is stretched out is directly related to the extent that the structure was stretched. In other words, stretch is proportional to stress. An understanding of this will enable you to understand how elastance and compliance change in the presence of disease, and how those changes affect both inhalation and lung emptying.

Elastance and compliance really need to be discussed together because they are reciprocals of each other. To be a reciprocal means to be the multiplicative inverse. Once we are finished discussing the forces that oppose lung inflation in this present section, we will then have a thorough discussion on lung compliance in the next section where we will also revisit elastance and compare and contrast it with compliance. Elastance and compliance are just different sides of the same coin. Whereas elastance is a measure of the resistance to stretch – compliance is a measure of the amount of force (stress) needed to overcome the elastance. Elastance cannot be measured directly, it is assessed indirectly as the reciprocal of compliance which can be effectively measured with an esophageal balloon.

B. Surface Tension

Surface tension is a phenomenon that occurs at a liquid – gas interface, and that is exactly what you have inside the alveoli. Just think of the alveoli as little gas filled balls, and the inner surface of those balls is lined with liquid. The resulting surface tension, which indeed can be thought of as a force, acts in such a way so as to promote the recoil or collapse of the alveoli. And therefore this is a force that must be overcome in order to inflate the lung.

In the last section on elastance we discussed how there are millions of elastic fibers that are part of the lung, and that the natural tendency of those fibers is to facilitate recoil. Well in similar fashion, surface tension is doing the same thing in that it too is acting in a way so as to promote the recoil or collapse of the lung – and therefore the force of surface tension must be overcome just like elastance has to be overcome in order to inflate the lung.

Don't forget that the alveoli have surfactant to modulate the effects of surface tension. Surfactant plays a significant role in enabling the alveoli to dynamically adjust their rates of inspiration and exhalation so as to equalize ventilation throughout the lung. Generally speaking however, surface tension is higher during rapid inspiration because the alveolar surface is expanding at a faster rate than what the surfactant can keep pace with. Thus, with rapid inspiration, the resistance to lung expansion due to surface tension is even greater.

2. Frictional Resistance

A. Tissue Viscous Resistance

Tissue viscous resistance is essentially the opposition of the movement of the of the lungs and thorax during ventilation. As the lungs and thorax expand and contract during inspiration and expiration, these tissues have to move over each other, and this movement generates frictional resistance which requires energy to overcome. Tissue viscous resistance is responsible for about 20% of the total frictional resistance to lung inflation.

B. Airway Resistance

Airway resistance is responsible for the other 80% of the frictional resistance to lung inflation. This is the friction that occurs between the flowing gas and the walls of the airways. If necessary, you may want to revisit the discussion on resistance to flow in section E of chapter one. Resistance in the airway is given by:

$$R_{AW} = \frac{\Delta P}{\dot{V}}$$

For a normal spontaneously breathing adult – R_{AW} ranges from $0.5 - 2.5$ cmH$_2$O/L/sec. Remember at the beginning of this chapter when we were discussing the various pressure gradients – recall that the P_{PL} at rest is around -5 cmH$_2$O, but that this was only enough to just keep the lung distended at FRC. In order to cause air to flow into the lungs the P_{PL} had to become even more sub-ambient. Well not only for that reason, but now you see that it must also become sub-ambient enough so as to establish a sufficient enough pressure differential to also overcome the R_{AW} of $0.5 - 2.5$ cmH$_2$O/L/sec just mentioned. And that is why it takes a P_{PL} of around -8 cmH$_2$O to not only get air to flow into the lungs, but to also be able to overcome the resistance to flow as well.

You also need to realize that anything that causes resistance to increase – (whether it is from an *obstruction in the airway* due to mucus plugs, tumors, or other foreign bodies - or a *narrowing of the airway* due to asthma or any other source of bronchoconstriction) –

is going to cause flow ($\dot{V}$) to become diminished. For a given pressure that is *constant*, if the resistance (the R_{AW} term – the quotient in the resistance equation) increases, then the flow term (the denominator) must decrease. Anything that would cause resistance to increase (thus making the quotient bigger) is going to make the denominator (flow) smaller.

As just mentioned, airway resistance is responsible for 80% of the total frictional resistance to lung inflation. Of this 80% - about 80% (or 64% of the total frictional resistance) is due to the resistance occurring in upper airway, trachea, bronchi, and larger bronchioles where flow is mostly turbulent. The other 20% (or 16% of the total frictional resistance) is due to the resistance in the small airways where flow is mostly laminar. In essence, the deeper you go in the airway, the less resistance you encounter. By the time gas reaches the smallest airways and alveolar ducts where flow has become *diffusional*, there is essentially no more resistance.

Some additional important thoughts

One of the overriding ideas of this chapter so far is that energy has to be provided to overcome resistance in order to enable the adequate flow of air. The KE (kinetic energy) of respiratory muscle contraction provides for the expansion of the thoracic cavity which thus causes the changes in pressure (the pressure gradients that are generated as a result of the muscles expanding the chest cavity). Chest expansion and the formation of the pressure gradients occurs because under conditions of normal breathing this muscle energy is sufficient enough to overcome the resistances to lung inflation. But realize that there is something else going on at the same time. Although the action of the muscles has expanded the chest cavity so as to create the pressure gradients that will ultimately drive the inspiration of air – that same muscle action has also served to impart PE (potential energy) to the lung tissue itself by virtue of having stretched it. The action of the respiratory muscles thus has a twofold effect. It expands the chest cavity so as to create the pressure gradients, but then at the same time, by virtue of stretching the lung tissue itself – PE is imparted to that tissue. When you stretch a structure that is inherently elastic such as the lungs, you are effectively increasing the amount of PE of that structure. Think of the elastic fibers of the lungs as a spring – when you stretch out a spring you are imparting potential energy to it. Just let go of that stretched out spring and it will return immediately to its resting state – it will have released that stored PE in the form of KE in the process of returning to its resting state. It's the same thing with the lungs. During exhalation, the stored PE (the energy imparted to the elastic fibers of the lungs by virtue of having been stretched during inspiration) is then released via the elastic recoil. The PE that was stored in the elastic fibers of the lungs as a result of having been stretched during inspiration now becomes KE in the form of the recoil – and the recoil motion of those elastic fibers is what decreases the volume of the lungs and thus simultaneously raises the pressure of the alveolar gas above ambient such that the gas is exhaled out of the lungs.

F. Compliance

Of all the concepts that you must have at your fingertips in order to be a great respiratory therapist, the concept of lung compliance is one of the most important. Understanding lung compliance is important because it comes into play in the understanding of various disease states as well as the strategies that are employed in the management of a patient – especially when the patient is being ventilated mechanically.

In the last section the concept of elastance was introduced, and it was described as the tendency of the lungs to resist a stretching force (inflation) and thus recoil or return to their original size or form after deformation (expansion). I then went on to say that compliance is the reciprocal of elastance. Whereas elastance is a measure of the resistance to stretch – compliance is a measure of the amount of force (stress) needed to overcome the elastance. Put another way – compliance is the ease with which the lungs can be inflated. It is the ease with which something can be stretched. It reflects the amount of force (energy) needed to expand the chest wall and inflate the lungs. Mathematically, compliance is represented by the following:

$$\text{Compliance} \ = \ \frac{\Delta V}{\Delta P}$$

Compliance is the reciprocal of elastance. Compliance and elastance are therefore reciprocals of each other.

Elastance: $E \ = \ \dfrac{\Delta P}{\Delta V}$ or $E = \dfrac{1}{C}$

Compliance: $C = \dfrac{\Delta V}{\Delta P}$ or $C = \dfrac{1}{E}$

The reciprocal relationship between compliance and elastance

Consider the following 2 graphs.

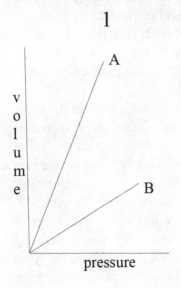

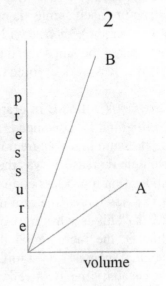

$$\text{Compliance} \ = \ \frac{\Delta V}{\Delta P} \qquad\qquad \text{Elastance} \ = \ \frac{\Delta P}{\Delta V}$$

Start by looking at line A in graph 1. It has a steep slope. That means that for incremental increases in pressure (ΔP) there are significant increases in volume (ΔV). This is good compliance – the numerator (ΔV) is high with respect to the denominator (ΔP), which gives you a large quotient. Line A in graph 1 is representing lungs with good compliance – they are easily inflated because the resistance to inflation (elastance) is low.

Now compare that to line A in graph 2 which is its reciprocal – elastance. The slope is much smaller, which is what you would expect since elastance is the reciprocal of compliance. If the lungs have high compliance as indicated by line A in graph 1 – then we would expect them to have low elastance as indicated by line A in graph 2. Line A in graph 2 shows you that for incremental increases in volume that the changes in pressure aren't as steep – this is indicating low elastance. It's telling you that it's not requiring significant increases in pressure in order to achieve increases in volume. When elastance is low, that means that the structure has less resistance to being stretched - which means that its reciprocal – compliance (the ease with which it can be stretched) is higher. If the structure itself (lungs) is not exhibiting a lot of elastance (resistance to stretching), then it will be easier to stretch (inflate). The more compliant the lungs are, the easier they are to inflate. In other words, it takes less work or force to inflate lungs that have good compliance.

Now look at line B in graph 1. The slope is much smaller than line A in graph 1. This means that for those same incremental increases in pressure that you are not getting anywhere near the same level of volume increase as was the case in line A. This is because line B is indicating much less compliant lungs. With line A, your numerator (ΔV) was increasing at a much quicker rate than your denominator (ΔP). This is why line A is much steeper line than line B. With line B, the incremental increases in pressure are not generating volume increases as significantly as was the case with line A. This is because line B is reflecting much less compliant lungs. Line B is representing lungs that are not as easy to inflate as the lungs represented by line A.

Look at the reciprocal graph for line B in graph 2 and see the steepness of the slope. Line B in graph 2 is showing lungs with high elastance, which is what we would expect for lungs whose compliance graph (line B in graph 1) showed low compliance. It's telling you that it's requiring significant increases in pressure in order to achieve increases in volume. When elastance is high, that means that the structure has more resistance to being stretched.

From this point forward – understand that the word elastance is almost never used clinically. In the clinical setting lungs are described in terms of their compliance. But now you know that they are just opposite sides of the same coin. When you hear it said that the patient has good lung compliance – you know that inherently means that elastance is low because you know that in order for compliance to be good that there can't be high resistance to lung inflation. Conversely – when the patient has low lung compliance you now know that means that elastance is high. In order for a patient to have low lung compliance there needs to be something going on that is causing a high resistance to lung inflation. From a clinical standpoint, there are various diseases and conditions that directly affect lung compliance. Pulmonary fibrosis is a condition that will greatly reduce the compliance of the lungs. With pulmonary fibrosis you end up with excessive amounts of fibrous connective tissue in the lung parenchyma which imposes serious restrictions on the ability to inflate the lung. ARDS, pulmonary edema, pneumonia, and other issues that cause lung consolidation will decrease pulmonary compliance because it is much harder to inflate the lungs when the alveoli are full of fluid. Lungs with low compliance are said to be "stiff" lungs, and in order to inspire an adequate tidal volume it requires a significant increase in the work of breathing. On the other hand, there are conditions that can affect the lungs that make pulmonary compliance too high. The best example of this is emphysema. The pathology of emphysema will be covered in depth in chapter 9, but understand for now that the reason why emphysema causes the lungs to be overly compliant is because one of the consequences of emphysema is that the lungs lose a significant amount of their recoil ability (hence elastance is super low). The extra high lung compliance associated with emphysema is due to the significantly reduced elastic recoil of the lungs. Patients with emphysema therefore have extreme difficulty with exhalation. Whereas exhalation is passive for a normal person, an emphysema patient often has to work to exhale.

Graphical example of the differences in lung compliance depending upon disease / condition:

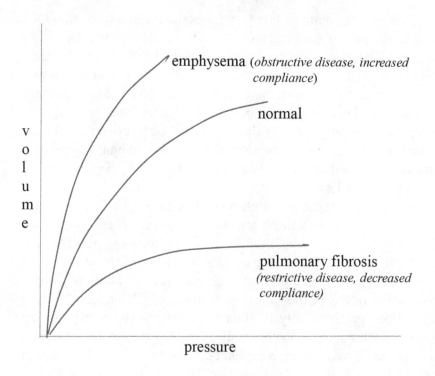

Compared to normal lungs, emphysematous lungs have much higher compliance (too high). The emphysema curve is the steepest curve with the greatest increases in volume per unit increase of pressure.

Fibrotic lungs on the other hand have much lower compliance than the normal lung. Not only is the curve less steep indicating smaller increases in volume per unit increase of pressure, but the curve itself eventually levels off which indicates that there is no more volume increase – no matter how much the pressure is increased.

As previously indicated, compliance is expressed as the change in volume divided by the change in pressure. The pressure we are speaking of in the compliance equation is the intrapleural pressure. The standard units used to express compliance are L/cmH_2O, and under normal conditions the lung/thorax compliance is 0.1 L/cmH_2O, or 100ml/cmH_2O (but note that normal values can range from 60 – 100ml/cmH_2O). Both the lungs and the thorax have a compliance of 0.1 L/cmH_2O, but remember that the forces of the lungs and the thorax oppose one another – so rather than being additive, the compliance of the lungs + thorax is simply 0.1 L/cmH_2O or 100ml/cmH_2O.

By way of example – consider a patient who inhales a tidal volume (V_T) of 500 mL (.5L). Let's say their P_{PL} before inspiration is – 5 cmH_2O and at the end of inspiration their P_{PL} is -10 cmH_2O.

Therefore:

$$\text{Compliance} = \frac{\Delta V}{\Delta P} = \frac{.5\ L}{-5\ cmH_2O - (-10\ cmH_2O)} = \frac{.5\ L}{5\ cmH_2O}$$

$$= 0.1\ L/cmH_2O, \text{ or } 100\ ml/cmH_2O$$

When a patient is receiving positive pressure mechanical ventilation, compliance is discussed in terms of either static compliance or dynamic compliance. I am discussing this now because I want you to have a thorough presentation of compliance, but there are going to be a couple of items in the equations that follow that you won't have full understanding of until you study mechanical ventilation. In the mechanical ventilation chapter, you will gain a thorough understanding of what is meant by plateau pressure (P_{PLT}), positive end expiratory pressure (PEEP), and peak inspiratory pressure (PIP), but for now it is sufficient for you to just realize that those terms are just the parameters that are used to determine ΔP – and by this point you are conceptually familiar with ΔP as it pertains to the basic lung compliance equation.

The two equations about to be presented for static and dynamic compliance *are used with mechanically ventilated patients*, and they are simply variations of the basic equation for pulmonary compliance that you already know and understand.

$$C_L = \frac{\Delta V}{\Delta P}$$

The L after the C is just designating it as the compliance of the lung.

Static Compliance - (C_{stat}) - *In mechanically ventilated patients*

Static compliance represents pulmonary compliance during periods when gas is not flowing, such as during an inspiratory hold. An inspiratory hold is a maneuver that is done when a patient is on mechanical ventilation in order to obtain the plateau pressure (P_{PLT}).

$$C_{stat} = \frac{V_T}{P_{PLT} - PEEP}$$

V_T is the tidal volume - it represents ΔV. With static compliance, P_{PLT} - PEEP represents ΔP for a patient that is receiving positive pressure mechanical ventilation. P_{PLT} is the plateau pressure and PEEP is the positive end expiratory pressure.

Dynamic Compliance (C_{dyn}) - *In mechanically ventilated patients*

$$C_{dyn} = \frac{V_T}{PIP - PEEP}$$

Dynamic compliance represents pulmonary compliance when gas is flowing. Dynamic compliance should always be $\leq$ static compliance because the denominator of C_{dyn} - (PIP - PEEP) should always be greater than the denominator of C_{stat} – (P_{PLT} - PEEP) – This is because PEEP is a constant and P_{PLT} is never greater than PIP. Again - V_T is the tidal volume and it represents ΔV. With dynamic compliance, PIP – PEEP represents ΔP for a patient that is receiving positive pressure mechanical ventilation. PIP is the peak inspiratory pressure and PEEP is positive end expiratory pressure.

The next important topic is the compliance *curve*. This curve is the graphical representation of lung compliance and you will see it often, both in school and throughout your clinical career. There are variations to this basic curve, but having a good understanding of this basic curve will enable you to interpret any of the various other forms this curve can assume. The curve is basically a graphical representation of the relationship between pressure and lung volume. You may also see it referred to as the pressure – volume curve or the pressure – volume loop.

The Compliance Curve

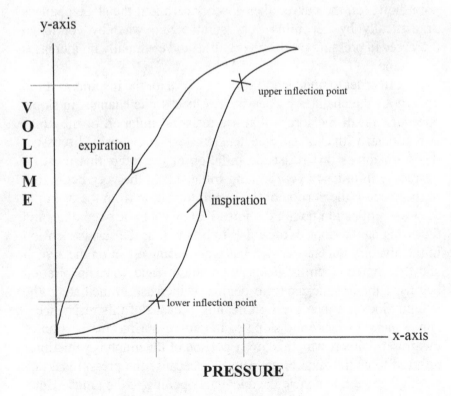

Looking at the compliance curve you will observe that there are 2 parts to the curve. There is an inspiratory limb and an expiratory limb. The inspiratory limb is showing the relationship between pressure and volume during inspiration, and the expiratory limb is showing the relationship between pressure and volume during expiration. Notice on the inspiratory limb that there are two points that are marked – the lower inflection point and the upper inflection point.

Let us begin our analysis of the graph by starting at the origin and working our way up the inspiratory limb. Notice that from the origin to the lower inflection point that the slope of the curve is rather minimal and that for incremental increases in pressure that there are only small and gradual increases in volume. But then – at the point of the lower inflection point, the slope of the curve changes drastically. It takes an upward turn and becomes a very steep curve all the way up to the upper inflection point. From the lower inflection point up to the upper inflection point, for incremental increases in pressure, there are significant increases in volume. At the upper inflection point however, the curve takes another turn and the slope changes dramatically by becoming very small again whereby continued increases in pressure produce very little and eventually no increases in volume.

In order to understand why the curve for the inspiratory limb undergoes the changes it does with respect to its changes in slope, one must recall the forces that are resisting inflation of the lungs – particularly that of surface tension. As previously discussed, there are forces that resist the inflation of the lungs that must be overcome in order to get the lung inflated. At the very beginning of inspiration (the portion of the inspiratory limb from the origin to the lower inflection point), the force that needs to be overcome, and thus causing the slope of the curve to be small, is the surface tension in the alveoli. Surface tension has a collapsing effect on the alveoli and thus makes them resistant to inflation - and when inspiration begins, although the pressure begins to increase immediately, the volume does not increase significantly because of this resistance – hence the very moderate slope of the curve during this portion of the graph. This is why this lower portion of the graph is sometimes referred to as the zone of atelectasis – because the pressures aren't yet high enough to enable the adequate opening of the lungs. But –

at the point of the lower inflection point, the pressure has become sufficient enough to overcome the resistance due to surface tension such that the alveoli then "pop" open and are then able to be much more easily inflated. This is why the pressure that corresponds to the lower inflection point is known at the *critical opening pressure*. It is the pressure needed to pop open the alveoli and thus the reason why the graph takes such a sharp upward turn at this point. From the lower inflection point up to the upper inflection point there are significant increases in volume for the incremental changes in pressure. Look at the graph – from the lower inflection point to the upper inflection point, the change in pressure (ΔP) along the x-axis of the graph is not that much. But the change in volume (ΔV) along the y-axis is significant during this portion of the graph. The two lines marked on the x-axis are indicating the pressures at the lower and upper inflection points respectively. ΔP is the change in pressure from what the pressure was at the lower inflection point to what it is at the upper inflection point. The two lines marked on the y-axis are indicating the volumes that correspond the to the pressures at the lower inflection point and the upper inflection point respectively. ΔV is the change in volume from what the volume was at the lower inflection point to what it is at the upper inflection point. Just a casual observation of the graph immediately shows you that the ΔV that occurs between the lower and upper inflection points is much larger compared to the corresponding ΔP that occurs between the lower and upper inflection points. This is because during this portion of the graph, surface tension has already been overcome such that the alveoli can fill much more readily.

At the point of the upper inflection point, the curve turns dramatically again – this time to the right, and the slope becomes very small again. This is showing that from the point of the upper inflection point – any further increases in pressure are only going to result in very minimal increases in volume. And if the inspiratory limb of the curve was to be extended at this point, it would show it eventually becoming flat - indicating that there would be no further volume increases regardless of any additional increases in pressure. This portion of the curve is telling you that the lungs have reached their limit – in other words they are full and cannot hold anymore volume. Further increases in pressure will not result in any further increases in volume – in fact, further increases in pressure at this point are going to cause damage due the trauma that would be caused by excessive pressures. The upper inflection point therefore is indicating the point beyond which is the overdistension of the lungs. This is why the upper portion of the graph beyond the upper inflection point is sometimes referred to as the zone of over-distension.

The expiratory limb does not have the two drastic curvature changes like the inspiratory limb. During expiration, there is nothing holding the lungs open except the gas contained within them, and under the conditions of normal expiration in the absence of any pathology, there is nothing resisting the flow of gas out of the airway – hence the uniformity and gradual decrease of the expiratory limb.

Hysteresis

If you look at the compliance curve, it is very obvious that there is space in between the inspiratory limb and the expiratory limb. The fact that this space exists is indicating to you that for any given pressure – the corresponding volume for that pressure on the inspiratory limb is different than the corresponding volume for that pressure on the expiratory limb. This difference in volumes for inspiration compared to expiration for a given pressure (or the difference in lung compliance) is what is known as hysteresis. For any given pressure, lung volume will always be greater on the expiratory limb than the inspiratory limb – or you could conversely say that for any given pressure, lung volume will always be less on the inspiratory limb than the expiratory limb.

In all likelihood, whether in your other reading or in your lectures, you will have encountered an example of the compliance curve showing no real hysteresis by virtue of the lungs having been filled with saline rather than air. In that example, the inspiratory and expiratory limbs essentially run right along one another with no appreciable space in between them, and there is no true lower inflection point. This is because when you fill a lung with saline solution rather than air, there is no surface tension to contend with. Surface tension occurs at a gas – liquid interface, and when you're filling a lung with a liquid, the surface tension issue is not a factor –

hence the two limbs are essentially the same with no hysteresis.

Hysteresis, or the difference in compliance between inspiration and expiration, occurs because of the additional energy that is required during inspiration in order to recruit and inflate the alveoli. Another way of looking at it is to say that it takes less energy or force to keep an already inflated lung open during expiration (deflation) than it does to inflate it initially during inspiration. The lungs dissipate energy during inspiration, which is to say that some of the energy that is expended in the inflation of the lungs is either not fully recovered, or there is delayed recovery of the energy during deflation. The lungs are not a perfectly elastic system in the sense of the energy that is imparted to them being immediately returned.

These ideas completely reinforce why it is so important to prevent atelectasis, as an atelectatic lung is so much more difficult to open. The actual mechanism by which the lung units (alveoli) are either inflated or deflated during inspiration and expiration respectively is through what is known as recruitment and decruitment. At the end of expiration, when the lungs are at FRC, some alveoli are open and others are closed, but those that are closed are for the most part recruitable. An atelectatic lung is one where there are more closed alveoli than what there normally should be – hence there are more closed units that need to be opened. This makes the recruitment effort more challenging and this is why you want to avoid atelectasis. When you look at the beginning of the compliance curve from the origin to the lower inflection point – the beginning of the recruitment of alveoli is what is going on during this part of the curve. Throughout this beginning part of the curve, as the pressure continues to increase, more alveoli are recruited and forced open. But when the critical opening pressure is reached at the lower inflection point, the alveolar recruitment rate begins to accelerate as indicated by the upward turn of the curve and the steep slope all the way up to the upper inflection point. Realize that the entire inspiratory limb of the compliance curve is an alveolar recruitment curve. Under normal conditions, at the end of inspiration the lungs are at TLC (total lung capacity), and the alveoli have all been recruited and are thus open. At the very beginning of expiration, with all the alveoli being open, deflation begins and proceeds along a gradual and uniformly descending slope until the lungs are emptied to FRC. As stated previously, the forces that resist the recruitment process during inflation (surface tension) are not a factor during expiration. During expiration there is nothing holding the lungs open except the gas contained within them, and under the conditions of normal expiration in the absence of any pathology, there is nothing resisting the flow of gas out of the airway – hence the uniformity and gradual decrease of the expiratory limb. During expiration, while the lungs are emptying and thus de-recruiting, they will have a greater volume for a given pressure than they did during inspiration. This is because hysteresis has shown us that it takes less energy or force to keep an already inflated lung open during expiration (deflation) than it does to inflate it initially during inspiration.

G. Pulmonary Time Constants

When a change in pressure (ΔP) is applied to the lungs, it takes a certain amount of time before a change in volume (ΔV) occurs. This applies to both inspiration and expiration. It is the compliance of the lung along with airway resistance that determine the rate (time) of alveolar filling (inspiration) and emptying (expiration). The combined effects of lung compliance and airway resistance can be determined as a physical property that is called the time constant. In other words – it is compliance and resistance that determine the time constant. Mathematically, the time constant (T_C) is defined as the product of compliance (C_L) and R_{AW}. This calculation allows you to assess the combined effect of resistance and compliance on gas flow.

$$T_C = R_{AW} \times C_L$$

- R_{AW} is expressed in $cmH_2O/L/sec$.
- C_L is expressed L/cmH_2O.
- All the units will cancel leaving T_C expressed in seconds.

NOW – <u>One time constant</u> is defined as the time in seconds that it takes to fill or empty about 63% of the volume of the lungs.

Consider the following:

Consider a patient with a normal airway resistance of 2.0 $cmH_2O/L/sec$, and a normal lung compliance of 0.1 L/cmH_2O. The time constant for this individual would be determined as follows:

$T_C = R_{AW} \times C_L$

$T_C = 2.0\ cmH_2O/L/sec \times 0.1\ L/cmH_2O$

$T_C = 0.2$ seconds

This means that after 1 time constant (0.2 seconds), the lungs will have either filled to 63% of their capacity (in the case of inspiration) OR emptied 63% of their volume (in the case of expiration).

After the second time constant (the second 0.2 seconds), another 63% of the *remaining* volume of gas will have been moved. Think about what this means – after the first time constant (the first 0.2 seconds), 63% of the gas volume was either inhaled or exhaled. That means that there is 37% left to go (remaining). During the time of the second time constant (the second 0.2 seconds), another 63% of the gas volume is moved – but since there was only 37% left to go at the beginning of the second time constant - that means the lungs either filled or emptied another 23% (63% of 37) such that after the second time constant the lungs will have either filled or emptied a total of 86% (63% + 23% = 86%).

After the third time constant (the third 0.2 seconds – a total of 0.6 seconds now), another 63% of the *remaining* volume of gas will have been moved. After the second time constant, 86 % of the gas volume was either inhaled or exhaled. That means that there is 14% left to go (remaining). During the time of the third time constant (the third 0.2 seconds), another 63% of the gas volume is moved – but since there was only 14% left to go at the beginning of the third time constant - that means the lungs either filled or emptied another 9% (63% of 14) such that after the third time constant the lungs will have either filled or emptied a total of 95% - (86% + 9% = 95%).

Summary: During each time constant, 63% of the *remaining* volume is moved – therefore:

After 1 T_C – the lungs are either filled or emptied 63%

After 2 T_C – the lungs are either filled or emptied 86%

After 3 T_C – the lungs are either filled or emptied 95%

After 4 T_C – the lungs are either filled or emptied 98%

After 5 T_C – the lungs are either filled or emptied 99%

THESE PERCENTAGES WILL ALWAYS REMAIN THE SAME BECAUSE 63% OF THE *REMAINING* VOLUME IS WHAT IS ALWAYS MOVED DURING EACH TIME CONSTANT.

THE EQUATION – $T_C = R_{AW} \times C_L$ SIMPLY DICTATES HOW LONG EACH TIME CONSTANT WILL BE.

Consider the following example:

Consider a 500ml tidal volume being moved (either inspired or exhaled) according to what was just described. The time constant is 0.2 seconds. For each time constant, 63% of the remaining volume is moved.

500ml – Total volume that is either inhaled or exhaled.

- 315ml – Volume moved during first time constant. 315 is 63% of 500.

185ml – Volume remaining after first time constant.

After the first time constant (the first 0.2 seconds), 315ml of gas will have been moved. This is because you started out with 500ml of gas, and 63% of 500ml (.63 x 500) is 315ml. Total gas moved at this point is 63% of 500ml. That leaves 185ml remaining.

185ml – Volume remaining after first time constant.

- 117ml – Volume moved during second time constant. 117 is 63% of 185.

68ml – Volume remaining after second time constant.

After the second time constant (the second 0.2 seconds), 117ml of gas will have been moved. Remember that for each time constant, 63% of the remaining volume is moved. If there was 185ml remaining after the first time constant, and .63 x 185ml = 117ml, then after the second time constant, another 117ml of gas will have moved. After the second time constant, 86% of the gas volume has been moved. 315ml + 117ml = 432ml, and 432ml is ≈ 86% of 500ml. The amount now remaining is 68ml.

68ml – Volume remaining after second time constant.

- 43ml – Volume moved during third time constant. 43 is 63% of 68.

25ml – Volume remaining after third time constant.

After the third time constant (the third 0.2 seconds), 43ml of gas will have been moved. If there was 68ml remaining after the second time constant, and .63 x 68ml = 43ml, then after the third time constant, another 43ml of gas will have moved. After the third time constant, 95% of the gas volume has been moved. 315ml + 117ml + 43ml = 475ml, and 475ml is 95% of 500ml. The amount now remaining is 25ml.

25ml – Volume after third time constant.

- 16ml – Volume moved during fourth time constant. 16 is 63% of 25.

9ml – Volume remaining after fourth time constant.

After the fourth time constant (the fourth 0.2 seconds), 16ml of gas will have been moved. If there was 25ml remaining after the third time constant, and .63 x 25ml = 16ml, then after the fourth time constant, another 16ml of gas will have moved. After the fourth constant, 98% of the gas volume has been moved. 315ml + 117ml + 43ml + 16ml = 491ml, and 491ml is ≈ 98% of 500ml. The amount now remaining is 9ml.

This is why it is said that it takes roughly 4 time constants to either inspire or exhale a complete tidal volume. In the case of the example just given, the total tidal volume to be moved (inhaled or exhaled) was 500ml, and it took 4 time constants (0.8 seconds – almost 1 second) to move 98% of that volume.

Ventilation throughout the lungs is not always evenly distributed due to differences in compliance and resistance in different areas of the lungs. Differences in compliance and resistance in different areas of the lungs will then cause variation in the time constant in different parts of the lungs.

- The TC can change, as C_L and R_{AW} can either improve or worsen.
- Lung units with high compliance and/or high airway resistance will have a longer than normal T_C. Think about it – if $T_C = C_L$ x R_{AW}, and if either C_L or R_{AW} is increased, then the product (T_C) is going to be bigger (meaning longer in duration since T_C is expressed in seconds.)
- Lung units with low compliance and/or low airway resistance will have a shorter than normal T_C because if either C_L or R_{AW} is decreased, then the product (T_C) will be smaller (shorter in duration.)

Insofar as you now know how to determine the time constant (T_C) as being the product of compliance (C_L) and resistance (R_{AW}), when you get to chapter 8 and study mechanical ventilation, you will be able to apply the concept of the time constant when it comes to manipulation of T_I and T_E. T_I is a parameter that you set in pressure control ventilation, and now you know that the T_I has to be set so as to be *at least* 3 time constants in length. Although T_E is not a parameter you directly set - it is manipulated by other means, but for all modes of ventilation you now know that the T_E also needs to be *at least* 3 time constants in length.

H. The Frequency Dependence of Compliance

Frequency dependence of compliance is something that is observed primarily in patients with COPD that have obstruction in the small airways. Frequency dependence of compliance means that as breathing frequency increases, compliance decreases. COPD patients tend to breath at increased rates, and lung compliance is considered frequency dependent when the dynamic compliance at any of those increased breathing rates becomes less than 80% of the static compliance. In normal individuals, the alveoli fill and empty in a fairly synchronous manner at all respiratory rates. As such, lung compliance is not usually dependent on respiratory rate. Frequency dependence of compliance, however, implies that there are regions of the lungs where the filling and emptying of the lungs is not happening synchronously – meaning that there are regions of the lungs that are moving out of phase with other regions.

The rate at which alveoli respond to a given change in pressure (ΔP) by undergoing a change in volume (ΔV) is determined by the time constant. The higher the resistance, or the greater the compliance of a lung unit – the longer it takes for gas to either fill or be emptied from that particular lung unit – thus a longer time constant. COPD is characterized by either increased resistance in the airways and/or increased lung compliance – and those areas of the lungs that are affected as such are therefore going to have longer time constants.

When different areas of the lungs have different time constants, they fill and empty at different rates. Having different time constants in different areas of the lungs, and thus different filling and emptying rates in those areas, is due to obstruction of the small airways. But despite this variation in filling and emptying rates in different parts of the lungs, when the respiratory rate is slower, gas can still be somewhat equally distributed such that dynamic compliance is not significantly altered. But during rapid breathing, which is often the case with COPD patients, gas moves less rapidly into the areas of the lung that have longer time constants – especially those with high airway resistance. Although that may seem like a contradiction at first, remember that if the time constant of a particular part of the lung is longer, it is because that part of the lung has either increased compliance or increased resistance to begin with. Lung units with increased compliance take longer to fill and gas takes longer to flow through airways with increased resistance. Rapid breathing also usually means shallow breathing with COPD patients. For any given breath, these patients are not taking in that great of a tidal volume – they're not moving a good volume of air anyway. That, along with the fact that most of their lung units have longer time constants due to their disease, is why rapid breathing doesn't enable them to sufficiently expand their lung units that have longer time constants. The lung units with longer time constants therefore fill less and empty much slower than lung units with normal compliance and resistance. In other words, it takes too long to get these lung units to expand – there is insufficient time to expand these lung units. As a result, greater pressure is needed to move the volume of gas in order to maintain alveolar ventilation, and dynamic compliance falls.

Furthermore, flowing gas will follow the path of least resistance if it can, and this means that gas will be diverted to the areas of their lungs that have shorter time constants. Frequency dependence of compliance is observed in patients with COPD when the small number of lung units that do have relatively normal time constants end up getting more ventilation than the abnormal lung units that have longer time constants. As the lung units with normal time constants fill – their compliance goes down.

I. The Equal Pressure Point & Dynamic Compression of the Airways

Understanding the concept of the equal pressure point is important because it enables you to understand what is going on with respect to limitations on expiratory flow under the conditions of *forced exhalation*. To reiterate - we are not talking about normal passive exhalation, but rather the situation of forced exhalation. In a healthy individual, forced exhalation usually only occurs during exercise or perhaps when they are undergoing pulmonary function tests where they are required to forcefully exhale as part of the PFT. An individual with obstructive lung disease (emphysema for example), however, often finds themselves exhaling forcefully in an attempt to adequately empty their lungs – and forced exhalation with these patients unfortunately causes even further limitations to expiratory flow.

Under conditions of normal spontaneous expiration, it is the recoil force of the lungs that is providing the energy to drive the flow of air out of the lungs. When expiration is forced, however, muscle energy is added and this causes some changes in lung dynamics so as to impose limitations on expiratory flow. Under conditions of forced expiration, these changes in lung dynamics cause the airways to narrow, and this in turn imposes limitations on expiratory flow because the narrowing of the airways in and of itself is an obstruction to flow. With healthy individuals, this doesn't usually present a problem because airway narrowing and collapse doesn't generally occur except at very low lung volumes, whereas with an emphysema patient the airway narrowing and collapse occurs at much higher lung volumes. In order to understand how this occurs, consider the following.

To begin with, you need to have a solid understanding of the anatomy of the lungs and be able to picture the lungs and the airways three dimensionally in your mind. As the airways course along through the lung parenchyma, there are certain factors that help to maintain their structural integrity and patency. With the larger airways, the cartilage that is part of the walls of the airways is the main factor in structural support, but with the smaller airways that lack cartilage in their walls, structural integrity is maintained by radial traction and transmural pressure. The exterior of the small airways is directly adhered to the surrounding lung tissue by connective tissue fibers. These fibers "tug" on the airways so as to help them remain patent - this is radial traction. Transmural pressure is the pressure across the wall of a tube (the airways). It is a ratio of the pressure inside the tube (which acts to distend the tube) to the pressure outside the tube (which acts to collapse the tube). As long as the pressure inside the airways is greater than the pressure outside the airways, the transmural pressure will favor keeping the airways open.

So, you have these two main factors helping to keep the small airways open – radial traction and transmural pressure. Now, picture the pleura three dimensionally. The pleural cavity is not a two-dimensional structure just occurring on the lateral borders of the lungs as depicted in a drawing in a book – it's a three-dimensional structure that completely surrounds and envelops the lungs. Having said that – let's continue to extend this train of thought by looking at the role of pleural pressure.

The pleural pressure (P_{PL}) that is reflected into the alveoli (the transpulmonary gradient), which under normal circumstances is negative – surrounds the small airways. This is why I said it is necessary to envision this in 3D in your mind. At the level that we are talking about (smallest airways, alveoli) – these structures are all right next to each other. The negative pressure in the pleural space that is reflected into the alveoli is also "felt" throughout the small airways. The P_{PL} is therefore the pressure felt on the outside of the airways, and the pressure of the gas inside the airways dictates the pressure inside the airways. The difference between these two is the transmural pressure just mentioned. Depending upon whether the pressure *inside* those airways is greater or less than the P_{PL} that is *outside* of those airways is what is going to determine whether those airways are distended or collapsed. And this is the crux of the issue regarding the issue of the equal pressure point.

During normal breathing, P_{PL} is sub-ambient. This means that P_{PL} is negative – it's less than atmospheric pressure. And P_{PL} stays negative during expiration. With normal passive expiration, gas does not exit the lungs as a result of the P_{PL} becoming positive – it exits the lungs because the elastic recoil of the lungs reduces the volume of the lungs such that the pressure of the gas in the alveoli becomes greater than ambient and thus flows out of the lungs according to Boyle's Law. But the P_{PL} is still negative, therefore the pressure outside the small airways is less than the pressure inside and thus they stay distended. The net outcome can be summarized as follows: During passive exhalation, the pressure driving gas out of the lungs is coming from increased alveolar pressure due to a reduction of lung volume because of elastic recoil – but P_{PL} remains negative throughout this process – and since P_{PL} remains negative throughout passive expiration, the transmural pressure favors the distension of the airways thereby keeping the small airways open – hence during normal passive exhalation, air flows out of the lungs without any collapse of the airways.

Under conditions of forced exhalation, however, the game changes. The muscle contraction that is associated with forced exhalation makes the P_{PL} positive, and this is what changes the dynamics. Now instead of just having elastic recoil driving the gas out of the lungs, you also have the added force of muscle contraction contributing to driving the gas out of the lungs. In this situation, since P_{PL} is positive, P_A is now a combination of elastic recoil energy + P_{PL}. But this in and of itself isn't the problem. Having additional muscle energy being added to the elastic recoil to drive the gas out of the lungs isn't inherently what causes the eventual collapse of the airways. The problem lies in the fact that the muscle contraction causes the P_{PL} *to become positive* – and as long as the patient is contracting their muscles in their effort to exhale, P_{PL} is going to remain positive. The reason why this is the fundamental problem can be explained as follows.

There are a few things that you need to keep in mind when trying to understand what is going on here. Remember the transmural pressure – it's the transmural pressure that is acting to help keep the small airways open. The transmural pressure is the difference between the pressure on the outside of the airways (P_{PL}) compared to the pressure inside the airways. When the P_{PL} is negative as in the case of passive exhalation, that negative P_{PL} is translated throughout the length of all the small airways. A negative P_{PL} is always going to result in a transmural pressure that favors distension of the small airways which in effect helps keeps them open. With passive exhalation, the reduction in lung volume due to elastic recoil raises the pressure of the gas in the alveoli so that the gas flows out of the lungs – but in terms of the dynamics of the airways themselves – this means that the pressure inside those tubes (airways) is always greater than the pressure outside of them (because P_{PL} is negative) – this is what enables the transmural pressure to favor airway distension. When you have a scenario like you do with passive exhalation where the pressure inside the tube is always greater than the pressure outside the tube - therein lies the reason why the tubes (airways) don't collapse in such a scenario. Even though the pressure inside the airways does indeed gradually decrease due to frictional resistance, it is still nonetheless positive, and since the P_{PL} outside the airways is negative, the airways will remain patent.

But when P_{PL} is positive as in the case of forced exhalation due to muscle contraction – and remember that P_{PL} is translated throughout the outside of all the small airways – then the dynamics of the transmural pressure changes dramatically. The pressure inside the airways is positive. Elastic recoil alone would have ensured this, but now with P_{PL} being positive, it is even more so. From the perspective of the airways, when expiratory flow begins, the pressure inside the airways is positive (above ambient) and thus gas is going to flow out of the lungs. Because of muscle contraction though, P_{PL} is also positive, and whatever amount of positive pressure P_{PL} is exerting is going to be exerted throughout the outsides of the small airways. As long as the positive pressure inside the airways that is driving the gas out of the lungs is greater than the positive P_{PL} that is being imposed upon the outside of the airways, the airways will not experience collapse. But remember that as the gas flows out of the alveoli and travels throughout the airways up to the mouth that it is losing pressure along the way due to frictional resistance along with the fact that the lungs are getting smaller during exhalation such that the recoil force diminishes. Because the pressure inside the airways is continually decreasing as the gas continues to progress towards the mouth, there is going to come a point where the pressure inside the airways becomes the same as the pressure being exerted on the outside of the airways by the positive P_{PL}. And the precise location along the airways where this occurs is called the equal pressure point. As the gas continues to flow beyond this point towards the mouth, the pressure inside the airways is going to continue to decrease, but the positive P_{PL} remains. From the point of the equal pressure point on up towards the mouth, the pressure outside the airways is greater than the pressure inside - hence the positive P_{PL} outside the airways that is now higher than the pressure inside the airways is going to compress and narrow those airways, and that is what is known as dynamic compression of the airways.

Starting from the alveoli and moving towards the mouth, the sooner the equal pressure point is reached, the more significant, or widespread the amount of dynamic airway compression there will be in all the remaining portions of the airways beyond the equal pressure point up towards the mouth. Think about the factors involved with this with an emphysema patient. First of all, their elastic recoil force is drastically diminished as a consequence of their disease. The architecture of their alveoli is destroyed, and as a result they lack many of the structural features that facilitate radial traction. Then they complicate the issue even further with forced exhalation involving muscle contraction that reverses the transmural pressure across their airways. The fact that their elastic recoil is already diminished greatly lowers the driving pressure they have to exhale gas. This means they are going to reach the equal pressure point sooner – and combined with the fact that they don't have adequate structures to help maintain patency of their small airways is why these patients experience dynamic compression and thus airway collapse during exhalation. With airway collapse comes air trapping, and when they trap air they raise the resting volume (FRC) of their lungs. Air trapping and inadequate lung emptying also translate into CO_2 retention which then becomes the source of their acidosis.

The issue of airway collapse often presents significant challenges in the management of COPD patients because of the myriad problems that arise due to this issue. You are going to encounter COPD patients more often than any other type of patient in your career. Having a good understanding of the nuances of their condition will enable you to better understand the treatment strategies that are employed to help them.

J. The Distribution of Ventilation

Realize that even in a normal, healthy individual, the distribution of air throughout the lungs for any given breath is not uniformly even. This is why the V/Q ratio (ventilation/perfusion ratio) is somewhat uneven in normal individuals. The V/Q ratio will be discussed in detail in chapter 3 and referenced throughout this text, but it has been introduced here as it is one of the ways that quantitatively illustrates the uneven distribution of ventilation throughout the lungs. In the case of chronic lung disease (COPD), the extent of the unevenness of gas distribution can be so severe that it contributes significantly to the inadequate exchange of oxygen and carbon dioxide.

A number of reasons exist for the uneven distribution of ventilation including gravity, thoracic shape, and diaphragmatic movement, but all of these reasons ultimately cause the following to occur:

1. Uneven resistances to the flow of gas in various different parts of the lungs.
2. Uneven compliances in different parts of the lungs.
3. Uneven pressures in different areas of the lungs (meaning that the transpulmonary pressure isn't exactly the same in all the alveoli throughout the lungs.

In general, the alveoli all have similar volume capacities and elastic characteristics. This is to say that they are all *similar* with respect to their *ability* to be stretched and in their size limits.

- Previously when P_{PL} was introduced and discussed, it was indicated to be between -3 to -6 cmH_2O at rest with -5 cmH_2O being the average. What you need to realize now is that -5 cmH_2O average is only for the middle level of the lungs. At the bases and apices of the lungs it is different – hence the first concrete example to illustrate the uneven distribution of gas.

Consider the following:

When an individual is in the upright position, the weight of the lungs pulls down on the apices while simultaneously pressing the bases up against the diaphragm. Remember that in this position (upright) that the bases are the dependent area of the lungs (the dependent area is always the area of the lungs that is at the lowest point where gravity has the most effect). In the upright position, the alveoli at the bases of the lungs are closer to the diaphragm and are thus exposed to a greater range of diaphragmatic excursion. As such, the lower thorax tends to expand about 50% more than the upper thorax.

Remember that the pleural space is the "space" between the visceral and the parietal pleura. The visceral pleura is directly adhered to the lung itself whereas the parietal pleura is adhered to the inner surface of the chest wall. If gravity is pulling the apices down, the visceral pleura that is attached to the apices is also pulled along as well. Insofar as the parietal pleura is not subject to the same movement, this means that the pleural space in the apical region of the lungs will be a bit wider – hence making the resting P_{PL} in the apical region of the lungs closer to -10 cmH_2O. Consider now the bases of the lungs – the same thing is going on with regards to gravity – it's just that now you're at the bottom of the lungs and they are being pushed against the diaphragm. In this context, the visceral pleura that is attached to the lung bases is being pushed rather than pulled like it was with the apices, therefore the pleural space at the bases will be a little narrower – hence making the resting P_{PL} in the bases of the lungs closer to -2.5 cmH_2O. This means that the alveolar distending pressure at the apices of the lungs is about four times more than it is at the bases of the lungs. It is at the middle portion of the lungs where the pleural space is at the right width to have a resting P_{PL} of -5 cmH_2O (average).

Consider now the implications of what has just been discussed:

- Since the apices have a more sub-ambient resting P_{PL} at around -10 cmH_2O – this means the apical alveoli are going to have a higher resting volume – therefore the apical alveoli have the least amount of room to expand during inspiration because their compliance is low. If a structure is almost full to begin with – then the ability to further distend it is minimalized – hence why apical alveoli are said to have low compliance (as compared to the rest of the lung).
- The lung bases, however, have a less sub-ambient resting P_{PL} at around -2.5 cmH_2O – this means that the alveoli at the bases are going to have a much lower resting volume – but they then have the most amount of room to expand during inspiration so they are therefore said to be much more compliant than the apices.

Realize that everything that was just discussed is applicable when a patient is in a position other than upright. They could be supine (laying on their back), or lateral (laying on their side) – it doesn't matter. The dependent area will always have the lowest resting volume and thus be able to experience the largest amount of ventilation.

Now let us revisit the compliance curve from the previous section on compliance and put what has just been discussed into the context of that curve. Recall the lower inflection point – the point where sufficient pressure has been reached such that the alveoli then "pop" open and begin to inflate with much more ease. Then note the steep part of the curve from the lower inflection point on up to the upper inflection point – it is during this steep part of the curve (particularly the beginning of the steep part) that ventilation is predominately occurring in the lung bases. Think about what was just said in terms of the difference in compliance between the apices and the bases of the lungs. The bases have a much lower resting volume and have much better compliance than the apices – therefore it is the alveoli in the bases that are filling during the steep of the curve. The middle portions of the lungs will also fill during the steep part of the curve as well (mostly during the middle of the curve). The apical alveoli, because of the fact that they already have a higher resting volume to begin with and are therefore much less compliant, are representative of the top of the compliance curve where you see only very small volume changes for given increases in pressure.

Other factors contributing to the uneven distribution of ventilation:

- P_{PL} is not evenly transmitted across the lungs as some of the pressure is lost overcoming tissue viscous resistance.

- Alveoli at the periphery of the lungs (closer to the visceral pleura) end up with higher distending pressures than the alveoli that are deeper within the lungs.

- Local differences in alveolar compliance will have an effect on the ventilation (filling and emptying) of different lung segments.
- Alveoli with higher compliance take longer to fill because they are able to take a larger volume – BUT they also have less elastance so therefore they also empty more slowly.
- Alveoli with lower compliance will fill more quickly because they are only able to take a smaller volume – BUT they also have more elastance so therefore they also empty faster.

- Local differences in R_{AW} also affects the filling and emptying of the lungs.
- R_{AW} determines the magnitude of the pressure drop in the airway.
- Pressure that is used up in order to overcome R_{AW} is no longer available to overcome elastic resistance and expand alveolar volume.

- The size (diameter) of the airways can be effected by:
  - local airway compression due to body posture
  - dynamic airway compression due to forced exhalation

- Airways can be blocked due to obstructions (mucus, secretions) that will then cause uneven distribution.

K. The Efficiency of Ventilation

Ventilation by definition is the process of moving gas from the atmosphere into the alveoli and then from the alveoli back to the atmosphere so as to meet the body's demands for oxygen uptake and carbon dioxide removal. Ventilation occurs primarily through spontaneous breathing; however, it can also be accomplished artificially through mechanical ventilation. In order to ensure survival, the process of ventilation must maintain normal concentrations of oxygen and carbon dioxide in the alveolar gas. In other words - the process of moving gas in and out of the lungs (ventilation) needs to be efficient in order to maintain life.

Minute Ventilation

In order to understand the efficiency of ventilation we need to start with the concept of minute ventilation. Ventilation is measured per minute and is called *minute ventilation* (V_E). There should be a dot above the V, and it is commonly referred to as V-dot-E. But as was indicated on the Note to the Reader page at the beginning of this book, because of formatting limitations, the dot will not always appear above the V in this book – just know that it is supposed to be there.

Minute ventilation ($\dot{V}_E$) is the amount of air moved in and out of the lungs in one minute. Mathematically it is expressed as follows:

$$\dot{V}_E = V_T \times f$$

where V_T is the tidal volume and f is the frequency (respiratory rate). V_E is expressed in liters per minute (LPM or L/min.).

Regulation of breathing

In healthy individuals, V_E is controlled by the central chemoreceptors that respond to the CO_2 level in the blood. As such, this is why we say that the principle drive for ventilation is CO_2 level. But the central chemoreceptors do not detect changes in the level of CO_2 directly. They are actually detecting changes in the pH of the CSF (cerebrospinal fluid).

CO_2 acts as an acid when in solution (plasma and/or cerebrospinal fluid for example). The CO_2 in the plasma or CSF reacts with water (remember that plasma and CSF are mostly water) to form carbonic acid (H_2CO_3). Carbonic acid then dissociates into H^+ and HCO_3^-, and it is the amount of H^+ (hydrogen ion) that determines the pH. The greater the amount of H^+ - the more acidic the solution and thus the lower the pH. Conversely, lower H^+ means the solution is more alkaline with a higher pH. When ventilation is inadequate, CO_2 levels in the blood rise (H^+ increases) and thus the pH decreases. Or conversely – if ventilation is excessive such that too much CO_2 is being removed, then CO_2 levels in the blood will fall (H^+ decreases) and thus the pH will increase.

The hydrogen ions (H^+) in the blood, however, cannot pass the blood-brain barrier, but CO_2 does traverse the blood-brain barrier, and it is the changes in the pH of the CSF that are detected by the central chemoreceptors. CO_2 reacts with the water in the CSF the same way it does with the water in the plasma. When the central chemoreceptors detect a drop in the pH of the CSF (which correlates to elevated CO_2 in the blood), they will then send the appropriate neural signals whereby the body will respond by increasing the rate and/or depth of breathing so as to remove the excessive amount of CO_2 and thus restore the pH to within normal range. If the central chemoreceptors detect a rise in the pH of the CSF (which correlates to lower than normal levels of CO_2 in the blood), they will send the appropriate neural signals whereby the body will respond by decreasing the rate and/or depth of breathing so that less CO_2 is removed such that the pH is restored to within normal range.

When the body responds by either increasing or decreasing the rate and/or depth of breathing in response to changes in the pH, this corresponds to f and V_T of the minute ventilation equation. Rate is f, and depth is V_T.

- V_E is actually referring to the volume of air *exhaled* over one minute. Exhaled air is easier to measure, and it obviously reflects the volume of air that was inhaled.

- Normal values for minute ventilation ($\dot{V}_E$) are 5 – 6 L/min.

- Acceptable values are those under 10 L/min.

- If V_E falls below 5 L/min., the patient is not adequately ventilating. If V_E is above 10 L/min., this is also cause for concern because it indicates that their WOB is too high and they are going to become exhausted.

- When you are manipulating $\dot{V}_E$ in mechanical ventilation – the variables that you can manipulate are either V_T or f. You manipulate them one at a time – but never change them both at the same time.

Alveolar Ventilation

Whereas minute ventilation ($\dot{V}_E$) tells you the amount of total ventilation over the course of a minute – alveolar ventilation (V_A) tells you the amount of ventilation per minute that actually makes it into the alveoli to participate in gas exchange. Alveolar minute ventilation (V_A) is expressed mathematically as follows:

$$\dot{V}_A = (V_T - V_D) \times f$$

where V_T is the tidal volume, V_D is the dead space ventilation, and f is the respiratory rate.

Now – when we consider V_E – even though V_E is talking about the total amount of ventilation over the course of a minute – realize that not all of that gas makes it to the level of the alveoli in order to participate in gas exchange. This is why we must then consider V_A – *because V_A is what is actually important.*

From the mouth all the way down the airway to the terminal bronchioles is what is known as the conducting airway. It is called this because there is no gas exchange in this part of the airway. Gas exchange begins right after the terminal bronchioles when you reach the respiratory bronchioles and see the first appearance of alveoli. The conducting airway therefore is what is referred to as anatomic dead space. Dead space in the sense that it is "wasted" ventilation because it does not participate in gas exchange. Think about it – the V_D is the portion of the V_T that stays in the conducting airway. The V_D is the portion of the V_T that does not participate in gas exchange. If you want to know how much of the tidal volume (V_T) that makes it to the alveoli – you subtract V_D from V_T, i.e. ($V_T - V_D$). When you multiply that difference by f, you then have the alveolar minute ventilation (V_A).

$\dot{V_A}$ is therefore <u>always</u> less than $\dot{V_E}$

<u>Dead Space Ventilation</u>

Let us now look at some specifics regarding dead space.

V_D typically amounts to being 1ml/lb. of IBW. Obviously the anatomic dead space cannot be measured directly. The 1ml/lb. is derived from calculations using a mathematical technique known as Fowler's equal area method. If a patient's IBW was calculated to be 175 lbs., then their V_D would be 175ml. This means for example that if they took a breath, and the tidal volume of that breath was 500ml – then 175ml of that V_T was dead space ventilation (i.e. V_D – the air remaining in the conducting airways), and the other 325ml made it to the alveoli to participate in gas exchange.

Now let us extend this further. Let's say that patient who is breathing a V_T of 500ml has a f (respiratory rate) of 12 breaths per minute.

Their $\dot{V}_E = V_T$ x f
Therefore $\dot{V}_E$ = 500ml x 12 breaths/min. = 6000ml/min. or 6 LPM.

Since 175 ml of that ventilation is wasted (V_D), then the total wasted ventilation is 175ml x 12 bpm = 2100ml/min. or 2.1 LPM.

Therefore, the alveolar ventilation ($\dot{V}_A$ – the ventilation that effectively makes it to the alveoli) is determined as follows:

$\dot{V}_A = (V_T - V_D)$ x f
$\dot{V}_A = (500ml - 175ml)$ x 12 bpm
$\dot{V}_A =$ 325ml   x 12 bpm = 3900 ml/min. or 3.9 LPM

Notice that the sum of $\dot{V}_A$ and $V_D = \dot{V}_E$. 3.9 LPM + 2.1 LPM = 6 LPM. You would expect this because $\dot{V}_E$ is the total ventilation per minute which includes both alveolar ventilation ($\dot{V}_A$) and dead space ventilation (V_D).

NOW – THIS IS REALLY IMPORTANT. If you find yourself in a clinical situation where you are needing to increase your patient's minute ventilation ($\dot{V}_E$) – you will accomplish this much more efficiently by increasing their V_T. Obviously you can increase $\dot{V}_E$ by increasing either the V_T or f, but increasing f contributes to increasing dead space ventilation which is of no value. Remember that it is $\dot{V}_A$ that you are more concerned with, and $\dot{V}_A = (V_T - V_D)$ x f. $\dot{V}_A$ changes in response to changes in either V_T or f because V_D is relatively fixed (anatomical dead space is what it is based on 1ml/lb. IBW– it doesn't really fluctuate). But after you consider the following example you will see the impact that changes in either V_T or f have on the amount of dead space ventilation.

Consider this example using the same patient as above:

Instead of breathing a V_T of 500ml for each breath, let's say they were only taking in a V_T of 250ml. But they increased their f (respiratory rate) to 24 breaths per minute. In this scenario they would still achieve a V_E of 6 LPM because $V_E = V_T$ x f, and 250ml x 24 bpm = 6000ml/min. or 6LPM. But let us consider the *quality* of this ventilation.

Their dead space is still 175ml because that is based on their IBW which has not changed. If they are breathing a V_T of only 250ml, and 175ml of that is dead space ventilation, then that means that only 75ml of that V_T is making to the alveoli for gas exchange. Look how this changes the math with respect to their alveolar ventilation.

V_D stays the same because it's based on IBW – it's 175ml. But when you increase the rate from 12 to 24 – the amount of dead space ventilation goes from being 175 x 12 to 175 x 24. And 175 x 24 = 4200ml/min. or 4.2 LPM compared to 2.1 LPM when the rate was only 12 bpm.

In this scenario, when you now figure out their V_A (alveolar ventilation) you'll see that has decreased dramatically. $V_A = (V_T - V_D)$ x f. If their V_T has dropped to 250ml, but yet their V_D is the same at 175ml, then (250ml – 175ml) x 24 = 1800ml/min. or 1.8 LPM compared to 3.9 LPM when the rate was only 12 bpm.

Remember this later on when you get into mechanical ventilation. V_E is something you always have to be mindful of when you have a patient that is being mechanically ventilated because you always have to ensure that V_E is adequate. Obviously V_E can be manipulated in mechanical ventilation by changing either the V_T or f since V_E is the product of V_T and f. If you have a patient whose V_E is not adequate such that you need to increase it – you now know that the best way to accomplish this is by increasing the V_T – not f – because you now know that even though you may be able to get the V_E where you want it to be numerically by raising the frequency, you know that V_E will be of poor quality because increasing the frequency increases the amount of dead space ventilation while simultaneously decreasing the amount of alveolar ventilation – and you never want to decrease the amount of alveolar ventilation.

- *Breathing patterns at high respiratory rates and/or low tidal volumes are inefficient. It results in a greater proportion of wasted ventilation per minute – i.e. - a low V_A.*
- *The most efficient breathing pattern is slow, deep breathing.*

<u>Anatomical Dead Space</u>

Dead space as it has been discussed thus far is the anatomical dead space. It is the volume of gas that is in the conducting airways and thus not involved with gas exchange. It is wasted ventilation. When referring to anatomic dead space specifically, it is designated as V_{Danat}.

<u>Alveolar Dead Space</u>

This one is a new concept. Alveolar dead space is when you have alveoli that are indeed ventilated – but there is no perfusion. There are problems with the Q part of the V/Q ratio. V/Q was mentioned earlier in section J, and will be covered in more detail in chapter 3. V represents ventilation and Q represents perfusion. V/Q essentially is showing the relationship between ventilation and perfusion, and it is a relationship that will be referred to throughout this text. In this instance, however, you can appreciate that if there is no perfusion of blood through the capillaries that surround the alveoli – then the ventilation that is in those alveoli is wasted and therefore considered dead space. In a normal individual, there should be no alveolar dead space. When there are significant amounts of alveolar dead space, it is pathologic and usually related to defects in the pulmonary circulation. Consider a patient with a pulmonary embolism. Here you have a situation where an embolus is causing a blockage somewhere in the pulmonary arterial circulation. The exact location of the embolus in the pulmonary arterial circulation will determine just how many lung units will be affected, but in any case, lung units that are distal to the embolus are going be denied blood circulation and thus there will be no blood for those lung units to have gas exchange with – hence the ventilation to those lung units is wasted and you end up with alveolar dead space. When referring to alveolar dead space specifically, it is designated as V_{Dalv}.

Physiologic Dead Space

Physiological dead space is simply the anatomic dead space + the alveolar dead space. When referring to physiologic dead space, it is designated as V_{Dphy}.

Therefore:

In normal individuals without lung disease – the dead space in consideration is anatomic dead space (V_{Danat}).

In patients with lung disease where a condition such as a pulmonary embolism causes increased alveolar dead space - the dead space in consideration is physiologic dead space (V_{Dphys}), which is the sum of anatomic dead space and alveolar dead space (V_{Danat} + V_{Dalv}).

Dead Space to Tidal Volume Ratio (V_D/V_T)

Earlier in this chapter, tidal volume (V_T) was defined as the volume of gas that is inhaled and exhaled with each normal breath. You now know that a tidal volume consists of gas that remains in the conducting airway (dead space) along with gas that makes it to the alveoli. Tidal volume therefore can be expressed as follows:

$V_T = V_D + V_A$ (Tidal Volume = Dead Space Volume + Alveolar Volume)

- The larger the V_D, the less efficient the V_T is in eliminating CO_2.

- CO_2 removal is less for a given V_T as V_D increases. This is because for a given V_T, if V_D increases, that means that V_A has decreased – and if V_A is decreased, the amount of CO_2 removed is decreased.

- Therefore, the estimation of dead space ventilation is essential in assessing the efficiency of ventilation – and the way that is done is by determining what is known as the dead space/tidal volume ratio (V_D/V_T).

The dead space/tidal volume ratio (V_D/V_T) is a measure of the amount of wasted ventilation per breath. In order to calculate the V_D/V_T ratio you need to know the following:

1. $PaCO_2$ ($PaCO_2$ is derived from an ABG – or you can use the $EtCO_2$ and still have a good estimate of $PaCO_2$)

2. P_ECO_2 (this is mixed expired CO_2 – the amount of which is usually determined by collecting it in a sampling bag or estimating it from capnography).

Note – the difference between $EtCO_2$ and P_ECO_2.

$EtCO_2$ can be used as a rough estimate of $PaCO_2$ because it is measured towards the end of exhalation. Remember that when exhalation begins, the first gas to be exhaled is the gas in the conducting airway (the anatomical dead space), and being that the gas in the conducting airway has not participated in gas exchange, the amount of CO_2 in that gas is the same as it is in the atmosphere – essentially nothing (a miniscule amount). But in the latter part of exhalation at the end (when $EtCO_2$ is measured), you're exhaling gas from the alveoli where gas exchange did occur. This is why $EtCO_2$ is a reliable estimate of $PaCO_2$. P_ECO_2 on the other hand is measuring mixed CO_2 – meaning that it is a sample of gas that is a mixture of gas from the anatomical dead space along with gas from the alveoli. It is determined from exhaled gas much earlier in the exhalation phase.

The dead space/tidal volume ratio (V_D/V_T) is calculated as follows. This is the main V_D/V_T equation, and it accounts for both anatomic and alveolar dead space – hence V_D in this equation is representing physiologic dead space (V_{Dphy}). V_{Dphy} is the preferred measure of ventilation efficiency.

$$\frac{V_D}{V_T} = \frac{PaCO_2 - P_ECO_2}{PaCO_2}$$

- The normal range for V_D/V_T is $0.2 - 0.4$, or $20 - 40\%$. The threshold of what would be considered acceptable is 60%. A V_D/V_T beyond 60% is not acceptable.
- When a patient is on mechanical ventilation, the normal range of V_D/V_T is $40 - 60\%$. This accounts for the fact that the endotracheal tube itself adds to the amount of dead space.

Consider the following example with a normal patient. The normal value for $PaCO_2$ is 40mmHg and the normal value for P_ECO_2 is 28mmHg.

$$\frac{V_D}{V_T} = \frac{PaCO_2 - P_ECO_2}{PaCO_2}$$

$$\frac{V_D}{V_T} = \frac{40 - 28}{40}$$

$$= \frac{12}{40} = 0.3 \text{ or } 30\%$$

This therefore shows that 30% of the ventilation (30% of the tidal volume) is wasted. When you solve $PaCO_2 - P_ECO_2/PaCO_2$, it gives you the percentage of physiologic dead space. You can then take that percentage and multiply it by the V_T and the result will tell you the actual amount of wasted ventilation. If the tidal volume was

500ml for example, then 150ml is wasted ventilation because 500 x 0.3 = 150. In general, the physiologic dead space is about one third of the tidal volume.

- V_D/V_T decreases with exercise. With exertion, tidal volume increases – that makes the denominator larger and thus results in a smaller quotient – hence the V_D/V_T ratio decreases.

- V_D/V_T increases with pulmonary conditions that cause an increase in dead space (e.g. pulmonary embolism). For a given tidal volume, if V_D increases, that makes the numerator bigger and thus results in a bigger quotient – hence the V_D/V_T ratio increases.

End Tidal CO_2 (EtCO$_2$) and the Basic Capnogram

As just mentioned, EtCO$_2$ can be used as a rough estimate of PaCO$_2$ because it is measured towards the end of exhalation. When exhalation begins, the gas that is exhaled first is the gas in the conducting airway (the anatomical dead space). This gas has not participated in gas exchange - therefore the amount of CO$_2$ in that gas is essentially the same as it is in the atmosphere – virtually nothing (a miniscule amount). But in the latter part of exhalation at the end (when EtCO$_2$ is measured), you're exhaling gas from the alveoli where gas exchange did occur. This is why EtCO$_2$ is a reliable estimate of PaCO$_2$.

Capnography is the monitoring of the concentration (partial pressure) of CO$_2$ in the respiratory gases (both expired and inspired). A capnogram (or capnograph) is a graphical representation of this monitoring. By paying attention to the monitoring of the CO$_2$ during exhalation, capnography enables you to objectively evaluate a patient's ventilatory status – remember that CO$_2$ level is the best indicator of ventilation. When you have a patient that is having their EtCO$_2$ monitored, you will see the following curve being displayed on the monitor.

The Basic Capnographic Curve

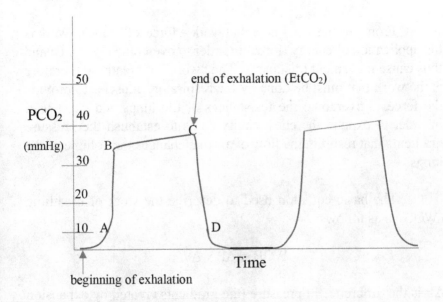

Phase 1 – from the beginning of exhalation to point A. This represents dead space gas at the beginning of expiration that contains virtually no CO_2.

Phase 2 – from point A to point B. This shows a rapid rise in in CO_2 as alveolar gas begins to mix with dead space gas.

Phase 3 – from point B to point C. This "plateau" portion of the curve is showing exhaled gas that is coming mostly from ventilated and perfused alveoli. Point C at the end of exhalation represents the end tidal gas, and the CO_2 at point C is the end tidal CO_2 (EtCO$_2$).

From point C to point D is the inspiration of the next breath. The steep downward slope of the curve (indicating a significant drop in CO_2) is because virtually no CO_2 is inhaled.

L. The Work of Breathing (WOB)

From physics you know that work = force x distance. Work is the application of energy (force) in order to overcome resistance and thus cause movement (distance). The "work" of breathing therefore is the work that must be done by the respiratory muscles to provide the force to overcome the resistances of the lungs and chest wall in order to expand the chest cavity so as to establish the pressure gradients that result in the flow of air that changes the volume of the lungs.

The basic equation used to describe the work of breathing (WOB) is as follows:

$$WOB = \Delta P \times \Delta V$$

ΔP is the difference in pressure (the gradients created by expansion of the chest cavity) – this is the force. ΔV is the change in volume of the lungs as a result of air flowing into them and thus increasing their size – this is the "distance" that the lungs are moved.

original equation for
work from physics:

$$Work = Force \times Distance$$

that equation now
specifically applied to WOB:

$$WOB = \Delta P \times \Delta V$$

The normal value for WOB is 0.5 ± 0.2 joules/L. This is for you to know. It would be extremely rare if you were ever asked to do a WOB calculation on an exam, and you will never be calculating WOB at the beside in clinical practice. You need however to conceptually understand WOB as it is something that you will encounter constantly.

In normal spontaneous breathing the respiratory muscles do the work and the process is under autonomic control. In mechanical ventilation, the ventilator takes over the work of breathing (inspiration only – expiration is always passive, even during mechanical ventilation). The factors that determine how much air is able to be inspired are:

- Lung and chest wall compliance
- Airway resistance
- The stimulation level of the nervous system
  - determined by CO_2 level

The WOB can be broadly divided into 2 categories – the mechanical WOB and the metabolic WOB.

Mechanical WOB

This is the energy expended to overcome frictional and elastic resistance. In a normal patient, 2/3 of the mechanical WOB is utilized to overcome elastic resistance and the other 1/3 is to overcome frictional resistance.

With normal individuals:

- When they increase their V_T, it increases the elastic WOB.
- When they increase their RR, it increases the frictional WOB.

With sick patients:

- Restrictive disease – patients with restrictive lung disease have increased elastance, which means their elastic WOB is increased. With increased elastance it is going to take much more work to inflate the lungs. They will therefore achieve the lowest WOB by breathing at higher respiratory rates and lower tidal volumes. They spend less energy on lung inflation (V_T) since this is where they meet with the most resistance due to the increased elastance, but they'll offset that by spending additional energy on increasing their rate. This is why these patients tend to assume rapid, shallow breathing patterns.

In restrictive disease, it is the inspiratory WOB that is the hardest because in restrictive disease the patient needs to overcome the high elastance of the lungs.

- Obstructive disease – patients with obstructive lung disease have increased compliance. They don't have issues with increased elastance as is the case with restrictive disease. These patients will therefore achieve the lowest WOB with a breathing pattern that minimalizes frictional resistance - which is breathing at lower respiratory rates with higher tidal volumes. This is why these patients tend to assume slow breathing with pursed lips.

In obstructive disease, it is the expiratory WOB that is the hardest because patients with obstructive disease use muscle energy to exhale (forced exhalation) in order to try to overcome the frictional resistance to flow. The consequences of forced exhalation that further complicates their problems was discussed in detail in the last section on the equal pressure point and dynamic airway compression.

Note that in either case – if the patient also is suffering from muscle weakness, it is going to be even more difficult for them to sustain the work of breathing. Respiratory muscle weakness can result from:

- Acidosis
- Sepsis
- Shock
- Electrolyte disorders
- Muscle disease
- Neurological disease

Metabolic WOB

- The metabolic WOB is the OXYGEN COST OF BREATHING. It is the amount of energy expended by the respiratory muscles themselves in order to move air. In other words, the oxygen cost of breathing is the amount of oxygen consumed by the respiratory muscles in the course of doing their work.

- Oxygen consumption (VO_2) by the respiratory muscles is $\approx$ 0.5 – 1ml O_2 per liter of increased ventilation (V_E).

- This represents substantially less than 5% of total O_2 consumption, however, at extremely high levels of ventilation during vigorous exercise the oxygen consumption by the respiratory muscles can increase to the point of exceeding 30% of the body's total O_2 consumption. During vigorous exercise, an individual's minute ventilation can become > 100 L/min. When V_E becomes that high, oxygen consumption by the respiratory muscles is extremely high. At this level of exercise, the respiratory muscles are essentially working at maximal levels to sustain such a high level of ventilation – hence the dramatic increase in oxygen consumption by the respiratory muscles. There is a limit, however, where the cardiopulmonary system will simply no longer be able to keep up with such a demand – and this is a major limiting factor in athletic performance.

- In cases of obstructive lung disease (COPD), the patient's diaphragm is often not working optimally, or perhaps not working at all. Their diaphragm becomes flattened as a result of the hyperinflation of their lungs, and this lessens the diaphragm's ability to contract properly. The diaphragm is the primary respiratory muscle for inspiration, and when the diaphragm is not working properly, these patients then must resort to using the accessory muscles of breathing which are not nearly as efficient as the diaphragm.

- COPD patients also have greatly decreased efficiency in getting oxygen from the alveoli into the capillaries. This is due in large part to the structural damage done to the alveolar-capillary membrane that is a consequence of their disease.

- For reasons like the last two just mentioned, the oxygen cost of breathing for a COPD patient can be as high as 10ml O_2 per liter of ventilation – and this is just for their "normal" breathing – this does not involve any exercise.

Chapter 3

Selected Topics in Gas Exchange

A. Introduction

Whereas ventilation is the mechanical process by which gas is moved in and out of the lungs, gas exchange is the diffusion of gas (both O_2 and CO_2) between the alveoli and the blood, and between the blood and the cells of the body. Gas transport on the other hand, involves the precise means by which the blood transports oxygen from the lungs to the body's cells and carbon dioxide from the body's cells back to the lungs in order that it may be expired. Gas exchange and gas transport must be efficient because the body's cells not only have a continuous need for oxygen in order to function; there is also a continuous need to be able to remove the carbon dioxide that is a product of cellular metabolism.

Let us begin by gaining an understanding of carbon dioxide production by the body's cells and how that relates to alveolar ventilation (V_A) and the partial pressure of alveolar CO_2 ($PACO_2$).

- $\dot{V}CO_2$ is the minute production of CO_2. At rest it is normally about 200ml/min. Remember this.

- $\dot{V}_A$ is alveolar minute ventilation. You already know this from the last chapter. $V_A = (V_T - V_D) \times f$. Average V_A at rest is about 4200ml/min.

Now:

$$PACO_2 = \frac{\dot{V}CO_2 \times 863}{\dot{V}_A}$$

*   *Note on the 863 in the equation: The number 863 is a correction factor. VCO_2 is expressed at STPD whereas V_A is expressed at BTPS. The correction factor reconciles these incompatibilities along with also reconciling units of flow to be able to be expressed as units of pressure.*

Realize that $PACO_2$ is the partial pressure of CO_2 in the alveoli. That CO_2 is coming from the pulmonary capillaries – it is NOT coming from inspired gas – there is virtually no CO_2 in inspired gas. Average $PACO_2$ is 40mmHg.

What this equation is telling you is that $PACO_2$ is inversely related to V_A, and directly related to VCO_2. The difference between an inverse and a direct relationship was discussed at length at the beginning of chapter 1 if you need to review these ideas. These relationships between the variables in the equation have the following implications:

$PACO_2$ will increase:

*   If $\dot{V}CO_2$ increases with $\dot{V}_A$ remaining constant.

*   If $\dot{V}_A$ decreases with $\dot{V}CO_2$ remaining constant.

*   If there is an increase in dead space (V_D), then there will be an increase in $PACO_2$. Remember that when there is an increase in V_D, that reduces V_A, and if V_A is decreased then $PACO_2$ will increase. *V_A is in the denominator – when you make the denominator smaller, the quotient ($PACO_2$) gets bigger.*

$PACO_2$ will decrease:

*   If $\dot{V}CO_2$ decreases with $\dot{V}_A$ remaining constant.

*   If $\dot{V}_A$ increases with $\dot{V}CO_2$ remaining constant.

B. Pulmonary Pressure Gradients

At the beginning of the last chapter you learned about the pressure gradients that were needed to move air in and out of the lungs. Pressure gradients are what enable gases to move, and this section will identify the gradients that enable oxygen in the alveoli to diffuse across the A/C membrane into the blood, and carbon dioxide in the blood to diffuse across the A/C membrane into the alveoli. Those gases are able to diffuse across the A/C membrane the way they do because of the differences in the partial pressures of those gases in the alveoli and pulmonary capillaries. Remember that gas will always flow from an area of higher partial pressure to an area of lower partial pressure.

Consider the following model of an alveolus and a pulmonary capillary. Blood is moving from left to right.

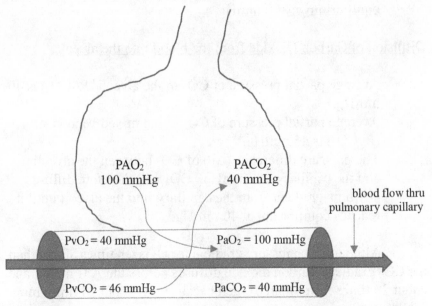

PAO$_2$
100 mmHg

PACO$_2$
40 mmHg

blood flow thru
pulmonary capillary

PvO$_2$ = 40 mmHg

PaO$_2$ = 100 mmHg

PvCO$_2$ = 46 mmHg

PaCO$_2$ = 40 mmHg

blood coming from
the pulmonary artery.
It is venous blood coming
from the right heart.

blood going to the pulmonary vein
on its way back to the left heart.
It is now oxygenated arterial blood
that will be pumped out into the
systemic circulation.

* PvO$_2$ & PvCO$_2$ are
mixed venous O$_2$ & CO$_2$

Diffusion of Oxygen from the alveoli into the blood

- Average partial pressure of O_2 in the alveoli (PAO_2) is 100 mmHg.
- Average partial pressure of O_2 in the mixed venous return (PvO_2) is 40 mmHg. This is the blood that has been returned to the right heart from the body, and has been pumped into the pulmonary artery (*remember the anatomy of the pulmonary vasculature*) in order to participate in gas exchange in the lungs.
  - as a side note: If you ever see a $PvO_2 > 60$ mmHg
    - suspect cyanide poisoning. Cyanide prevents the mitochondria from utilizing O_2, so if this is the case, you'll see elevated O_2 in the venous return blood.
- The pressure difference (ΔP) of O_2 between the alveoli and the capillary is 60 mmHg. O_2 will therefore diffuse down its gradient from the alveoli into the capillary until it reaches equilibrium at 100 mmHg.

Diffusion of Carbon Dioxide from the blood into the alveoli

- Average partial pressure of CO_2 in the alveoli ($PACO_2$) is 40 mmHg.
- Average partial pressure of CO_2 in the mixed venous return ($PvCO_2$) is 46 mmHg.
- The pressure difference (ΔP) of CO_2 between the alveoli and the capillary is 6 mmHg. CO_2 will therefore diffuse down its gradient from the capillary into the alveoli until it reaches equilibrium at 40 mmHg.

Although the pressure gradient for O_2 is ten times higher than the CO_2 gradient, carbon dioxide diffuses across the A/C membrane about 20 times faster than oxygen because it is about 20 times more soluble in plasma than oxygen.

Carbon dioxide is continuously diffusing into the alveoli (CO_2 excretion) at a rate of 200ml/min. This is consistent with VCO_2 being 200ml/min. That constant diffusion of CO_2 from the capillaries into the alveoli explains the normal $PACO_2$ of 40 mmHg.

Oxygen is continuously diffusing out of the alveoli (O_2 uptake) at a rate of 250ml/min.

NOW – Dalton's Law enables us to know that the sum of the PaO_2 and the $PaCO_2$ is about 140 mmHg. It is extremely useful for you to recognize that in light of how it can help you discern an ABG.

- If PaO_2 + $PaCO_2$ is significantly > 140 mmHg, and the PaO_2 is greater than 120 mmHg – then the patient must be on an FiO_2 > 21%. If the patient is not on an FiO_2 > 21% and they are just breathing room air – and you're getting a PaO_2 and $PaCO_2$ reading from the ABG where their sum is > 140 mmHg, then it is a lab error.

- If the sum is between 110 – 130 mmHg, that is indicating hypoxemia secondary to hypoventilation.

- If the sum is < 110 mmHg, this is indicating V̇/Q̇ mismatching, shunting, or a diffusion defect.

Another point to realize from this is that for a constant FiO_2, PAO_2 and $PACO_2$ are inversely related. Increased CO_2 will take up more room in the alveolus and will displace O_2.

The A/C Membrane – the barrier to diffusion

In order for oxygen to diffuse from the alveoli into the blood – or for carbon dioxide to diffuse from the blood into the alveoli, either of these gases must cross the A/C (alveolar-capillary) membrane. The A/C membrane is the "barrier" to diffusion, and the A/C membrane consists of the:

- Alveolar epithelium
- The interstitial space
- The capillary endothelium

Furthermore – in the blood, both O_2 and CO_2 must diffuse across another barrier – namely the cell membrane of the red blood cell.

Fick's Law

Fick's Law describes the bulk movement of a gas across a biological membrane.

$$\overset{\cdot}{V}_{gas} = \frac{\text{surface area} \times \text{solubility coefficient} \times \Delta P}{\sqrt{mw} \times \text{thickness}}$$

* mw is the molecular weight of the gas

$\overset{\cdot}{V}_{gas}$ is the bulk flow of gas

- $\overset{\cdot}{V}_{gas}$ is directly related to surface area, the solubility coefficient, and ΔP.

- $\overset{\cdot}{V}_{gas}$ is inversely related to membrane thickness and mw.

Normal diffusion time of oxygen in the pulmonary capillaries

- The normal transit time of a RBC in the pulmonary capillaries is ¾ (0.75) seconds. This is the amount of time that oxygen has to diffuse from the alveoli into the capillaries. The RBC is usually oxygenated within ¼ - ½ of a second, but definitely by ¾ of a second.

- During heavy exercise, cardiac output can increase such that the total transit time for the RBC is only ¼ of a second. From what I just said, this is still an adequate amount of time for the diffusion of oxygen - provided there are no other issues that would interfere with diffusion.

- There are certain conditions – septic shock for example, where the heart rate is increased, but yet adequate diffusion is not able to be accomplished within the reduced transit time because the pathology itself (e.g. pneumonia) is impairing the diffusion process – hence oxygenation will be diminished. *To reiterate – it's not the increased cardiac output in and of itself causing the impaired diffusion, but rather the pathology that is causing the septic shock.*

C. The Respiratory Quotient and the Ventilation/ Perfusion (V/Q) Ratio

The respiratory quotient (R), also referred to as the respiratory exchange ratio, is the ratio between VCO_2 and VO_2. It is the quotient of minute CO_2 production (VCO_2) divided by minute O_2 uptake (VO_2). As mentioned already in the last section, CO_2 diffuses out of the pulmonary capillaries into the alveoli at a rate of about 200ml/ min., and O_2 diffuses out of the alveoli into the pulmonary capillaries at a rate of about 250ml/min. The normal value for R at rest is 0.8.

$$R = \frac{\dot{V}CO_2}{\dot{V}O_2} = \frac{200ml/min.}{250ml/min.} = 0.8$$

The ventilation/perfusion ratio (V/Q), is the ratio between $\dot{V}_A$ and $\dot{Q}$. It is the quotient of minute alveolar ventilation (V_A) divided by cardiac output (Q). The normal value for V_A at rest is about 4 LPM, and normal cardiac output at rest is about 5 LPM. Therefore, the normal value for V/Q at rest is 0.8.

$$\frac{\dot{V}}{\dot{Q}} = \frac{4\ LPM}{5\ LPM} = 0.8$$

You should immediately notice that at rest, R and V/Q are the same. They both equal 0.8. In order to maintain R and V/Q at 0.8, the cardiopulmonary system must be functioning properly in order that it can adjust the level of alveolar ventilation (V_A) and cardiac output (Q) in response to the different levels of CO_2 production (VCO_2) and O_2 consumption (VO_2) during exercise, illness, or being at a high altitude.

D. The Alveolar Air Equation and PAO$_2$

Knowing the partial pressure of oxygen in the alveoli (PAO$_2$) is the first step in assessing the adequacy of oxygen transfer across the A/C membrane into the capillary blood. Remember that the PAO$_2$ provides the driving pressure for O$_2$ to diffuse across the A/C membrane into the blood. There are 5 components that go into determining the PAO$_2$.

1. FiO$_2$ (the fractional percentage of inspired oxygen) – when a patient is breathing ambient air (room air), the FiO$_2$ is ALWAYS 0.21 or 21%.

2. P$_B$ (the barometric pressure) – at sea level it averages 760 mmHg. If you are in Denver it will be around 640 mmHg. The point is that if your location is not at sea level, then you need to find out what P$_B$ is for where you are.

3. P$_{H2O}$ (water vapor pressure) – this is the pressure exerted by the water vapor in the lungs. Remember from chapter 1 that P$_{H2O}$ is a function of body temperature. At normal body temperature (37°C), P$_{H2O}$ is 47 mmHg.

   These first 3 – FiO$_2$, P$_B$, and P$_{H2O}$ are what enable you to determine PIO$_2$ (partial pressure of inspired O$_2$). This was covered thoroughly in chapter 1. Remember (P$_B$ - P$_{H2O}$) x FiO$_2$ = PIO$_2$? Think about this when you see the alveolar air equation on the next page and you'll realize the subtle connection of how it is PIO$_2$ that is the most important factor in determining PAO$_2$ – even though PIO$_2$ isn't listed directly on this list.

4. PaCO$_2$ (partial pressure of CO$_2$ in the arterial blood) – for the CO$_2$ term in the alveolar air equation we are obviously looking at the CO$_2$ in the alveoli, but it is difficult to measure PACO$_2$ directly. From what was previously discussed, however, we can assume that PACO$_2$ is the same as PaCO$_2$ – therefore it is PaCO$_2$ that is used in the alveolar air equation, and you get the PaCO$_2$ value from an ABG.

5. R (respiratory quotient) – covered in the last section. It is essentially a constant – (0.8), and serves as a correction factor that corrects for the difference between CO_2 and O_2 diffusion in and out of the alveoli. In the alveolar air equation about to be presented, R is in the denominator. You can either divide by 0.8, or if you prefer, you can multiply by the reciprocal of 0.8 – which is 1/0.8, or 1.25. It's your choice – either divide by 0.8 or multiply by 1.25 – your answer will be the same.

When I was in respiratory school, my particular program did not allow calculators during exams – and that is because you can't use a calculator on the boards – so get used to it now. When doing math long hand without a calculator I generally prefer to multiply, but the choice is yours as either way will give the same exact answer.

<u>THE ALVEOLAR AIR EQUATION</u>

$$PAO_2 = FiO_2 (P_B - 47) - \frac{PaCO_2}{R}$$

The form of the equation just given above is the general form of the equation. But as I just said – you have 2 choices of how you may handle R – hence the reason why I will give you two versions of the alveolar equation to pick from. Pick one and stick with it because the alveolar air equation is something that you will always need to know – not just for school and boards, but in real life practice.

<u>Version 1</u>: $PAO_2 = FiO_2 (P_B - 47) - (PaCO_2 \times 1.25)$

OR

<u>Version 2</u>: $PAO_2 = FiO_2 (P_B - 47) - (PaCO_2 \div 0.8)$

See the $FiO_2 (P_B - 47)$ part of the equation – that's the PIO_2 that I mentioned in the italics under #3 on the previous page. It is subtle perhaps until pointed out, but now you see it.

Important Note:

- When the $FiO_2 \geq 60\%$ - you drop the R term from the equation. At this level of FiO_2, the correction factor is no longer necessary as the need for correction is insignificant. In this case the alveolar air equation becomes:

$$PAO_2 = FiO_2 (P_B - 47) - PaCO_2$$

E. Regional Variations in $\dot{V}/\dot{Q}$

- Variations in $\dot{V}_A$ impacts $PACO_2$, which in turn affects PAO_2.

- Variations in perfusion will also affect $PACO_2$ and PAO_2.

  - An increase in perfusion to an area of the lung will enable CO_2 to be excreted faster. Therefore – in the context of V_A being constant, if CO_2 is being excreted faster, then $PACO_2$ will increase and PAO_2 will thus decrease.

  - Conversely – a decrease in perfusion to an area of the lung will cause CO_2 to be excreted slower. Therefore – in the context of V_A being constant, if CO_2 is being excreted slower, then $PACO_2$ will decrease and PAO_2 will increase.

Let us now look more closely at the relationship between ventilation (V) and perfusion (Q), and the consequences of what could be described as a somewhat less than perfect relationship.

Generally speaking:

A High $\dot{V}/\dot{Q}$ * ventilation > usual and/or perfusion < usual
is when: * PAO_2 > usual (i.e. PAO_2 > 100 mmHg)
                  * $PACO_2$ < usual (i.e. $PACO_2$ < 40 mmHg)

A Low $\dot{V}/\dot{Q}$ * ventilation < usual and/or perfusion > usual
is when: * PAO_2 < usual (i.e. PAO_2 < 100 mmHg)
            * $PACO_2$ > usual (i.e. $PACO_2$ > 40 mmHg)

      Specifically, there are variations in the $\dot{V}/\dot{Q}$ ratio depending upon what part of the lungs you are considering. Ventilation and perfusion vary from the apices of the lungs to the bases. In the apices of the lungs, there is more ventilation than perfusion (V/Q ratio is higher in the apices - V is higher than Q), whereas in the bases, there is more perfusion than ventilation (V/Q ratio is lower - Q is higher than V).

Apices:	ventilation – lower	* at the lung apices, both V & Q are lower,
wasted	perfusion – lower	but Q is much lower than V – therefore the
ventilation	$V/Q \approx 3.3$	V/Q ratio is higher at the apices.
V/Q > 1	$PAO_2 \approx 130$ mmHg	
	$PACO_2 \approx 30$ mmHg	

Middle:	ventilation – moderate (roughly equal to perfusion)	
optimal	perfusion – moderate (roughly equal to ventilation)	
ventilation &	$V/Q \approx 1$ *(0.8)*	
perfusion	$PAO_2 \approx 100$ mmHg	
V/Q ≈ 1	$PACO_2 \approx 40$ mmHg	

Bases:	ventilation – higher	*at the lung bases, both V & Q are higher,
wasted	perfusion – higher	but Q is much higher than V – therefore
perfusion	$V/Q \approx 0.66$	the V/Q ratio is lower at the bases.
V/Q < 1	$PAO_2 \approx 89$ mmHg	
	$PACO_2 \approx 42$ mmHg	

*When $\dot{V}/\dot{Q} > 1$, or $\dot{V}/\dot{Q} < 1$ – then $\dot{V}/\dot{Q}$ is "mismatched",
and gas exchange is impaired.*

- Alveoli in the lung bases with lower V/Q ratios tend towards shunting. Pulmonary shunting is attributed to alveoli with a V/Q < 1.

- Alveoli in the lung apices with higher V/Q ratios tend towards dead space. Alveolar dead space is attributed to alveoli with a V/Q > 1.

If you revisit and review the discussion on the distribution of ventilation in the last chapter, you will recall that it is gravity that is the main reason for the variations that exist in the V/Q ratio of the different areas of the lungs. The effect of gravity becomes more pronounced as you move from the apices to the bases of the lungs. Visualize the lungs in the upright position and you will be able to understand how the effect of gravity becomes more pronounced as you descend down the lungs from the apices to the bases. Even though the distance from the apices to the bases is rather small insofar as gravity exerting an effect, remember that the pressure in the pulmonary circulation is very low, hence gravity can and does enable greater perfusion at the lung bases. As also explained in the discussion on the distribution of ventilation in the last chapter, it is the effect of gravity that causes the differences in pleural pressure between the apices and the bases, and this also contributes to the reason why there is regional variation in ventilation.

The means by which the body maintains a normal V/Q ratio

The following are two ways in which the body will attempt to compensate for mismatches in the V/Q ratio.

Hypocapnic Bronchoconstriction

It's called hypocapnic bronchoconstriction because in this case it is a response to a high V/Q. With a high V/Q you have an area of the lung with wasted ventilation and a lower than normal $PACO_2$ (hypocapnia). The body's response in this situation will be to induce bronchoconstriction in those areas so as to increase the resistance in the airway so that it decreases the amount of ventilation that is going to an area that is otherwise not well perfused. This will reduce the amount of dead space (wasted) ventilation and bring more balance between V and Q and thus compensate for the V/Q mismatching.

<u>Hypoxic Vasoconstriction</u>

It is called hypoxic vasoconstriction because in this case it is a response to a low V/Q. With a low V/Q you have an area of the lung with wasted perfusion and a lower than normal PAO_2 (alveolar hypoxia). The body's response in this situation will be to induce pulmonary vasoconstriction in those areas so as to redirect that blood to other parts of the lungs that are better ventilated. This will reduce shunting and bring more balance between V and Q and thus compensate for the V/Q mismatching.

F. Oxygenation

$P(A - a)O_2$

The $P(A - a)O_2$ is commonly known as the A – a gradient, but in reality it is NOT a diffusion gradient. It should actually be referred to as the A – a *difference* because it is telling you the difference between the PAO_2 and the PaO_2. The difference between alveolar and arterial oxygen should be very small, and being able to determine the difference between the two enables you to detect abnormalities in gas exchange.

You derive the PAO_2 from the alveolar air equation and the PaO_2 from an ABG.

Then you look at the difference: $PAO_2 - PaO_2$

- For a normal patient breathing room air, the difference should be no more than 5 – 10 mmHg, but this does increase with age. The following formula will enable you to approximate what the expected difference should be as a function of a patient's age.

$$\text{Expected (A - a) difference} = \frac{\text{patient's age}}{4} + 4$$

The difference should be < 4 mmHg for every 10 years of age.

e.g.:   age 10   expected (A - a) difference is 6.5 mmHg
         age 20   expected (A - a) difference is 9 mmHg
         age 30   expected (A - a) difference is 11.5 mmHg

* The (A - a) difference between these 10 yr. periods < 4 mmHg.

If the (A - a) difference is greater than expected (including accounting for age), then there are problems with the A/C membrane and oxygen transfer across the membrane.

- If the patient is on 100% oxygen (FiO_2 = 100%), then the (A - a) difference should be no more than 65 mmHg.

  - when a patient is on an FiO_2 of 100% - every 50 mmHg difference in (A - a) approximates a 2% shunt.

  e.g.: the PAO_2 calculated from the alveolar air equation is 673 mmHg. This is based on an FiO_2 of 1 (100%), a normal $PaCO_2$ of 40 mmHg, and a normal P_B of 760 mmHg. R is not used in the calculation because the $FiO_2 \geq 0.6$ (60 %).

$$
\begin{aligned}
PAO_2 &= FiO_2 (P_B - 47) - PaCO_2 \\
      &= 1 (760 - 47) - 40 \\
      &= 1 (713) - 40 \\
      &= 713 - 40 \\
      &= 673 \text{ mmHg}
\end{aligned}
$$

And let's say the PaO_2 from the ABG is 173 mmHg

Therefore, the $P(A - a)O_2$ difference is 673 − 173 = 500 mmHg.

This is a huge (A - a) difference. For every 50 mmHg of difference there is a 2% shunt. You have a difference of 500. 500 ÷ 50 = 10, and 10 x 2% = 20%. A 20% shunt is significant, and it is telling you why there is such disparity between the alveolar and arterial oxygen. A shunt is when there is perfusion to the alveoli, but there is very little or no ventilation in those alveoli. In terms of the V/Q ratio, V is extremely low with respect to Q. The quotient of V/Q in this case is no longer 0.8 - it is much lower. Cardiac output (Q) is fine and maintaining perfusion, however V is drastically diminished. A significant lowering of V with respect to Q remaining normal is going to make the V/Q ratio much smaller. This could be due to atelectasis, or more than likely pulmonary consolidation. When the alveoli become consolidated they are full of fluid and therefore aren't ventilated with gas. This drastically alters V/Q because even though you have blood perfusing the alveoli, there is no ventilation in the alveoli. The blood is not able to pick up any oxygen because there is no gas in the alveoli, and this is why the PaO_2 is nowhere near what it should be. This is why there is such a huge difference between the PAO_2 and the PaO_2. When you have shunting – it is representing that there are areas in the lungs that are not participating in gas exchange. This is why using 100% oxygen isn't able to help with the hypoxemia – because the O_2 isn't getting through to the blood. In fact – if you want to know if the hypoxemia that your patient is experiencing is due to pulmonary shunting – raise their FiO_2 to 100% for 10 minutes and draw an ABG and compare the PaO_2 from that ABG to the PAO_2 that you calculated from the alveolar air equation. You'll know right then and there if the hypoxemia is secondary to shunting.

Why the normal $P(A – a)O_2$ difference exists

The $P(A – a)O_2$ difference, when small and within the limits previously discussed, is normal. One may ask - why is the PaO_2 always slightly less than the PAO_2? The reason is due to the following considerations.

- Normal right to left *anatomic* shunts in the bronchial and cardiac circulation. Although shunting by definition is perfusion without ventilation, ultimately it is indicating that there is perfused blood in the pulmonary circulation that is not getting oxygenated. Just a minute ago alveolar shunts were discussed. This was the case of blood perfusing the pulmonary capillaries, but yet not picking up any oxygen because there was no gas in the alveoli due to a situation such as atelectasis or pulmonary consolidation. This type of shunting is pathological – in other words the shunting is occurring because of a problem with the alveoli (i.e. – they were atelectatic or consolidated). When we talk about a *normal* right to left anatomic shunt, however, we are not talking about the shunting that occurs because of problems with the alveoli - we are talking about a portion of the cardiac output that has returned to the left heart without having ever been oxygenated because of bypassing the right heart - and thus having never been exposed to ventilated alveoli.

A. Some of the cardiac output goes to the bronchial arteries in order to perfuse the lungs themselves. This isn't the pulmonary circulation, but rather the bronchial circulation. The bronchial arteries arise from the aorta and go to the lungs in order to provide the lungs themselves with oxygen and nutrition. Once the blood in the bronchial arteries has delivered O_2 and nutrition to the lungs, it is returned to the heart via the bronchial veins. The issue here is that some of the blood in the bronchial veins is drained into the pulmonary veins, and the pulmonary veins go directly to the left heart (left atrium). The portion of blood from the bronchial veins that drains directly into the pulmonary veins never goes through the right heart and therefore never gets oxygenated. As such, there is a portion of deoxygenated blood that came from the bronchial veins that has been mixed with the oxygenated blood in the pulmonary veins. And this will obviously cause a slight lowering of the PaO_2.

B. The Thebesian veins are the smallest of the cardiac veins. The Thebesian veins are located within all 4 heart chambers and serve as part of the venous drainage of the myocardium itself. Although most of the venous drainage through the Thebesian veins goes into the right atrium, there is a portion of it that goes to the left heart as well. The portion of deoxygenated blood from the Thebesian veins that drains into the left heart never goes through the right heart and therefore never gets oxygenated. This deoxygenated blood from the Thebesian veins is mixed with the oxygenated blood that is in the left heart and it will contribute to slightly lowering the PaO_2.

Therefore – the deoxygenated blood from the bronchial veins and the Thebesian veins that ends up in the arterial circulation (this is called a venous admixture) is what slightly reduces the PaO_2.

These two normal anatomic shunts (the bronchial and Thebesian veins) account for about 75% of the normal $P(A - a)O_2$ difference.

- The other 25% is accounted for by normal variations in pulmonary ventilation and perfusion (i.e. regional differences in ventilation and perfusion).

a/A ratio

The a/A ratio is the ratio between PaO_2 and PAO_2. It is the fraction PaO_2/PAO_2. It is another tool that is used to evaluate the efficiency of O_2 transfer from the alveoli into the blood. This ratio should be as close to 1 as possible - at least 0.9 (90%) - because under normal conditions, at least 90% of alveolar O_2 diffuses across the A/C membrane into the blood. This ratio is telling you the percentage of oxygen that is getting from the alveoli into the blood. It goes hand in hand with the $P(A - a)O_2$ just discussed.

- If $\dfrac{PaO_2}{PAO_2}$ < 0.15 (15%), this is considered critical *(very bad)*

- When you have a HIGH $P(A - a)O_2$ difference *and* a LOW a/A ratio – it is indicative of a diffusion defect.
  - A diffusion defect is a condition that "thickens" the A/C

membrane. Pulmonary edema, ARDS, and pulmonary fibrosis are examples of conditions that will cause a diffusion defect.

G. O_2 Transport

Oxygen is carried in the blood in two ways:

1. A very small amount is *dissolved* in the plasma and the intracellular fluid of the red blood cells (RBC's).

2. Most of the oxygen is carried by being *bound* to hemoglobin (Hb).

Dissolved Oxygen

The PaO_2 is the partial pressure of the O_2 that is dissolved in the plasma and the intracellular fluid of the RBC's. It is the dissolved O_2 that you are seeing on an ABG. When O_2 is bound to Hb, it no longer contributes to the partial pressure of oxygen being exerted in the plasma. Therefore, the O_2 that is bound to Hb does not contribute the PaO_2 that you see on the ABG.

Whereas the PAO_2 is the *driving pressure* to get oxygen across the A/C membrane from the alveoli into the blood, the PaO_2 is the *driving pressure* to get oxygen across the cell membrane of the erythrocyte so it can bind with Hb.

Henry's Law (chapter 1) enables us to know how much O_2 is dissolved in the plasma.

$$\text{Amount of gas dissolved} = PaO_2 \times SC$$

- using the normal value for PaO_2 of 100 mmHg, and the SC being 0.003, the amount of dissolved O_2 is determined as follows:

Amount of dissolved O_2 $= PaO_2 \times SC$
$= 100 \text{ mmHg} \times 0.003\text{ml}/100\text{ml}$
$= 0.3\text{ml}/100\text{ml}$ *or* $0.3\text{ml}/\text{dl}$ *or* 0.3 vol%

* you may see the units of dissolved oxygen expressed as volume per cent (vol%). *Vol% is just another way of expressing ml/dl.* The answer above for the amount of dissolved O_2 was 0.3ml/100ml. 100ml is the same thing as 1 deciliter – so you could also say the answer is 0.3ml/dl or 0.3 vol%.

NOW – even though the amount of dissolved oxygen is obviously small (< 2% of the total amount of oxygen that is being carried), it is nonetheless highly significant because the dissolved oxygen functions as a reserve to keep the hemoglobin saturated as the blood perfuses the systemic capillaries.

Oxygen Bound to Hemoglobin (Hb)

The low solubility of oxygen in plasma makes it impossible for the plasma to carry enough dissolved oxygen to meet the body's normal demand of about 250ml/min. Hemoglobin makes sufficient transport of oxygen possible. This section assumes that you already have an understanding of the structure and function of hemoglobin.

- The average total amount of Hb in the blood is 15g/100ml, or 15g/dl, with a normal range from 11 – 16g/dl.

- Each gram of Hb can carry 1.34ml of oxygen (1.34ml O_2 per gram Hb).

If that was all there was to it – you could say that the amount of O_2 bound to hemoglobin is 15g/dl x 1.34ml/g = 20.1ml/dl. Although we can say that 20.1ml/dl is the capacity for bound Hb – it will never be quite that high because not all the available Hb gets oxygenated. Consider the following discussion on hemoglobin saturation in order to understand how the actual amount of oxygenated hemoglobin (HbO_2) is determined.

Hemoglobin saturation

Hb saturation is a measurement of the percentage of total hemoglobin that is actually carrying oxygen. Not all of the hemoglobin in the blood will have oxygen bound to it. Recall from the last section that there are two normal anatomical shunts (the bronchial and Thebesian veins) where some of the blood in those vessels gets delivered into the left heart without having been oxygenated. Remember that this is what accounted for the normal difference in the $P(A - a)O_2$. There could also be some hemoglobin that is defective and thus unable to properly carry oxygen. The percentage of saturated Hb is therefore the ratio of the amount of Hb that actually has O_2 bound to it (HbO_2) over the total amount of hemoglobin in the blood. The percentage of saturated Hb is what you know as either the SaO_2 (obtained from an ABG) or the SpO_2 (derived from a pulse oximeter). It is expressed as follows:

$$\% \ SaO_2 \ = \ \frac{HbO_2}{Total \ Hb} \ x \ 100$$

where: HbO_2 is the amount of Hb that is bound with O_2
  - this is the actual *content* of Hb that has oxygen bound (g/dl)
  Total Hb is the total amount of hemoglobin in the blood
  - this is the *capacity* – the total amount of Hb (g/dl)

- Normal SaO_2 is 95 – 100% (varies with age)

the equation above is written the way it is to show you how SaO_2 is derived. In real life you will get the SaO_2 from an ABG (or you can use the SpO_2 from a pulse oximeter). The total Hb will come from a CBC. With those two values - you'll then be able rearrange the equation and solve for HbO_2. HbO_2 is expressed in g/dl.

You know that the average total Hb in the blood is 15g/dl. You know that each gram of Hb can carry 1.34ml of oxygen. But you also know that some of the hemoglobin has not been oxygenated because it was either defective or it was in the circulation that was part of one of the normal anatomical shunts – hence the need to know the percentage of total Hb that is actually saturated with O_2. By knowing these three things, you can then determine the amount of oxygen in ml/dl that is bound to Hb by applying the following formula:

Total Hb x SaO_2 x 1.34 = Amount of bound O_2 (ml/dl)

look at the previous equation – this is HbO_2 expressed in g/dl

15g/dl x 0.97 x 1.34ml/g = 19.5ml/dl   * an SaO_2 of 97% (0.97) was
                                         used for this example

Consider the following:

If 0.3 ml/dl is the amount of oxygen transported as dissolved O_2 in the plasma, and 19.5 ml/dl is the amount of oxygen that is transported by being bound to Hb – that tells you that 65 times more oxygen is being transported by way of being bound to hemoglobin than is transported by just being dissolved in the plasma.

Clinical correlation between PaO_2 and SpO_2

You always want to keep a patient's $PaO_2 \geq 60$ mmHg because at 60 mmHg you have an SpO_2 of at least 90%. At a PaO_2 of 50 mmHg, the SpO_2 drops to 80%. And at a PaO_2 of 40 mmHg, the SpO_2 drops to 70%. *As the PaO_2 drops, Hb has less affinity for oxygen.* By memorizing what follows below, you will always be able to know a patient's approximate PaO_2 by knowing their saturation, or know their saturation by knowing the PaO_2. What follows is known as the 40, 50, 60 – 70, 80, 90 rule.

PaO_2	SpO_2
40 mmHg	70 %
50 mmHg	80 %
60 mmHg	90 %

Oxygen Content (CaO$_2$)

Oxygen content (CaO$_2$) is simply the sum of dissolved oxygen and the oxygen bound to hemoglobin. It is the content of oxygen in the arterial blood.

Dissolved O$_2$ = PaO$_2$ x 0.003

Bound O$_2$ = Total Hb x SaO$_2$ x 1.34

Oxygen Content = (PaO$_2$ x 0.003) + (Total Hb x SaO$_2$ x 1.34)
   (CaO$_2$)

   = (100 x 0.003) + (15 x 0.97 x 1.34)

   = (0.3ml/dl) + (19.5ml/dl)

CaO$_2$ = 19.8ml/dl or 19.8 vol%
   *the range for normal CaO$_2$ is 16 – 20ml/dl
   or 16 – 20 vol%*

Summary in chart form:

	Arterial blood (ml/dl)	Venous blood (ml/dl)
Dissolved O$_2$ PaO$_2$ x 0.003	0.3	0.1
Bound O$_2$ Total Hb x SaO$_2$ x 1.34	19.5	14.7
Oxygen Content Dissolved O$_2$ + Bound O$_2$	19.8 (CaO$_2$)	14.8 (CvO$_2$)

Notice on the right-hand side of the chart that I also included the values for dissolved O$_2$, bound O$_2$, and O$_2$ content for venous blood. I included the values for venous blood so you can easily reference them as we now extend this discussion to the next idea of what is known as oxygen loading and unloading – the C(a – v)O$_2$.

Oxygen Loading and Unloading: $C(a - v)O_2$

Oxygen loading and unloading refers to the reversible loading and unloading of hemoglobin with oxygen. As blood circulates through the pulmonary capillaries, hemoglobin is loaded with oxygen. Oxygenated hemoglobin is then transported to the systemic tissues where blood perfuses the systemic capillaries and unloads oxygen to the cells according to their metabolic needs. The difference between the oxygen content at the arterial end of the capillaries (CaO_2) and the oxygen content at the venous end of the capillaries (CvO_2) is the amount of oxygen that was unloaded and actually taken up by the cells.

$CaO_2 - CvO_2$, or $C(a - v)O_2$, is the amount of oxygen taken by the cells. It is the arterial – mixed venous content difference. The difference between CaO_2 and CvO_2 is about 5ml/dl. This means that on average – the cells uptake about 5ml/dl, or 5 vol% of oxygen. With $C(a - v)O_2$ being expressed as ml/dl – just remember that this means that for every 100ml of blood that perfuses the systemic capillaries, 5ml of O_2 is released to the cells.

19.8ml/dl is the O_2 content on the arterial side of the systemic capillaries (CaO_2). As that blood perfuses through the systemic capillaries, it will give up 5ml/dl to the cells for their metabolic needs. Having given up 5ml/dl to the cells – the O_2 content on the venous side of the systemic capillaries (CvO_2) is therefore now only 14.8ml/dl.

Calculating cardiac output (Q_t) based upon knowing $C(a - v)O_2$

Besides telling you the amount of O_2 given up to the tissues, $C(a - v)O_2$ is also a part of the Fick equation that enables you to calculate cardiac output (Q_t). The Fick equation is as follows:

$$Q_t = \frac{\dot{V}O_2}{C(a - v)O_2 \times 10}$$

where: - Q_t is cardiac output
- $\dot{V}O_2$ is minute consumption oxygen (250ml/min.)
- $C(a - v)O_2$ is 5ml/dl
- multiplying the denominator by 10 converts ml/dl to ml/L

$$Q_t = \frac{250\text{ml/min.}}{5\text{ml/dl} \times 10} = \frac{250\text{ml/min.}}{50\text{ml/L}} = 5\text{ L/min.}$$

* 4 – 8 L/min. is the normal range for Q_t

For a constant VO_2 of 250ml/min.:

- If Q_t is decreased, then $C(a - v)O_2$ will increase.

This is obvious enough just based on the math alone – if you make the quotient smaller and keep the numerator the same, then the denominator had to have been increased. However – to explain it physiologically - if there is less cardiac output, there is less perfusion to the systemic capillaries in the tissue. A consequence of reduced perfusion is that the blood moves slower through the systemic capillaries such that the tissue has more time to extract O_2. Since cardiac output is reduced, the tissue compensates for this by extracting more O_2 per pass because it still has to meet its consumption demand of 250ml/min. Rather than taking the normal 5ml/dl, under conditions of reduced cardiac output the tissue will take more oxygen. This makes the blood leaving the systemic capillaries (CvO_2) lower in oxygen content than its normal 14.8ml/dl – hence the difference between CaO_2 and CvO_2 will increase.

- If Q_t is increased, then $C(a - v)O_2$ will decrease.

If there is more cardiac output, there is more perfusion to the systemic capillaries in the tissue. This scenario is just the opposite of what was just discussed. With more perfusion, less oxygen will be extracted by the tissue on each pass (they don't need to take as much per pass because they are being perfused more) – therefore the blood leaving the systemic capillaries (CvO_2) will be higher in oxygen content than its normal 14.8ml/dl, and the difference between CaO_2 and CvO_2 will decrease.

H. The Oxyhemoglobin Dissociation Curve

The oxyhemoglobin dissociation curve is a graph that shows the relationship between PO_2 and the percentage of hemoglobin saturation. In order to understand the curve, it is first necessary to understand some important characteristics of hemoglobin.

- Hb can modify its affinity for oxygen.

- Hb displays *cooperative* binding and unbinding of oxygen.

As each molecule of O_2 binds or unbinds to Hb, it becomes easier for the next molecule of O_2 to bind or unbind.

When O_2 binds to the first heme group of Hb, it causes a slight conformational change of the molecule. A conformational change is when the geometric structure of a molecule is slightly altered. This slight alteration in the shape of Hb makes it easier for oxygen to bind.

With the binding of oxygen to the first heme group, that heme group changes its conformation from the tense (T) state of Hb to the relaxed (R) state of Hb. This conformational change from (T) to (R) is then translated to the other three heme groups such that the binding of O_2 to the other three heme groups becomes easier - hence the cooperative nature of hemoglobin's binding of oxygen. *The conformational changes that occur that make it easier for O_2 to bind are the essence of the cooperative nature of the hemoglobin molecule.*

During O_2 unloading (unbinding), the same cooperativity is in effect. The unloading of the first oxygen molecule facilitates the unloading of the second and so forth. The cooperativity displayed by the hemoglobin molecule is really important because it is what allows for the loading (binding) and unloading (unbinding) of relatively large amounts of oxygen at physiological oxygen pressures.

- The 2 states of hemoglobin – the relaxed (R) state, and the taut or tense (T) state.

R state (oxyhemoglobin): The R state is the form of Hb when blood is perfusing through the pulmonary capillaries. The R state of Hb has high affinity for oxygen and therefore favors the binding of O_2. This makes perfect sense as it is during the perfusion of the pulmonary capillaries that Hb would want to bind the O_2 that is in the alveoli. The conditions of higher pH, decreased 2,3 DPG, decreased CO_2, and decreased temperature at the level of the pulmonary capillaries are what enable hemoglobin to have greater affinity for O_2 and thus favor the R state. *The Hb in the deoxygenated blood coming from the right heart that is pumped through the pulmonary artery into the pulmonary circulation is in the T state. Once that blood gets down to the pulmonary capillaries where gas exchange occurs – and that first O_2 molecule binds to Hb – then the molecule changes to the R state so that oxygen can then easily bind to the remaining heme groups of each Hb molecule.*

T state (deoxyhemoglobin): The T state is the form of Hb when blood is perfusing through the systemic capillaries of the tissue. The T state of Hb has low affinity for oxygen and therefore favors the release (unbinding) of O_2. This also makes perfect sense as it is during the perfusion of the systemic capillaries that Hb would want to release O_2 so that it can be taken by the cells. The conditions of lower pH, increased 2,3 DPG, increased CO_2, and increased temperature at the level of the systemic capillaries are what enable hemoglobin to have less affinity for O_2 and thus favor the T state. *The Hb in the oxygenated blood coming from the left heart that is pumped through the aorta into the systemic circulation is in the R state. Once that blood gets down to the systemic capillaries where gas exchange occurs – and that first O_2 molecule is released (unbinds) from Hb – then the molecule changes to the T state so that oxygen can then easily unload from the remaining heme groups such that the O_2 is released to the tissue.*

The Oxyhemoglobin Dissociation Curve

If you were to look at the graph that showed the relationship between PO_2 and *dissolved* oxygen – it would be linear. For incremental increases in PO_2, you would see function values (dissolved O_2) that produced a straight line (a linear relationship).

The graph that shows the relationship between PO_2 and the percentage of hemoglobin saturation – the oxyhemoglobin dissociation curve – is an S-shaped, or sigmoidal curve. It has this S-shaped curvature because of the cooperative way that O_2 binds to hemoglobin along with the fact that saturation reaches a maximum that causes the curve to level off. The affinity of Hb for O_2 increases as successive O_2 molecules continue to bind – this is the result of the cooperative behavior of Hb. As the PO_2 continues to increase, more O_2 will bind to Hb and the percentage of Hb saturation will continue to increase – but to a limit. There is only so much Hb to begin with (total Hb) that can be saturated, and as this maximum saturation level is reached – the curve levels off. Thus, the reason why the oxyhemoglobin curve is sigmoidal in shape.

Let us examine the features of the curve.

- The plateau portion – this is the top of the curve where it levels off. If you look at the PO_2, you'll see that for PO_2's > 60 mmHg, there is no significant increase in saturation because at this point the limit for saturation has nearly been reached. As this limit is approached, very little additional binding of O_2 occurs and the curve levels off as the Hb is becoming saturated with O_2. No matter how much the PO_2 is increased beyond 60 mmHg, you can't saturate something beyond its limit, and the limit is defined by the amount of Hb that is available. The top (plateau) part of the curve where the Hb saturation levels are 90 – 100% correlates to the Hb in the pulmonary capillaries, and this is consistent with what you would expect as it is in the pulmonary capillaries where Hb has the highest affinity for O_2 and would thus be saturated with O_2.

- <u>The steep portion</u> – this is the large middle portion of the curve with the very steep slope. Looking again at the PO_2 at the point of 60 mmHg, you can see that for incremental decreases in the PO_2 below 60 mmHg that the hemoglobin saturation drops dramatically – hence the steepness of the curve in the area where the PO_2 < 60 mmHg. The steep portion of the curve where the Hb saturation levels are significantly lower correlates to the Hb in the systemic capillaries, and this is consistent with what you would expect as it is in the systemic capillaries where Hb has the lowest affinity for O_2. The graph is telling you that at PO_2's < 60 mmHg, small drops in the PO_2 in the systemic capillaries results in the release of large amounts of oxygen to the cells. In other words – the lower the PO_2 in the systemic capillaries, the more unsaturated Hb becomes because it is giving up the oxygen to the tissue and thus becoming deoxygenated Hb in the process.

Remember from section B at the beginning of this chapter that PvO_2 is 40 mmHg. This reflects equilibrium with the partial pressure of oxygen inside the cells – hence 40 mmHg is the typical partial pressure of oxygen inside the cells. When arterial blood with a PaO_2 of 100 mmHg arrives at the systemic capillaries, O_2 is unloaded to the cells and therefore the partial pressure of O_2 in the capillaries drops and thus the venous side of the systemic capillaries ends up with a PvO_2 of 40 mmHg. The oxygen that was delivered to the cells, and thus momentarily raising the partial pressure of oxygen inside the cells, is quickly used up such that the partial pressure of O_2 inside the cells is back to 40 mmHg by the time of the next pass of blood thru the systemic capillaries.

Careful examination of the oxyhemoglobin dissociation curve indicates that only about 25% of the hemoglobin gives up its oxygen in the systemic capillaries under normal resting conditions. This is important because it means that there is a significant amount of oxygen that is available in reserve.

Hemoglobin doesn't unload the same exact amount of O_2 to all the tissues, nor does it pick up the same exact amount of CO_2 from all the tissues. Realize that the more metabolically active any particular tissue is, that tissue will have a higher local temperature, a lower local partial pressure of O_2, a higher local CO_2 level, and thus a lower local pH. All of these factors favor enhanced O_2 unloading to the cells (hence Hb becomes more unsaturated at the tissue level). Hemoglobin has a remarkable ability to adjust the amount of gas exchange according to the particular needs of the tissues. By way of example - during periods of activity (exercise), the partial pressure of oxygen in the cells (muscle for example) will drop to below 40 mmHg and the other factors (higher local temperature, higher local CO_2, lower local pH) will also be present. When this happens – the curve drops significantly – Hb becomes much less saturated, indicating that Hb is unloading much more oxygen to those metabolically active cells that have increased oxygen demand.

- P50 – P50 is the partial pressure of oxygen in the blood when the hemoglobin saturation is 50%. In a normal, healthy individual, P50 is about 27 mmHg with a normal range of 24 – 30 mmHg. P50 is a measure of the amount of affinity that hemoglobin has for oxygen. A higher than normal P50 reflects a shifting of the curve to the right, indicating that Hb has lower affinity for O_2 and therefore requiring a higher PO_2 to maintain 50% saturation of Hb. A lower than normal P50 reflects a shifting of the curve to the left, indicating that Hb has higher affinity for O_2 and therefore enabling a lower PO_2 to maintain 50% saturation of Hb. Shifting of the curve to the right or the left will be discussed next.

Oxyhemoglobin Dissociation Curve

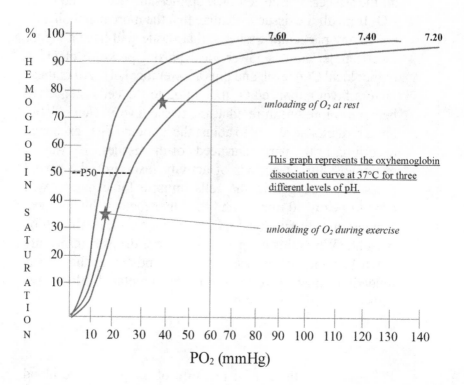

This graph represents the oxyhemoglobin dissociation curve at 37°C for three different levels of pH.

There are 3 curves in the graph above. The standard curve is in the middle, and then there is a curve to the right and the left of the standard curve. All three curves are normal. The shifted curves (the one to the right and the left) are showing how hemoglobin's affinity for oxygen changes in response to those changes in the local environment that I spoke of earlier. The values for PO_2, PCO_2, pH, temperature, and 2,3 DPG in the local environment of the pulmonary capillaries are different from what they are in the local environment of the systemic capillaries. The difference in the values of these factors are what affect hemoglobin's affinity for oxygen and therefore determine whether Hb will be loading or unloading oxygen.

Factors that affect the oxyhemoglobin curve

As I just said – all three curves are "normal". The curve shifts back and forth as the blood circulates between the pulmonary capillaries and the systemic capillaries.

SHIFT TO THE LEFT

- Occurs in the LUNGS (pulmonary capillaries)

  - when venous blood returns to the lungs (pulmonary capillaries), CO_2 is excreted and thus the pH goes back up again. The higher local pH now raises hemoglobin's affinity for O_2 thus facilitating the binding of O_2 to hemoglobin.

- Hb is in the R form – it therefore has higher affinity for O_2.

- In the local environment of the pulmonary capillaries:
  * pH is increased – due to CO_2 being decreased
  * 2,3 DPG is decreased
  * temperature is decreased

  * *all of these factors favor increasing hemoglobin's affinity for O_2.*

- P50 is lower.

SHIFT TO THE RIGHT

- Occurs in the CELLS/TISSUES (systemic capillaries)

  - blood in the systemic capillaries of the tissues is higher in CO_2 because CO_2 is being continuously produced as a byproduct of metabolism and therefore the local pH is lower. The lower local pH now decreases hemoglobin's affinity for O_2 such that Hb then releases its O_2 to the cells.

- Hb is in the T state – it therefore has lower affinity for O_2.

- In the local environment of the systemic capillaries:
  * pH is decreased – due to CO_2 being increased
  * 2,3 DPG is increased
  * temperature is increased

  * *all of these factors favor decreasing hemoglobin's affinity for O_2.*

- P50 is higher.

A word about pH – The Bohr Effect

The beauty of Hb is in its ability to adapt its affinity for O_2 according to the environment in which it finds itself. The word environment in this context is referring to the particular local capillary network where the blood happens to be perfusing. The differences in PO_2, PCO_2, pH, 2, 3 DPG, and temperature between the environment of the pulmonary capillaries and the environment of the systemic capillaries have already been discussed – these are the factors that dictate the degree of affinity that Hb will have for O_2. The Bohr Effect is simply a statement that describes the relationship between hemoglobin's affinity for oxygen and the degree of acidity and PCO_2 (degree of acidity and PCO_2 go hand in hand). The Bohr Effect states that hemoglobin's affinity for O_2 is inversely related to the concentration of carbon dioxide (PCO_2) and thus the acidity. This is consistent with everything you have learned in this section. When the PCO_2 increases (as is the case with the blood in the systemic capillaries), the level of acidity increases (as indicated by a lower pH) – and the affinity of Hb for O_2 decreases. This is an inverse relationship. When the PCO_2 decreases (as is the case with the blood in the pulmonary capillaries), the level of acidity decreases (as indicated by a higher pH) – and the affinity of Hb for O_2 increases. This too is an inverse relationship.

In the last chapter in the section on the regulation of breathing, it was explained how CO_2, when in solution (plasma), dissociates into H^+ and HCO_3^-. At the level of the systemic capillaries, when CO_2 diffuses out of the cells into the systemic capillaries, some of that CO_2 dissociates into H^+ and HCO_3^-. The amount of CO_2 diffusing out of those cells is high – so therefore the amount of H^+ is going to be high. This is why the environment of the systemic capillaries is more acidic and thus has a lower pH. Those H^+ ions contribute to causing Hb to change its conformation to the T state and thus lower hemoglobin's affinity for O_2 such that the O_2 is released to the cells.

Just the opposite happens in the pulmonary capillaries. In the pulmonary capillaries, CO_2 is diffusing out of the blood into the alveoli – therefore the amount of CO_2, and consequently the amount of H^+ in the blood of the pulmonary capillaries becomes much lower. The environment of the pulmonary capillaries is therefore much less acidic and thus has a higher pH. Having less H^+ in the environment of the pulmonary capillaries causes Hb to change its conformation to the R form and thus increases hemoglobin's affinity for O_2 such that O_2 binds to the hemoglobin.

A word about 2, 3 Diphosphoglyceric Acid (2, 3 DPG)

2, 3 DPG is a molecule that is synthesized by red blood cells. It plays a role in the production of ATP by the RBC, but it also plays another role by being what is known as an allosteric effector with regards to regulating hemoglobin's affinity for oxygen. Being an allosteric effector means that the 2, 3 DPG binds to Hb at a site other than the active site. The heme group is the active site of Hb where O_2 binds. 2, 3 DPG does not bind at the heme group, but rather binds elsewhere on the globin chains of the Hb molecule. By binding to the protein chains, however, 2, 3 DPG plays a role in assisting with the conformational changes that enable Hb to assume the T state.

2, 3 DPG essentially binds preferentially to Hb when Hb is in the deoxygenated state in the systemic capillaries in the tissues. As blood enters the systemic capillaries and Hb starts to become deoxygenated by virtue of having started to give up its O_2 to the cells, 2,3 DPG then readily binds to the protein chains of Hb and further decreases hemoglobin's affinity for O_2 by stabilizing the T state of Hb. By stabilizing the T state of Hb, 2,3 DPG therefore allosterically promotes the release of the remaining O_2 to the cells.

Therefore:

- Increased 2, 3 DPG enables Hb to be more efficient at unloading O_2 to the cells.
  - 2, 3 DPG production increases with chronic hypoxemia and anemia.

- Decreased 2, 3 DPG enables Hb to be more efficient at picking up O_2 in the lungs.
  - 2, 3 DPG production decreases with chronic acidosis

I. Abnormal Hemoglobin

There are four globular protein subunits that are part of the structure of hemoglobin. The primary structure of a protein is determined by the sequence of the amino acids that comprise the protein. It is the primary structure (amino acid sequence) that ultimately determines the shape of a protein. The amino acid sequence of a protein is determined by the sequence of the nucleic acid molecules that serve as the template for protein synthesis. When the nucleic acid molecules are not in the proper sequence, the amino acid sequence ends up not being correct – therefore the gene product (protein) is not made correctly and the result is a protein with an altered shape. Changes in the amino acid sequence of the proteins that comprise hemoglobin will alter the geometry of the hemoglobin molecule, and this altered geometry will then affect hemoglobin's affinity for oxygen.

Methemoglobin (metHb)

- Methemoglobin is when the normal ferrous iron (Fe^{2+}) in the heme group loses an electron and becomes ferric iron (Fe^{3+}).

- Fe^{3+} cannot bind O_2.

- Although O_2 can't bind to the heme group with Fe^{3+} - remember that there are 4 heme groups within a hemoglobin molecule. Any of the other 3 heme groups that are in the ferrous (Fe^{2+}) state can bind O_2. When O_2 binds to methemoglobin (not the heme group with Fe^{3+}, but one of the other heme groups that are Fe^{2+}), it results in the remaining heme groups within that Hb molecule that are in the Fe^{2+} state having increased affinity for oxygen. The greater affinity for oxygen brought about by this situation results in this variant form of Hb having much less ability to release the oxygen that it does have to the cells – hence the oxyhemoglobin dissociation curve will be shifted to the left, and at elevated levels of metHb, tissue hypoxia can certainly occur.

- Normal amounts of metHb are around 1 – 2% of the total Hb. At greater amounts of metHb, methemoglobinemia (a special type of anemia) will manifest. Methemoglobinemia is characterized by dyspnea, changes in LOC, cyanosis, and headache. Individuals often may not show any symptoms until metHb% ≥ 15%.

- metHb will cause the color of the blood to become brown, which in turn gives the skin an ashen/slight azure appearance that can mimic cyanosis.

- Methemoglobinemia can be congenital or acquired. Acquired methemoglobinemia can often be due to certain drugs.

* local anesthetics (benzocaine)
* nitrate medications (nitric oxide, nitroglycerin, nitroprusside)
* certain antibiotics (sulfa drugs)

- Methemoglobinemia is treated with methylene blue and oxygen therapy.

Carboxyhemoglobin (HbCO)

Carboxyhemoglobin (HbCO) is the complex that is formed when carbon monoxide binds to hemoglobin. Hemoglobin's affinity for carbon monoxide is roughly 230 times greater than its affinity for oxygen. Because of hemoglobin's greater affinity for carbon monoxide, HbCO forms much more readily than HbO_2. This poses a serious problem because even the lowest levels of carbon monoxide (PCO of 0.12 mmHg) are enough to cause significant interference with the binding of oxygen. Carbon monoxide binds to the same site as O_2 – in other words, it binds at the same location on the heme group as oxygen does. Since the affinity for carbon monoxide is so much greater - in the presence of carbon monoxide, not only will Hb preferentially bind carbon monoxide rather than oxygen, but it will also hold on to that carbon monoxide much more tightly. With Hb holding onto carbon monoxide tightly, the problem is further complicated in that it is also difficult to get the carbon monoxide released from the hemoglobin.

When carbon monoxide binds to hemoglobin – for any one particular hemoglobin molecule, carbon monoxide may not necessarily bind to all four heme groups. But the binding of carbon monoxide to one of the heme groups increases hemoglobin's affinity for oxygen at the other three groups. It's not that carbon monoxide prevents O_2 from binding – it just competes better for the site on the heme group. But for the oxygen that does get bound to the hemoglobin, the presence of carbon monoxide on one of the heme groups causes any oxygen that is bound on the other groups to be held more tightly. So not only is the carbon monoxide itself held tightly to the Hb, that carbon monoxide causes whatever oxygen that may be bound to also be held tightly. This presents a problem at the tissue level as it means that the oxygen that is being held tightly will not be released to the cells. This situation effectively describes the oxyhemoglobin curve being shifted to the left, the result of which is that the cells are denied oxygen and thus tissue hypoxia ensues.

To summarize – with carbon monoxide poisoning you have less oxygen bound to Hb to begin with because carbon monoxide competes better for the binding sites on the heme groups, and whatever oxygen that did manage to be able to bind – it's affinity for Hb has been increased by the presence of the carbon monoxide to the point where that O_2 is not going to be released to the cells. The net result of this is that the tissues will be denied oxygen, and the consequence of this if not corrected quickly is death.

With carbon monoxide (CO) poisoning, it normally takes the body 5 hours to remove ½ of the carboxyhemoglobin if just room air is being breathed. This obviously is probably not going to be adequate.

Therefore - The treatment of CO poisoning is oxygen therapy (FiO₂ 100%) and/or hyperbaric oxygen.

* 100% O_2 reduces the ½ life of CO to 80 minutes.
* 3 ATM of HBO (hyperbaric oxygen) reduces the ½ life of CO to 23 minutes.

J. CO_2 Transport

Carbon dioxide is produced by the cells as a byproduct of cellular metabolism. Recall from the beginning of this chapter that carbon dioxide production (VCO_2) is about 200ml/min. The CO_2 that is produced by the cells diffuses into the blood and is carried by the blood to the alveoli where it is excreted (exhaled). About 45 – 55ml/dl of CO_2 is normally carried in the blood via 3 different methods.

3 different methods for transporting CO_2

Method 1. Dissolved in solution
Method 2. Bound to protein (carbamino compounds)
Method 3. Ionized as bicarbonate

The 3 different methods of transporting CO_2 occur in **both** the plasma and within the erythrocyte. Overall – approximately 10% of the CO_2 is transported in the plasma, and approximately 90% of the CO_2 is transported within the RBC. To reiterate - in both the plasma and the RBC – all 3 methods of CO_2 transport are employed.

The 10 % of the CO_2 that is transported in the plasma

Of this 10% that is transported in the plasma:

- Method 1: 5% is transported simply as dissolved CO_2. Remember that CO_2 is roughly 22 times more soluble in plasma than oxygen, so it stands to reason that this is why 5% of the CO_2 can be carried as dissolved CO_2 in the plasma.

- Method 2: $< 1\%$ is transported as a carbamino compound. There are protein molecules in the plasma (albumins, globulins, fibrinogen, etc.), but as you can see, very little CO_2 is transported by way of being bound to a plasma protein. Of the CO_2 that is transported as a carbamino compound, most of it occurs within the RBC where it is transported as carbaminohemoglobin.

- Method 3:   5% is transported as ionized bicarbonate. Remember that CO_2 in solution (plasma) reacts with water to form bicarbonate (HCO_3^-).

$$CO_2 + H_2O \leftrightarrow H_2CO_3 \leftrightarrow H^+ + \underline{HCO_3^-}$$

This reaction is what is referred to as the SLOW REACTION. It is considered slow because of the slower rate at which this reaction occurs.   It is slow because the reaction is not catalyzed by an enzyme. In the next section where the other ninety percent of CO_2 is discussed, you'll see that the bicarbonate reaction is a fast reaction because it is catalyzed by an enzyme.

The 90 % of the CO_2 that is transported in the RBC

Of this 90% that is transported in the RBC:

- Method 1: 5% is transported simply as dissolved CO_2. In this instance it is dissolved in the intracellular fluid of the RBC. This is in addition to the 5% that is dissolved in the plasma.

- Method 2: 21% is transported as a carbamino compound. In the RBC, carbon dioxide binds to Hb to form the carbamino compound called carbaminohemoglobin.   Although CO_2 is carried by Hb, it does not compete with O_2 for the iron-binding position in the heme group, but rather it is bound to the protein chains of the Hb molecule.

- Method 3: 63% is transported as ionized bicarbonate (HCO_3). Inside the RBC, CO_2 undergoes the same reaction with water as it did in the plasma.

$$CO_2 + H_2O \leftrightarrow H_2CO_3 \leftrightarrow H^+ + \underline{HCO_3^-}$$

When this reaction occurs inside the RBC, however, it is a FAST REACTION because inside the RBC there is an enzyme called carbonic anhydrase – and carbonic anhydrase catalyzes this reaction such that is proceeds very quickly.

Totals of CO_2 transport according to the method of transport

Method 1. Dissolved in solution

   5%   dissolved in plasma
+ 5%   dissolved in intracellular fluid of RBC
  10%

Method 2. Bound to protein (carbamino compounds)

  < 1% transported as a carbamino compound in plasma
+ 21% transported as carbaminohemoglobin in the RBC
≈ 22%

Method 3. Ionized as bicarbonate (HCO_3-)

  5%   ionized in plasma (SLOW RXN.)
+ 63% ionized in the intracellular fluid of the RBC (FAST RXN.)
  68%

The Hamburger Phenomenon and The Haldane Effect

The Hamburger Phenomenon (the chloride shift)

      With respect to the reaction that occurs in the RBC between CO_2 and H_2O that is catalyzed by carbonic anhydrase (the fast reaction) – note the following:

$$CO_2 + H_2O \leftrightarrow H_2CO_3 \leftrightarrow H^+ + HCO_3^-$$

As this reaction is occurring within the RBC, several things happen:

- Hb buffers the H^+ that is being formed from this reaction – thereby removing the H^+ from solution such that they don't accumulate. *This buffering is occurring as Hb is releasing O_2 to the tissue as deoxygenated Hb acts as a better buffer than oxygenated Hb.*

- The buffering of H+ helps to accelerate the reaction such that HCO_3^- begins to accumulate in the RBC. HCO_3^- accumulates to the point where the concentration of HCO_3^- inside the RBC exceeds the HCO_3- concentration in the plasma. When this happens, HCO_3- moves out of the RBC into the plasma by means of facilitated diffusion through an anion exchanger protein (Cl-HCO_3 exchanger) located in the cell membrane of the RBC.
- When HCO_3- is moved out of the RBC into the plasma, in terms of the balance of charge (remember that HCO_3^- is a negative ion), the inside of the RBC ends up being *positive* with respect to the plasma. It's actually less negative, but being less negative has the same effect as being positive when being considered in terms of the balance across a membrane (the plasma membrane of the RBC in this case which is what separates the inside of the RBC from the plasma.)
- In order to restore the balance of charge between the RBC and the plasma, chloride ion (Cl-) moves from the plasma into the RBC by means of facilitated diffusion through the same anion exchanger protein (Cl-HCO_3 exchanger) located in the cell membrane of the RBC. When Cl- moves into the RBC it compensates for the negative charge that was lost from the HCO_3^- leaving the RBC. In so doing, the movement of Cl- into the RBC restores electrical neutrality.
- This movement of Cl- from the plasma into the RBC is what is known as the chloride shift – also referred to as the Hamburger Phenomenon.

The Haldane Effect

The Haldane Effect essentially describes the effect that oxygen has on carbon dioxide. Blood that is deoxygenated is able to carry more CO_2, whereas oxygenated blood is less able to carry CO_2.

The Haldane Effect describes how the binding of O_2 to hemoglobin promotes the release of CO_2. This therefore describes how oxygen concentrations affect hemoglobin's affinity for carbon dioxide. High oxygen concentrations enhance the unloading of carbon dioxide, but conversely, low oxygen concentrations enhance the uploading of carbon dioxide. In many respects, the Haldane Effect and the Bohr Effect work together to achieve the uptake of O_2 and release of CO_2 in the lungs, and the release of O_2 and uptake of CO_2 in the tissue. The Bohr Effect states that hemoglobin's affinity for O_2 is inversely related to the concentration of carbon dioxide (PCO_2) and thus the acidity. The Bohr effect therefore is describing how CO_2 and H^+ affect the affinity of hemoglobin for oxygen. High CO_2, and thus high H^+ concentrations cause hemoglobin's affinity for oxygen to decrease, whereas low CO_2, and thus low H^+ concentrations cause hemoglobin to have a high affinity for oxygen.

In the environment of the pulmonary capillaries where the concentration of CO_2 and thus H^+ are low (CO_2 is diffusing out of the capillaries into the alveoli), hemoglobin's affinity for oxygen will be high. Realize that the diffusion of O_2 out of the alveoli into the blood and binding to hemoglobin – and the diffusion of CO_2 out of the blood into the alveoli are happening simultaneously. As oxygen diffuses into the pulmonary capillary blood and binds to hemoglobin – that binding of O_2 to Hb promotes the release of CO_2 as oxygenated blood is less able to carry CO_2. This is the Haldane Effect. In the pulmonary capillaries – the decreased CO_2 and H^+ levels promote the loading of O_2 to hemoglobin (Bohr). But then the binding of O_2 to hemoglobin promotes the unloading of CO_2 (Haldane). This is how the Haldane Effect and the Bohr Effect complement one another regarding the uptake of oxygen and the release of carbon dioxide in the lungs.

In the environment of the systemic capillaries, the CO_2 and H^+ concentrations are high (CO_2 is diffusing out of the cells into the capillary blood). The high CO_2 and H^+ causes the local environment to be acidic (low pH). This high CO_2 acidic environment causes hemoglobin to have much less affinity for oxygen and therefore hemoglobin gives up its oxygen to the tissue. This is the Bohr Effect – the inverse relationship between PCO_2 and hemoglobin's affinity for O_2. But in the course of giving up its oxygen, hemoglobin is becoming deoxygenated – and deoxygenated blood is able to carry more carbon dioxide, and this is the Haldane Effect. In the systemic capillaries – the increased CO_2 and H^+ levels decrease hemoglobin's affinity for oxygen and thus promote the unloading of O_2 to the cells (Bohr). But the unloading of oxygen from hemoglobin then causes hemoglobin to become deoxygenated and that promotes the uptake of carbon dioxide (Haldane).

K.   Gas Exchange Abnormalities

Adequate ventilation requires a sufficient enough $\dot{V}_A$ to ensure that enough O_2 is inspired and enough CO_2 is expired to meet the physiological needs of the body. The purpose of ventilation therefore is gas exchange. One must realize, however, that sufficient ventilation does not necessarily guarantee adequate oxygenation.

Hypoxemia (an inadequate level of oxygen in the arterial blood – in other words a lower than normal PaO_2). Hypoxemia is defined as a PaO_2 that is lower than the predicted value for a patient's age.

* PaO_2 normally decreases with age. The expected PaO_2 as a
  function of a patient's age is given as follows:

In supine position: $PaO_2 = 103.5 - (0.42 \times \text{age in years})$

Standing upright: $PaO_2 = 104 - (0.27 \times \text{age in years})$

Hypoxemia can be classified as follows:

Mild: $PaO_2 = 60 - 79$ mmHg. Although at 60 mmHg there would
       still normally be an oxygen saturation of 90%, a PaO_2 of 60 -
       79 mmHg is still considered mild hypoxemia.

Moderate: $PaO_2 = 41 - 59$ mmHg

Severe: $PaO_2 \leq 40$ mmHg

Hypoxemia (lower than normal PaO_2) can be caused by:

1. An inadequate amount of oxygen reaching the alveoli.

    -   Hypoventilation (e.g. – a drug overdose)
        - hypoventilation lowers V_A which lowers PAO_2 which in turn lowers PaO_2.

    -   Tachypnea – rapid, shallow breathing increases deadspace ventilation.   With rapid, shallow breathing, a greater proportion of the V_T is in the anatomical deadspace – hence V_A is diminished which lowers PAO_2 which in turn lowers PaO_2.

    -   Low ambient PO_2 (being at high altitude)
        - remember that the FiO_2 of ambient air is 21% throughout the Earth's atmosphere – even at high altitude. But at high altitude, the P_B is lower. With a lower P_B, PAO_2 will be reduced according to the alveolar air equation – which will result in a lower PaO_2.

        *   Recognize something here: Remember the $P(A - a)O_2$ from section F? The $P(A - a)O_2$ is used to be able to tell how well a patient is oxygenating. It tells you how much of the O_2 in the alveoli is getting into the blood. In this present example of a low PAO_2 due to being at high altitude - the PaO_2 will also be correspondingly lower due to the lower PAO_2, but the $P(A - a)O_2$ will still be normal because in the absence of any diffusion defects, the oxygen that is in the alveoli will still make it into the arterial blood – so the (A – a) difference will remain normal. Be conscientious that a "normal" $P(A – a)O_2$ in a situation like this is not reflective of adequate oxygenation.

        *   The same thing applies in the case of hypoventilation. With hypoventilation, V_A is lowered. PAO_2 is lowered not only because of a reduced V_A in and of itself, but with a reduced V_A, PAO_2 will be reduced because of an increase in $PACO_2$. PAO_2 and $PACO_2$ are inversely related. CO_2 is still

continuously diffusing out of the capillaries into the alveoli
– if V_A is not adequate enough to remove that CO_2, then the
$PACO_2$ is going to increase and the PAO_2 will thus decrease.
But the $P(A - a)O_2$ difference will still appear normal in this
case because in the absence of any diffusion defects, whatever
oxygen is in the alveoli will still make it into the blood and
thus the $P(A - a)O_2$ will appear to be normal. So also be
conscientious that a "normal" $P(A - a)O_2$ in a situation like
this is not reflective of adequate oxygenation.

2. An inadequate amount of oxygen crossing the A/C membrane.

- Impaired diffusion (diffusion defect)
  - disorders of the A/C membrane
    - e.g. pulmonary fibrosis
    - e.g. pulmonary edema

3. V/Q imbalances (dead space ventilation and/or shunting)

- *The #1 cause of hypoxemia in patients with pulmonary
  disease is V/Q mismatching.*

  - Lower V/Q ratios tend towards shunting. Pulmonary
    shunting is attributed to alveoli with a V/Q < 1.

  - Higher V/Q ratios tend towards dead space. Alveolar
    dead space is attributed to alveoli with a V/Q > 1.

* Whether it is a low V/Q where you have perfusion but yet inadequate
ventilation (shunting), or a high V/Q where you have ventilation but
yet inadequate perfusion (dead space ventilation) – in either case you
end up with inadequate gas exchange with diminished oxygenation
and thus hypoxemia.

50/50 Rule

Although not as specific as calculating the $P(A - a)O_2$ - if you want to know if a patient's hypoxemia is from a V/Q imbalance or a physiological shunt – apply the 50/50 rule.

If the FiO_2 > 50% AND the PaO_2 < 50 mmHg

Then the patient has remarkable shunting occurring

if not, the hypoxemia is predominantly due to V/Q mismatching.

4. Hemoglobin deficiencies

- Absolute Hb deficiency
  - [Hb] lower than normal

- Relative Hb deficiency
  - oxygen displacement from normal hemoglobin
  - presence of pathological Hb variants
    - pathological variants of hemoglobin will result in a variety of hemoglobinopathies that will interfere with Hb's ability to properly load and unload oxygen.

Hypoxia (an inadequate amount of oxygen at the tissue level)

Adequate amounts of oxygen at the tissue level depend upon adequate oxygen delivery (DO_2), which is the product of CaO_2 and cardiac output ($\dot{Q}_t$).

Oxygen delivery (DO_2) = CaO_2 x $\dot{Q}_t$

$$\dot{D}O_2 = \underbrace{CaO_2}_{\text{dissolved } O_2 \mid \text{bound } O_2} \quad x \quad \dot{Q}_t$$

$$\dot{D}O_2 = [(0.003 \text{ x } PaO_2) + (Hb \text{ x } 1.34 \text{ x } SaO_2)] \quad x \quad \dot{Q}_t$$

Normal $\dot{DO_2}$

$\dot{DO_2}$ = [(0.003 x 100) + (15 x 1.34 x .97)]   x   5 L/min

    = (0.3ml/dl + 19.5ml/dl)   x   5L/min

    = *19.8ml/dl x 5 L/min   *you have to multiply 19.8 ml/dl by 10 to get it expressed as ml/L

    = *198ml/L x 5 L/min = 990 ml/min, or $\approx$ 1 LPM.

If $\dot{DO_2}$ is not adequate, which means that either CaO_2 or Q_t (or both) are not adequate, then gas exchange will not be adequate at the tissue level and hypoxia will ensue.

Hypoxia can also be caused by:

1. Any of the issues that cause hypoxemia

2. Reduction in blood flow (shock, ischemia)

3. Dysoxia – Dysoxia, also known as histotoxic hypoxia or hypoxidosis, is a condition when the cells are unable to take up and use oxygen. When Dysoxia occurs, PaO_2, CaO_2, SaO_2, and O_2 transport are all normal. What is abnormal is that the PvO_2 of the blood returning to the heart is essentially the same as what the PaO_2 was – in other words, the cells didn't take any oxygen – the $C(a - v)O_2$ is drastically decreased (essentially zero). The classic illustration of Dysoxia is cyanide poisoning. Cyanide binds to and inhibits mitochondrial cytochrome c oxidase. This prevents the binding of O_2 and thus prevents the cells from being able to make ATP aerobically.

Chapter 4

Selected Topics in Physical Assessment

The ability to competently examine a patient so as to be able to render a proper diagnosis is largely a matter of clinical experience. It takes time to develop these skills and to acquire the clinical judgement necessary to interpret your findings. You will begin your acquisition of these skills when you enter into your clinical rotations. Even though it is through experience that you solidify your knowledge and skills, you need to have a solid academic understanding of the basics before you enter into your rotations. You are probably already starting to realize that there are many factors that go into figuring out what is wrong with a patient and how to treat them. The physical examination is a big part of that process. There are all sorts of lab tests and blood tests and ABG's and x-rays, etc. that play a role in determining the medical condition of a patient by providing you with data, but the physical examination is unique in that it requires your skillset to be able to discern what is going on. Data derived from tests is absolutely valuable and essential, but make no mistake about the fact that your ability to examine and observe your patient with complete understanding about what is going on is of a level of importance that is second to none. Learn well and hone your skills so as to become an excellent diagnostician and you will have served your patients well.

Performing a proper physical assessment requires that you have the requisite knowledge of the various cardiopulmonary symptoms that you will encounter, and have memorized the appropriate sequence of steps that guide you through the process of examining a patient in order to be able to properly assess the various parts of the body that are relevant to your practice as a respiratory therapist. Insofar as much of that is simply a matter of memorizing factual information, the focus of this chapter will be to address only a limited number of particular areas of physical assessment that warrant further consideration and/or clarity.

Assessing and examining a patient is a combination of talking to them (provided that they are able to converse with you), and then actually examining them. The talking part is what is known as the interview. When it is possible, you should review the patient's chart and their medical history before you interview them. This will enable you to have a good base of understanding from which you can proceed in your evaluation. The actual examination itself consists of four parts as follows:

1) Inspection   2) Palpation   3) Percussion   4) Auscultation

Textbooks like to present the interview and examination of a patient as a sequence of events that follows a fairly outlined format, and that may be well and good so as to give you structure as you are learning, but the plain fact is that many of these events are happening simultaneously, and in real life clinical practice you are not going to be dealing with your patients according to a prescribed outline whereby you do one thing after the next in sequence. You have to learn to be able to multi-task. Obviously if your patient is awake and orientated and can talk to you, then the first thing you'll be doing is interviewing them, and that interview will be enhanced by the fact that you will have already read their chart first so that you have a good background as to what is going on. But while you are interviewing them you will also be doing an inspection. That means that while you are asking them questions you are also checking their appearance, color, and sensorium. You'll also use this time to check their respiratory rate. Do you see that while you were talking with them you also figured out their LOC and got part of their vitals (their respiratory rate)? As you continue the interview process and discuss their symptoms and their medical and family history, you may also be simultaneously taking their pulse (palpation), performing diagnostic chest percussion (percussion), and/or taking their temperature. Hopefully you are beginning to realize that all of the various components of interviewing and examining a patient are occurring within a fluid dynamic. The only time that you probably would not be talking to them is when you are performing auscultation of the lungs, heart, or blood pressure because when you are auscultating you need to be paying attention to the sounds you are hearing. So yes – learn and remember all the various elements that pertain to the proper interviewing and examination of a patient, but realize that it is occurring within the context of a fluid dynamic because in actual clinical practice there is no such thing as a perfect world. What is important is that you know *what* you are supposed to be asking them and *what* you are supposed to be assessing – and to accomplish that in a timely and orderly fashion within the dynamics of a clinical environment that is not always going to be conducive to allowing you to follow a textbook outline format.

A. The Medical History

Respiratory therapists must be familiar with the medical history of their patients.

1) Begin in the chart with current problems

    A. What is the chief complaint?

    B. History of the present illness.

2) Review the past medical history

    A. Previous illnesses
    B. Previous injuries
    C. Previous surgeries
    D. Known allergies
    E. Rx medications and/or OTC drugs being taken
    F. Smoking history
       - Assessment of pulmonary health requires an accurate assessment of the patient's smoking history.
       - You need to obtain the number of pack years of smoking history.
       - (# packs/day x # years = # pack years).

3) Review the family and social/environmental history.

- Look for possible genetic or occupational links that could be related to the patient's illness.

  * cystic fibrosis
  * COPD (α-1)
  * inhalation exposures

4) Review of systems/labs/imaging/etc.

- Review all relevant findings.

  - previous and/or current physician's notes
  - progress notes
  - findings of previous and/or current examinations
  - results of blood work, ABG's, x-rays, PFT's, etc.

5) Check for any advance directives – DNR, DNI

- Be certain of any limits to the extent of care that is to be given in the event of a cardiac or respiratory arrest.

B. Cardiopulmonary Symptoms

DYSPNEA

Most patients don't know the word dyspnea so the way they will describe what is going on is by saying they have shortness of breath (SOB) or breathlessness. What you need to understand from a physiological standpoint regardless of whether it is being called dyspnea, shortness of breath, or breathlessness - is that their WOB (work of breathing) has increased either from either a reduction in lung compliance and/or increased airway resistance, or a decrease in respiratory muscle strength. It could be from any one or all three of these things. Feeling short of breath is normal during vigorous exercise, but this is not how you are usually going to see it presented. Having shortness of breath can be brought on when a patient is hypercapnic (and therefore acidotic), or hypoxemic – and this is how you will usually see it - so when you encounter a patient experiencing shortness of breath – get an ABG and check to see if they are either hypercapnic or hypoxemic.

Positional Dyspnea

Orthopnea – This is dyspnea that occurs when a patient assumes a reclining or supine position. It is usually relieved by sitting up. When orthopnea occurs at night, generally when the patient is sleeping, it is known as paroxysmal nocturnal dyspnea. Paroxysmal nocturnal dyspnea is usually not relieved by sitting up.

- Orthopnea is often associated with CHF (congestive heart failure).
- Orthopnea can occur with bilateral diaphragmatic paralysis.

Platypnea – This is dyspnea that occurs when the patient is in the upright position. It is relieved by laying down. Platypnea is often accompanied by orthodeoxia. Orthodeoxia is when the oxygen saturation (SpO_2) drops when the patient is in the upright position. Orthodeoxia also is usually relieved by laying down. The combination of both platypnea and orthodeoxia is known as platypnea-orthodeoxia syndrome and it is considered rare.

- Platypnea is usually caused by either hepatopulmonary syndrome or when a patient has cardiac issues that increase right to left shunting.

Dyspnea on exertion (DOE)

This is just as it says – the dyspnea is occurring as a result of the patient exerting themselves. Exertion in this case does not mean vigorous exercise – it could be as simple as just walking across the room or going up a flight of steps. DOE is seen in patients with CHF and/or severe pulmonary disease.

COUGH

Type of cough:	What it is often related to:
non-productive (no sputum)	bronchospasm, viral illness, allergies, asthma
productive (with sputum)	acute infections, inflammation, viral illness, COPD
Acute (sudden onset)	upper airway infection
Chronic (> 8 weeks)	chronic bronchitis, asthma infections, ACE inhibitors

Sputum Terminology

Sputum – mucus that has passed through the mouth. It has been contaminated by the oral secretions in the mouth.

Phlegm – mucus that has not passed through the mouth, and therefore is *not contaminated* with oral secretions.

Purulent – sputum that contains pus. It is thick, colored   (green/ yellow), sticky, and suggestive of an infection.

Fetid – fetid sputum is sputum that is foul smelling – often seen with bronchiectasis and infections

Mucoid – mucoid sputum is clear and thick. It is often associated asthma and bronchitis.

CHEST PAIN

With chest pain, the first thing you want to determine is whether it is cardiac or non-cardiac in origin. Once you determine that, then you will want to determine if it is pleuritic or non-pleuritic. If the chest pain is cardiac in origin, then it will also be non-pleuritic. If the chest pain is not cardiac in origin, then it could be either pleuritic or non-pleuritic.

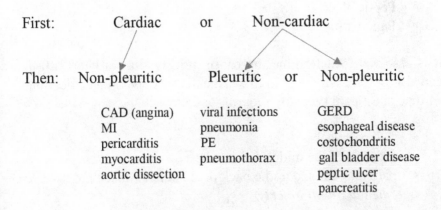

First: Cardiac   or   Non-cardiac

Then: Non-pleuritic   Pleuritic   or   Non-pleuritic

CAD (angina)	viral infections	GERD
MI	pneumonia	esophageal disease
pericarditis	PE	costochondritis
myocarditis	pneumothorax	gall bladder disease
aortic dissection		peptic ulcer
		pancreatitis

Some of the most serious problems associated with chest pain are an acute MI (myocardial infarction), PE, aortic dissection (a tear in the wall of the aorta), or a pneumothorax. You need to evaluate the patient's chest pain in combination with their other signs and symptoms in order to determine the cause.

Non-Pleuritic Chest Pain (cardiac)

The most common example of non-pleuritic cardiac chest pain is angina. Angina is the uncomfortable sensation of pressure in the chest upon exertion that is secondary to CAD (coronary artery disease - occlusion of the coronary arteries). The occlusion of the coronary arteries causes ischemia which the patient then feels as the non-pleuritic chest pain known as angina pectoris. This pain is therefore cardiac in nature as it pertains to the heart itself, and it is non-pleuritic because it does not involve the pleura.

Non-Pleuritic Chest Pain (non-cardiac)

Non-pleuritic chest pain can also be non-cardiac in nature when it is caused by:

- GERD
- Esophageal disease
- Costochondritis
- Gall bladder disease
- Peptic ulcer
- Pancreatitis

It is essential to determine the cause quickly since a heart attack can also present with pain in this same manner. Non-pleuritic, non-cardiac chest pain typically presents as follows:

- dull pain, ache
- presents in the middle of the chest
- pain may radiate to the back or shoulders *(hence the need to rule out an MI quickly)*
- unaffected by breathing

Pleuritic Chest Pain (non – cardiac)

Pleuritic chest pain can only be non-cardiac in nature. There is no heart involvement in pleuritic chest pain. Pleuritic chest pain is associated with conditions of inflammation of the pleural lining of the lung (particularly the parietal pleura). Pleuritic chest pain presents as follows:

- sharp pain
- presents laterally or posteriorly
- made worse with deep breathing and/or coughing

Pleuritic chest pain is often seen with viral infections as well as pneumonia, PE, and pneumothorax.

FEVER

Fever, also known as pyrexia, is an elevation in body temperature in response to a pathogen or disease. Fever is induced by substances known as pyrogens, which are either endogenous (from inside the body – e.g. immunological disease, etc.), or exogenous (from outside the body – e.g. infectious disease). Regardless of whether the pyrogen is from an exogenous or endogenous source, they act to increase the body's thermoregulatory set point in the hypothalamus. Endogenous pyrogens inherently exist as cytokines whereas exogenous pyrogens do not. But exogenous pyrogens undergo some cellular interactions that result in the release of cytokines. Cytokines then activate the arachidonic acid pathway which in turn causes the production and release of PGE2 (prostaglandin E2). It is PGE2 that acts on the hypothalamus to raise the set point, and this results in the systemic response of generating heat to raise the temperature to the new set point. In this respect the hypothalamus is functioning as a thermostat, but PGE2 is the ultimate regulator of the fever response. The set point will remain elevated until the levels of PGE2 go back down, and this in turn is dependent upon the causative factors being resolved.

Classifications of fever

Remittent (most infections) – fever varies around 2° per day but doesn't return to normal.

Intermittent – fever with wide swings in temperature with profuse night sweats (common with sepsis).

Sustained – fever with continuous elevation with little fluctuation.

Relapsing – bouts of fever interspersed with afebrile periods.

PEDAL EDEMA

Pitting edema – when you press on the skin and it leaves an indentation.

Weeping edema – edema that is so bad that the fluid literally seeps out of the skin.

Patients with COPD are very susceptible to right sided heart failure, and this results in edema. Although COPD means chronic obstructive pulmonary disease - it still results in chronic hypoxemia which in turn often leads to pulmonary vasoconstriction that results in pulmonary hypertension. This places increased stress on the right ventricle. In response to the increased resistance and pressure in the pulmonary circulation, the right ventricle enlarges over time so as to be able to meet the demand of being able to pump against this increased resistance and pressure. Eventually the right ventricle will not be able to keep up with this increased demand and it will start to fail. This right sided heart failure that is being caused by the increased resistance of the pulmonary circulation due to chronic hypoxemia is called *cor pulmonale*. With right sided heart failure, blood begins to back up in the systemic circulation, and it will result in pedal edema.

The presence of pedal edema should always prompt you to find out if the patient already has diagnosed heart failure. If they do not, then obviously they need further evaluation to determine the nature and extent of the cardiopulmonary issues that are causing the edema.

* The height of the edema up the leg above the ankle is suggestive of the extent of the heart failure – the higher the edema, the more severe the heart failure.

C. The Physical Examination

LOC (level of consciousness)

A conscious patient should be assessed for their orientation to the following:

1) Time (& date)
2) Place
3) Person
4) Situation

> evaluating the sensorium

Appropriate responses to the questions above indicate that the patient is orientated x 4.

If the patient is not awake and alert, then assess the LOC as follows:

There are 6 levels of impaired consciousness

1) Confused – disorientated, slow responses/slow thinking, unable to respond quickly to the questions regarding being orientated x 4

2) Delirious – restless, highly agitated, disorientated, illogical thinking

3) Lethargic – excessive drowsiness, may not respond to stimulus at all, or response may be disorganized or incoherent

4) Obtunded – very sleepy, diminished alertness, very slow responses

5) Stuporous – lowest level of consciousness just before coma, virtually no response to stimuli except pain,

6) Comatose – not arousable, unconscious, no gag or corneal reflex

<u>Two rating scales are used to assess a consciousness deficit:</u>

1) AVPU (In the field, this is assessed every few minutes)

Alert – orientated x 4
Verbal – awakens or responds to verbal stimuli, follows simple
          commands
Pain – responds to pain
Unresponsive – no response to pain or verbal stimuli

2) Glasgow Coma Scale

GCS uses a point scale for three areas:

- spontaneous eye opening   scored from 1 – 4
- verbal response   scored from 1 – 5
- motor response   scored from 1 – 6

The *total* GCS is the sum of the three individual scores. From a respiratory therapy perspective, total GCS means the following:

- GCS 13 – 15   low risk of airway compromise
- GCS 9 – 12   moderate risk of airway compromise
- GCS 3 – 8   high risk of airway compromise

* A total GCS < 8 is indicative that the patient my need urgent airway support (intubation).

Observable postural deficits and what *they indicate*:

When observing the patient to see if they are exhibiting either decorticate or decerebrate posturing, they are in the supine position.

Decorticate posturing

- *Damage to the corticospinal tract*
- Body is rigid
- Arms are flexed with hands on the chest

Decerebrate posturing

- *Severe brain (upper brainstem) injury*
- Body is rigid
- Rigid extension of arms & legs
- Arms are flat along the body

Pulsus Paradoxus

Pulsus paradoxus is when you have a significant (> 10mmHg) decrease in pulse pressure during spontaneous inspiration. Pulse pressure is (systolic BP – diastolic BP). During spontaneous inspiration, the thoracic pressure drops resulting in negative intrathoracic pressure with respect to the outside of the body. This is normal and is part of the normal mechanics of how a breath is inspired. When the pressure in the thorax becomes negative with respect to the outside – two things happen:

1) Temporary pooling of blood in the pulmonary circulation which then impedes the filling of the left side of the heart.

2) Temporary increased venous return to the right side of the heart which increases right ventricular volume and pressure that limits expansion of the left heart during diastole.

Now – these events (1 & 2) briefly reduce left ventricular stroke volume and decrease systolic blood pressure during inspiration, BUT not usually to the point where it would cause pulsus paradoxus. In other words – in a normal patient, when you auscultate the heart, the beats you hear should correlate with the beats you palpate at the radial pulse. The "paradox" is when you are auscultating the heart and you are able to hear beats that you are NOT able to palpate at the radial pulse. The reason why you can auscultate the beats but not palpate them at the radial pulse is because there has been a larger than normal drop in systolic blood pressure. You can hear the beats with your stethoscope, but the systolic pressure has dropped enough such that you're not able to palpate them. There are several reasons that can cause pulsus paradoxus, and because of the seriousness of some of them, it is very important to determine the cause.

Respiratory related reasons that can cause pulsus paradoxus:

- COPD
- Asthma
- Tension pneumothorax
- PE

Hypovolemia, an obstruction in the superior vena cava, and certain cardiac issues can also cause pulsus paradoxus - so if you have this as a finding upon examination you need to inform the physician right away and determine the cause.

Postural Hypotension

Postural hypotension, also known as *orthostatic hypotension,* is when there is an abrupt drop in blood pressure when the patient has either been sitting or lying down and then assumes the upright position (standing). In order to qualify as being postural or orthostatic hypotension, there should be a drop in the systolic blood pressure of at least 20 mm Hg or a drop in the diastolic blood pressure of at least 10 mm Hg when the patient assumes the upright position.

When a patient stands up after having been lying down, there is pooling of blood in the lower extremities due to gravity which will lead to less venous return to the heart which will then lead to reduced cardiac output and lowered blood pressure. But this drop in blood pressure is usually not significant because the body immediately responds with vasoconstriction in order to maintain an adequate amount of blood flow to the heart. When you do see a significant drop in blood pressure as in the case with postural hypotension, it is because there is a secondary issue going on that is preventing the body's normal vasoconstriction response from being able to quickly restore blood pressure to normal. Although there could be a couple of things causing this, hypovolemia (low blood volume) is often the issue. With hypovolemia, you'll not only end up with postural hypotension, but the reduced cardiac output from the hypovolemia will also lead to a reduction in cerebral blood flow which can then result in syncope.

EXAMINING THE HEAD & NECK

Cyanosis

- Cyanosis is the bluish discoloration of the skin and/or mucous membranes that results from having low oxygen saturation in the tissues near the skin.
- Cyanosis occurs when the amount of unsaturated (or deoxygenated) Hb in the capillary beds > 5 g/dl.
  - normal is 2.5 g/dl.
- Central cyanosis – bluish discoloration around the lips and tongue – indicative of a respiratory (ventilatory) or cardiac problem.
- Peripheral cyanosis – bluish discoloration seen in the extremities and fingers – indicative of a circulation problem.
- Cyanosis implies arterial hypoxemia, however it is not a perfectly reliable sign due to variations in skin tone.

Inspect and palpate the neck for:

1) Tracheal shift – a tracheal shift occurs as a result of a difference in pressure – and the trachea will shift (move) away from an area of high pressure and towards an area of lower pressure.

- The trachea will shift TOWARDS an area of lower pressure – i.e. a collapsed lung (atelectasis).
- The trachea will shift AWAY from areas with increased pressure – i.e. increased pressure from air – pneumothorax, or increased pressure from fluid - pleural effusion).

2) JVD (jugular venous distension) – assess the internal jugular for JVD as this is indicative of the volume and pressure in the right heart.

- In the supine position, the internal jugular should be normally distended.

- When the patient is placed in semi-Fowler's (45°), the blood column should only be 3 – 4 cm above the sternal angle, but when there is increased pressure in the right heart the column could be as high as the angle of the jaw.

  - Chronic hypoxemia will cause pulmonary vasoconstriction and hypertension which then increases the pressure in the right heart. This increased pressure in the right heart makes venous return to the right heart more difficult and you observe this difficulty by the presence of JVD. JVD is simply blood backing up in the internal jugular because of it being more difficult to enter the heart because of the increased pressure in the right heart.

JVD and breathing

- JVD should decrease (descend) during spontaneous inspiration. Remember that the overall pressure in the thorax decreases during inspiration so you should see the JVD descend.

- JVD should increase (ascend) during exhalation because during exhalation the pressure in the thorax is higher.

Therefore: Always assess JVD at the *end* of exhalation.

If JVD increases during inspiration – this is abnormal and rare. If this happens, it is a known as a Kussmaul's Sign and can be indicative of cardiac tamponade, a large pericardial effusion, or impairment of the pumping ability of the heart.

EXAMINING THE THORAX & LUNGS

Inspection

Thoracic configuration – normal thoracic configuration is when the AP diameter < transverse diameter.

- AP diameter increases in COPD patient's due to the hyperinflation of their lungs that is characteristic of their disease.

Other thoracic abnormalities to note:

- Pectus Carinatum - protrusion of the sternum
- Pectus Excavatum – depression of the sternum
- Scoliosis – abnormal lateral curvature of the spine
- Kyphosis – abnormal AP curvature of the spine
- Kyphoscoliosis – a combination of kyphosis & scoliosis

Pectus Excavatum and Kyphoscoliosis can restrict the expansion of the thorax and thus limit lung inflation.

Abnormal breathing patterns

1. Type: rapid & shallow
   Cause: restrictive issues – diseases/conditions that cause a
              loss of lung volume and/or increase lung stiffness.
   Examples: pulmonary edema, severe pneumonia, atelectasis,
              pulmonary fibrosis, ARDS

2. Type: relatively brief inspiration with abnormally
              prolonged exhalation – the I:E can go from 1:3 to
              1:4 or more
   Cause: obstructive issues – diseases/conditions that cause
              the airways to narrow
   Examples: asthma, bronchitis, COPD

3. Type: rapid and deep (Kussmaul's)
   Cause: metabolic disorders
   Examples: diabetic ketoacidosis

4. Type: prolonged inspiratory phase
   Cause: obstruction or narrowing of the upper airway
   Examples: epiglottitis, croup

Other abnormal breathing patterns

*Apneustic breathing: deep gasping inspiration with a pause after
inspiration followed by a brief and incomplete exhalation. Indicative
of brain damage, hypoglycemic coma, or severe hypoxia.

*Ataxic breathing: a completely irregular pattern with irregular
periods of apnea. Indicative of brain damage.

*Biot's breathing: characterized by groups of rapid and shallow
breathing followed by regular or irregular periods of apnea. Also
indicative of brain damage.

*Cheyne-Stokes: characterized by an increase in rate & depth, then
a decrease in rate & depth – then apnea. Seen with brain damage,
CHF, and encephalopathy.

*Paradoxical breathing:

  *Abdominal paradox: characterized by observation of the abdomen going inward during inspiration and going outward during exhalation. Seen in diaphragmatic fatigue or diaphragmatic paralysis.

  *Chest paradox: characterized by observation of the chest going inward during inspiration and going outward during exhalation. Seen in chest trauma and rib fractures.

*Periodic breathing: fluctuation between rapid & deep to slow & shallow without any periods of apnea. Also seen with brain damage.

Respiration (rate, depth, & rhythm)

* Eupnea: normal tidal breathing

* Apnea: cessation of breathing

* Bradypnea: rate < 10, normal depth, normal rhythm

* Tachypnea: rate > 20, normal depth, normal rhythm

* Hypoventilation: slow rate & depth, does not meet metabolic demands – results in increased $PaCO_2$ and decreased pH (acidosis).

* Hyperventilation: fast rate & depth, exceeds metabolic demands – results in decreased $PaCO_2$ and increased pH (alkalosis).

Palpation – palpation is used to assess and evaluate:

- vocal fremitus
- expansion of the thorax
- skin and subcutaneous tissue of the thorax

1) Vocal/Tactile fremitus

Vocal fremitus describes the vibrations generated by the vocal cords while speaking. Those vibrations travel down through the lungs and can be palpated on the chest wall where they are called tactile fremitus.

To assess for fremitus, have the patient repeat the word "blue balloons" or "99" while you are palpating the thorax. Palpate the anterior, posterior, and lateral thorax with the palmar aspect of your fingers.

Increased fremitus intensity – indicative of increased lung density - noted when there is lung consolidation (pneumonia)

Decreased fremitus intensity - noted when there is fluid or air in the pleural space (pleural effusion, pneumothorax), or with decreased lung density as seen with hyperinflation (emphysema).

2) Estimation of thoracic expansion

Place your hands on the patient's chest. On the anterior chest, place your thumbs at the xiphoid process. For the posterior chest, place your thumbs at T8. In each instance have the patient inhale. When the patient inhales, each thumb should move equally about 3 – 5 cm.

Symmetrical reductions in chest expansion may be noted with:

- Diseases affecting the respiratory muscles
- COPD.
  - With COPD, the FRC is already very high and doesn't allow for much more chest expansion.

Asymmetrical reductions in chest expansion may be noted with:

- atelectasis
- pneumothorax
- pleural effusions

3) Assessment of skin and subcutaneous tissue

Subcutaneous emphysema – SE is the presence of air or gas inside the subcutaneous tissue. It presents as small air bubbles on the surface of the skin that result from gas leaking out of the lungs into the subcutaneous tissue. It will usually present on the chest, face, or neck. Palpation of these air bubbles produces a crackling sound known as subcutaneous crepitation (crepitus). This sound is similar to what one would hear when squeezing bubble wrap. SE can arise from anything that would cause a puncture of the lung, so it could be indicative of a pneumothorax. If a patient is on mechanical ventilation, SE can be an indication of excessive airway pressures that are causing barotrauma.

Percussion

General clinical implications of percussion

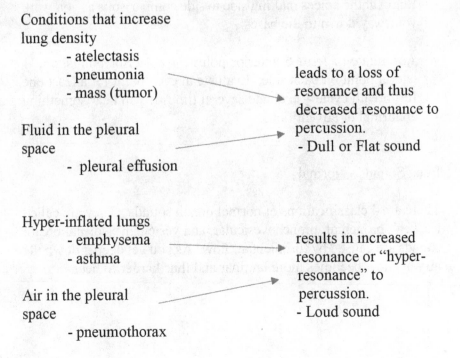

Conditions that increase
lung density
    - atelectasis
    - pneumonia
    - mass (tumor)

leads to a loss of resonance and thus decreased resonance to percussion.
- Dull or Flat sound

Fluid in the pleural
space
    - pleural effusion

Hyper-inflated lungs
    - emphysema
    - asthma

results in increased resonance or "hyper-resonance" to percussion.
- Loud sound

Air in the pleural
space
    - pneumothorax

- Percussion is limited in its diagnostic usefulness. Lesions smaller than 4 - 5cm are hard to detect, and lesions too deep (> 7cm) are hard to detect.

- Percussion is useful when considered along with other findings.

- Percussion however does enable rapid bedside assessment of abnormalities that may aid in the decision to order a chest x-ray.

Auscultation

Auscultation of the lungs *should* be done with the patient relaxed and sitting upright. Instruct the patient to take a deep breath through their mouth. Auscultation should be systematic and thorough as follows:

- Begin at the apices making side to side comparisons as you work your way down to the bases.

- Auscultate *at least* 6 anterior points, 4 posterior points, and 1 lateral point on each side. Evaluate at each point for a least one full breath cycle – evaluate several times if you hear something abnormal or adventitious.

Lung Sounds - Normal

There are 4 classifications of normal breath sounds. They are called tracheal, bronchial, bronchovesicular, and vesicular. Normal breath sounds are caused by turbulent air flow. As you get deeper down the airway, flow becomes more laminar and thus harder to hear.

1. *Tracheal* – These are the highest pitched and loudest of the breath sounds. These sounds are heard over the trachea. They are harsh sounds that sound like air being blown through a pipe. The I:E ratio for this sound is usually 1:1.

2. *Bronchial* – These sounds are also high pitched and loud, but not as harsh as tracheal sounds. These sounds are heard over the large airways of the anterior chest near the 2nd and 3rd intercostal spaces. Bronchial sounds have a short pause between inspiration and expiration and the expiratory sounds are longer than the inspiratory sounds – The I:E ratio for this sound is around 1:1.25.

3. *Bronchovesicular* – These sounds are moderate pitched with moderate intensity. They are softer than bronchial sounds and have a tubular quality. These sounds are heard over the posterior chest between the scapulae, and the center of the anterior chest. Differences in pitch and/or intensity are usually more easily detected during expiration. The I:E ratio for this sound is usually 1:1.

4. *Vesicular* – These sounds are the lowest pitched with soft intensity. These soft rustling sounds are heard throughout most lung fields. They are normally heard throughout inspiration. They continue without pause into expiration. The I:E ratio for this sound is around 1:0.25.

Lung sounds – abnormal

An abnormal breath sound is when you hear a normal breath sound in a location where it is not supposed to be heard. An example of this would be when you hear bronchial or bronchovesicular sounds over the peripheral chest. You would expect to hear vesicular sounds over the peripheral chest. This abnormal finding is indicative of lung consolidation. Lung consolidation is when you have fluid in the alveoli rather than air – hence lung density becomes increased.

Disease processes that increase the density of lung tissue will decrease the sound filtering properties of the lung. Therefore, when you have increased lung density due to disease, more sound will be transmitted to the lung periphery and you will hear more high pitched, high amplitude sounds – and this is NOT normal.

Sounds with abnormal I:E ratios that are often auscultated in COPD patients could be said to be "abnormal". Diminished or absent breath sounds could also be said to be abnormal. Slow or shallow breathing will result in less turbulent air flow which you will note as "diminished". Breath sounds can also be diminished if the airway is clogged with mucus, or hyperinflated from COPD, or from a pneumothorax.

Lung sounds – adventitious

Whereas abnormal breath sounds are when a normal breath sound is heard in the wrong place, adventitious breath sounds are completely different sounds. They are additional sounds or vibrations that will be auscultated in the presence of a variety of conditions. Being able to accurately discern adventitious breath sounds is key to being able to diagnose a variety of lung conditions.

Adventitious breath sounds are classified broadly as being either continuous or discontinuous. The terms continuous or discontinuous have nothing to do with the duration of the sound. Those terms refer to the frequency range of the sound. Continuous sounds are of a narrower frequency range and they sound more musical. Discontinuous sounds have a broader frequency range and they sound more like noise.

Discontinuous Adventitious Sounds

1. Crackles (you will also hear crackles referred to as *Rales*)

   - Crackles are intermittent, crackling, bubbling sounds that can be auscultated during both inspiration and expiration. Early inspiratory and expiratory crackles are characteristic of chronic bronchitis. Early inspiratory crackles are indicative of severe airway obstruction because the sound you are hearing is the re-opening of the larger proximal bronchi that closed during the previous exhalation. Late inspiratory crackles can be indicative of pneumonia, CHF, or atelectasis.

1A. Fine Crackles

- Fine crackles occur as a result of the sudden opening of collapsed peripheral airways.
- They are a faint, high-pitched sound that resembles cellophane being crumpled in your hand.
- Late inspiratory fine crackles are indicative of restrictive disease or atelectasis.

1B. Coarse Crackles

- Coarse crackles are heard as a result of airflow moving secretions or fluid in the airway – i.e. there are excessive secretions.
- They are more pronounced and louder than fine crackles. They are a clear, popping, bubbling sound that resembles the rolling of your hair between your fingers next to your ear.
- They often clear after coughing or suctioning.

Continuous Adventitious Sounds

1. Wheezes (you may still hear the low pitch wheeze referred to as Rhonchi)
   - A wheeze is high velocity airflow through a narrow airway. It can be due to bronchospasm, airway edema, tumors and/ or foreign bodies, or pulmonary edema.
   - Wheezes can be either low pitched or high pitched. Low pitched wheezes (sometimes still called Rhonchi) sound like a moan whereas high pitched wheezes sound like a squeak.
   - The proportion of the respiratory cycle occupied by the wheeze varies directly with the degree of airway obstruction.
   - Low pitched wheezes can be heard during both inspiration and expiration. They are heard over the chest wall where the bronchi are located – they are not heard over the periphery. Low pitched wheezes often clear after coughing.

- Wheezes can be further classified as being either monophonic or polyphonic.

    Monophonic Wheeze
    - The wheezing is occurring in a *single airway*.
    - Can be heard during inspiration and/or expiration.
    - Monophonic wheezing is usually NOT indicative of asthma.

    Polyphonic Wheeze
    - The wheezing is occurring in *multiple airways*.
    - Only heard on exhalation.
    - Indicative of asthma, bronchitis, CHF, and pulmonary edema.

2. Stridor

- Stridor is a high pitched monophonic sound that is auscultated over the trachea and/or the larynx. In most cases you won't even need to auscultate because you will hear it plainly as it is that loud. It can be heard during inspiration or expiration, although it is usually during inspiration. Stridor is often heard in infants and small children with croup or epiglottitis, and it can also occur after a patient has been extubated after having been on mechanical ventilation for an extended period of time. Stridor indicates severe airway compromise and it is a medical emergency that needs to be treated immediately as maintaining patency of the airway is of the utmost priority.

Vocal resonance

Assessing vocal resonance is done the same way as assessing for fremitus except that you use a stethoscope to auscultate the sound rather than using your fingers to palpate the sound.

Increased vocal resonance – this is known as *bronchophony*. Increased vocal resonance is indicative of lung consolidation (increased lung density).

Decreased vocal resonance – is indicative of hyperinflation (decreased lung density).

As you are assessing your patient through the various techniques of inspection, palpation, percussion, and auscultation, the way you will know that your findings are correct is if they are consistent with each other. In other words, what you find through one method should be consistent with what you find with the other methods. The findings of the four different techniques of assessment (inspection, palpation, percussion, auscultation) should corroborate with one another so as to give credence to your findings. The more positive corroboration you have between your various assessment techniques, the more certainty you will have in the correctness of your findings.

Example 1:

- Palpation reveals increased vocal/tactile fremitus.
- Percussion reveals dull or flat sound.
- Auscultation reveals bronchial breath sounds over the lung periphery.
- Auscultation also reveals increased vocal resonance (bronchophony).

These findings are all consistent with one another in indicating that there is an issue with consolidation and/or increased lung density. In terms of making a diagnosis, the consistency of these findings enables you to narrow your focus to issues you know that cause lung consolidation and/or increased lung density such as pneumonia, atelectasis, pulmonary edema, tumors, etc.

Example 2:

- Palpation reveals decreased vocal/tactile fremitus.
- Percussion reveals hyper-resonance.
- Auscultation reveals diminished breath sounds.
- Auscultation also reveals decreased vocal resonance.

These findings are all consistent with one another in indicating that there is an issue with hyper-inflation and/or decreased lung density. The consistency of these findings enables you to narrow your focus to issues you know that cause hyper-inflation and/or decreased lung density such as emphysema, asthma, pneumothorax, etc.

Chapter 5

Selected Topics in Acid/Base Chemistry and the Arterial Blood Gas

The presentation of this chapter is with the understanding that you have already studied chemistry and sufficient mathematics either in high school or college – and that you also remember what you were taught in those courses. The aim of this chapter is to cover the acid/base concepts that are specific to the analysis and understanding of the arterial blood gas and thus the acid/base status of your patient.

A. Derivation of the Henderson-Hasselbalch Equation

The Henderson-Hasselbalch equation is important because it is the basis for how pH is determined.

Given the following 3 facts:

$pH = -\log[H^+]$

K_a = dissociation constant   (*increased temperature increases K_a*)

$pK = -\log K_a$ (*therefore increased temperature decreases pK*)
pK is just the logarithmic
expression of K_a

Follow the train of thought to see how the Henderson-Hasselbalch equation is derived.

The bicarbonate buffering system of the blood:

$$H_2CO_3 \longleftrightarrow H^+ + HCO_3^-$$
$$HCO_3^- \longleftrightarrow H^+ + CO_3^{2-}$$

The H^+ component is where you derive the pH from.

NOW – the K_a just mentioned is expressed as follows:

$$K_a = \frac{[H^+][HCO_3^-]}{[H_2CO_3]}$$ *the k_a as expressed here is simply the dissociation constant for the dissociation of H_2CO_3*

To get the pH from K_a – you solve the equation for H^+

Therefore:

$$K_a[H_2CO_3] = [H^+][HCO_3^-]$$

$$\frac{K_a[H_2CO_3]}{[HCO_3^-]} = [H^+]$$

which is the same as: *(rearrange it to get H^+ on the left)*

$$[H^+] = \frac{K_a[H_2CO_3]}{[HCO_3^-]}$$

We will now introduce logs into this equation:

$$\log[H^+] = \log k_a + \log \frac{[H_2CO_3]}{[HCO_3^-]}$$

Then multiplying by (-1) to get log[H$^+$] negative so as to express pH will yield:

$$-\log[H^+] = -\log K_a - \log \frac{[H_2CO_3]}{[HCO_3^-]}$$

$$pH = pK + \log \frac{[HCO_3^-]}{[H_2CO_3]}$$

This is the Henderson-Hasselbalch equation

therefore, since $H_2CO_3 = PCO_2 \times 0.03$

$$pH = pK + \log \frac{[HCO_3^-]}{PaCO_2 \times 0.03}$$

HCO_3^- is the renal control of pH

$PaCO_2$ is the respiratory control of pH

And thus you have the pH of the bicarbonate buffer system, which equates to being the pH of the plasma since all the buffer systems in the plasma are in equilibrium with one another.

Consider the following example of the Henderson-Hasselbalch equation:

$$pH = pK + \log \frac{[HCO_3^-]}{[H_2CO_3]}$$

Given that:

- The pK of H_2CO_3 is 6.1
- Normal plasma $[HCO_3^-]$ is 24 mEq/L
- Normal $PaCO_2$ is 40 mmHg
- $H_2CO_3 = PaCO_2 \times 0.03$

Then:

$$pH = pK + \log \frac{[HCO_3^-]}{[H_2CO_3]}$$

$$pH = 6.1 + \log \frac{24}{40 \times 0.03}$$

$$pH = 6.1 + \log \frac{24}{1.2}$$

THIS IS IMPORTANT

under normal conditions, you will have a 20:1 ratio of HCO_3^- to PCO_2. In other words – you have 20 times more bicarb than CO_2. The body wants to maintain this 20:1 ratio. Another way to think of this is to say that pH is normal when HCO_3^-:CO_2 is 20:1.

$$pH = 6.1 + \log 20$$

$$pH = 6.1 + 1.301$$

$$pH = 7.401 - \text{which is normal pH}$$

B. Normal ABG and Electrolyte Values

<u>Normal Adult Blood Gas Values</u>

pH   7.35 – 7.45

PaCO$_2$ 35 – 45 mmHg   *From $\dot{V}CO_2 = V_A\,PaCO_2$*

When PaCO$_2$ < 35 mmHg ⟶ **Hyperventilation** is occurring
When PaCO$_2$ > 45 mmHg ⟶ **Hypoventilation** is occurring

HCO$_3^-$ 22 – 26 mEq/L

PaO$_2$ 85 – 100 mmHg   *From $PaO_2 = P_B \times FiO_2$*

SaO$_2$ 97 – 98%

                                          BE > +2 - gain of base or loss of acid
Base Excess   0 to +/- 2 mEq/L   *BE < -2 - loss of base or gain of acid*

<u>Normal Electrolyte Values</u>

Na$^+$ 135 – 145 mEq/L

                                        This is how you will see the
K$^+$ 3.5 – 5.5 mEq/L   *electrolytes in the chart. This is*
                                        how physicians chart electrolytes.

Cl$^-$ 95 – 110 mEq/L

Na$^+$	Cl$^-$	BUN	
K$^+$	HCO$_3^-$	Cr	Glu

HCO$_3^-$ 22 – 26 mEq/L

BUN   7 – 20 mg/dl

                                        In the chart there will be values
Creatinine   0.5 – 1.4 mg/dl   *in the respective spaces. You*
                                        need to memorize what each
Glucose   60 – 110 mg/dl   *space in the grid represents.*

C. Acidemia and Alkalemia – General Ideas

Having established the Henderson-Hasselbalch equation as the basis for how pH is determined, and having looked at how Henderson-Hasselbalch is solved to obtain the value for a normal pH, let us now look at what is happening when pH is not normal.

Given that Henderson-Hasselbalch describes pH as follows:

$$pH = pK + \log \frac{[HCO_3^-]}{PaCO_2 \times 0.03}$$

And given that pK is constant at 6.1

Then, in order for Acidemia to occur, which is when pH < 7.35

The fraction $\dfrac{[HCO_3^-]}{PaCO_2 \times 0.03}$ had to become smaller.

which means:

- Either $[HCO_3^-]$ went down
- Or $PaCO_2$ went up
- Or both have occurred

When either, or both of these events occurs, the HCO_3:CO_2 ratio < 20:1 and you end up with a pH less than normal.

In order for Alkalemia to occur, which is when pH > 7.45

The fraction $\dfrac{[HCO_3^-]}{PaCO_2 \times 0.03}$ had to become bigger.

which means:

- Either $[HCO_3^-]$ went up
- Or $PaCO_2$ went down
- Or both have occurred

When either, or both of these events occurs, the HCO_3:CO_2 ratio > 20:1 and you end up with a pH greater than normal.

D. Paradigm for Blood Gas Interpretation

First look at the pH

> If it is less than 7.35, then you have acidemia
>
> If it is greater than 7.45, then you have alkalemia

If the pH indicates acidemia:

Then you expect to see one of two things – or both.

Either the $PaCO_2$ is above normal (> 45 mmHg)

Or the HCO_3^- is below normal (< 22 mEq/L)

Or both of these events are occurring

If it is from elevated $PaCO_2$, then you have respiratory acidemia.

If it is from decreased HCO_3^-, then you have metabolic acidemia.

If you have both an elevated $PaCO_2$ and decreased HCO_3^-, then you have a combined (or mixed) respiratory and metabolic acidemia.

If neither of these is happening – you have an impossible ABG.

If the pH indicates alkalemia:

Then you expect to see one of two things – or both.

Either the $PaCO_2$ is below normal (< 35 mmHg)

Or the HCO_3^- is above normal (> 26 mEq/L)

Or both of these events are occurring

If it is from decreased $PaCO_2$, then you have respiratory alkalemia.

If it is from elevated HCO_3^-, then you have metabolic alkalemia.

If you have both a decreased $PaCO_2$ and elevated HCO_3^-, then you have a combined (or mixed) respiratory and metabolic alkalemia.

If neither of these is happening – you have an impossible ABG.

E. The Concept of Compensation

The body will always attempt to maintain the pH within normal range. If either the HCO_3^- or the $PaCO_2$ increases or decreases, the other value will either increase or decrease in an effort to compensate. This is the manner in which the lungs and the kidneys work together in an effort to maintain a stable pH.

If hyperventilation is occurring that is causing the $PaCO_2$ to be too low and thus raising the pH (respiratory alkalemia), the kidneys will respond by lowering the HCO_3^- level. Conversely, if hypoventilation is occurring that is causing the $PaCO_2$ to be too high and thus lowering the pH (respiratory acidemia), the kidneys will respond by raising the HCO_3^- level.

If, however, it is an issue of high HCO_3^- that is causing the pH to be too high (metabolic alkalemia), the brain will direct the lungs to respond by reducing ventilation in order to raise the $PaCO_2$. Conversely, if the issue is one of low HCO_3^- that is causing the pH to be too low (metabolic acidemia), the brain will direct the lungs to respond by increasing ventilation in order to lower the $PaCO_2$.

These compensatory mechanisms are in place because the body wants to maintain the HCO_3^-/CO_2 ratio at 20:1. When it comes to interpreting an ABG, once you find the offending value, if there is compensation going on, the other value will be going in the same direction as the offending value. The offending value is the value (either the HCO_3^- or the $PaCO_2$) that is the primary culprit in causing the pH to be abnormal.

The best way to learn how all of this works together is to actually analyze and interpret of a variety of ABG's so that you can see how this all fits together – so to that end, the next section will be doing just that.

F. Basic ABG Analysis & Interpretation

In the 11 examples that follow, the pH, HCO_3^-, and $PaCO_2$ from a hypothetical ABG will be given. Step by step analysis will enable you to learn how to interpret an ABG.

Example 1.   pH = 7.27 $PaCO_2$ = 29 HCO_3^- = 13
partially compensated metabolic acidemia

A. The pH of 7.27 is indicating acidemia.

B. Could a $PaCO_2$ of 29 be causing the acidemia? The answer is no. A low $PaCO_2$ such as this would cause the pH to go up – not down. $PaCO_2$ therefore is NOT the offending value.

C. Could a HCO_3^- of 13 be causing the acidemia? The answer is yes. The normal HCO_3^- level is 22 – 26. With HCO_3^- being this low, there will certainly be a primary metabolic acidemia. The HCO_3^- value of 13, therefore, is the offending value. It is the low HCO_3^- of 13 that is causing the metabolic acidemia.

D. Notice, however, that the $PaCO_2$ of 29 "followed" the low HCO_3^- so as to compensate for the low HCO_3^-. It is the low HCO_3^- that is causing the low pH of 7.27 to begin with – a $PaCO_2$ of 29 doesn't cause a low pH. The pH is low because HCO_3^- is too low, which is why the pH is reflecting metabolic acidemia. The response of the lungs was to increase the ventilation so as to blow off more CO_2, thus getting rid of more acid in an effort to compensate for the low HCO_3^-.

E. So what you have here is what is known as partially compensated metabolic acidemia. You could also state it as metabolic acidemia that is partially compensated by respiratory alkalemia.

NOTE:

With partial compensation, the pH is not fully restored to within normal range – hence the reason why it's said to only be a partial compensation.

With full compensation, the pH is restored to within the normal range.

Example 2.   pH = 7.10 $PaCO_2$ = 50 HCO_3^- = 15
mixed respiratory/metabolic acidemia

A. The pH of 7.10 is indicating acidemia.

B. Could a $PaCO_2$ of 50 be causing the acidemia? The answer is yes. A $PaCO_2$ this high would certainly cause an acidic pH.

C. Could a HCO_3^- of 15 be causing the acidemia? The answer is also yes. 15 is well below normal and would cause acidemia.

D.   Therefore, in this case, rather than having an individual offending value, we have both components contributing to the acidemia such that we have what is called a mixed respiratory/ metabolic acidemia.

E. This is a typical ABG during a cardiac arrest. Bicarb (HCO_3^-) is low because it is getting used up to neutralize the acid that is being formed from anaerobic respiration since there is no oxygen available for aerobic respiration because the patient isn't breathing.

Example 3.   pH = 7.62 $PaCO_2$ = 35 HCO_3^- = 35
pure metabolic alkalemia

A. The pH of 7.62 is indicating alkalemia.

B. Could a $PaCO_2$ of 35 be causing the alkalemia? The answer is no. Although it's on the lower edge of normal, 35 is still within the normal range for $PaCO_2$.

C. Could a HCO_3^- of 35 be causing the alkalemia? The answer is yes. A bicarb of 35 is quite high and is indeed the offending value that is causing the alkalemia.

D. This therefore represents a pure metabolic alkalemia.

Example 4.   pH = 7.62 $PaCO_2$ = 24 HCO_3^- = 24
pure respiratory alkalemia

A. The pH of 7.62 is indicating alkalemia.

B. Could a $PaCO_2$ of 24 be causing the alkalemia? The answer is yes. A $PaCO_2$ of 24 is way below normal, and with this much CO_2 being blown off, it would clearly cause an alkalemic pH. Insofar as your bicarb is normal, $PaCO_2$ is the offending value that is causing the alkalemia.

C. Could a HCO_3^- of 24 be causing the alkalemia? The answer is no. A bicarb of 24 is normal. Bicarb is not the issue in this case.

D. This case represents a pure respiratory alkalemia.

Example 5.   pH = 7.50   PaCO$_2$ = 47   HCO$_3^-$ = 20
an impossible ABG

A. The pH of 7.50 is indicating alkalemia.

B. Could a PaCO$_2$ of 47 be causing the alkalemia? The answer is no. A PaCO$_2$ of 47 would cause the pH to be lower than normal – not higher than normal.

C. Could a HCO$_3^-$ of 20 be causing the alkalemia? The answer is no. A bicarb of only 20 would not cause an alkalemic pH. Lower than normal bicarb would cause the pH to go down, not up.

D. This therefore represents an impossible ABG. In other words, it is a lab error and you need to get a new ABG and run it again. Furthermore, it you plugged the given values for the CO$_2$ and the HCO$_3^-$ into the Henderson-Hasselbalch equation, you would have determined that the pH should have been 7.25 – not 7.50 – further confirming that these ABG results are wrong.

Example 6.   pH = 7.20   PaCO$_2$ = 58   HCO$_3^-$ = 22
pure respiratory acidemia

A. The pH of 7.20 is indicating acidemia.

B. Could a PaCO$_2$ of 58 be causing the acidemia? The answer is yes. A PaCO$_2$ of 58 is way above normal, and with this much CO$_2$ being retained, it would clearly cause an acidic pH. Insofar as your bicarb is normal, PaCO$_2$ is the offending value that is causing the acidemia.

C. Could a HCO$_3^-$ of 22 be causing the acidemia? The answer is no. Although it's on the lower edge of normal, 22 is still within the normal range for bicarb. Bicarb is not the issue in this case.

D. This case therefore represents a pure respiratory acidemia.

Example 7.   pH = 7.69 $PaCO_2$ = 30 HCO_3^- = 35
mixed respiratory/metabolic alkalemia

A. The pH of 7.69 is indicating alkalemia.

B. Could a $PaCO_2$ of 30 be causing the alkalemia? The answer is yes. A $PaCO_2$ of 30 is below normal and would certainly cause an alkalemic pH.

C. Could a HCO_3^- of 35 be causing the alkalemia? The answer is yes. A HCO_3^- of 35 is way above normal and would certainly cause an alkalemic pH.

D. Therefore, in this case, rather than having an individual offending value, we have both components contributing to the alkalemia such that we have what is called a mixed respiratory/metabolic alkalemia.

Example 8.   pH = 7.55 $PaCO_2$ = 20 HCO_3^- = 17
partially compensated respiratory alkalemia

A. The pH of 7.55 is indicating alkalemia.

B. Could a $PaCO_2$ of 20 be causing the alkalemia? The answer is yes. A low $PaCO_2$ such as this would indeed cause the pH to go up.

C. Could a HCO_3^- of 17 be causing the alkalemia? The answer is no. The normal HCO_3^- level is 22 – 26. An HCO_3^- of 17 would cause the pH to go down – not up. The $PaCO_2$ of 20, therefore, is the offending value. It is the low $PaCO_2$ of 20 that is causing the respiratory alkalemia.

D. Notice, however, that the HCO_3^- of 17 "followed" the low $PaCO_2$ so as to compensate for the low $PaCO_2$. It is the low $PaCO_2$ that is causing the high pH of 7.55 to begin with – an HCO_3^- of 17 doesn't cause a high pH. The pH is high because the $PaCO_2$ is too low, which is why the pH is reflecting respiratory alkalemia. The response of the kidneys was to cut back on HCO_3^- so as to reduce the amount of base in an effort to compensate for the low $PaCO_2$.

E. So what you have here is what is known as partially compensated respiratory alkalemia. You could also state it as respiratory alkalemia that is partially compensated by metabolic acidemia.

Example 9.   **pH = 7.32**   **$PaCO_2$ = 70**   **HCO_3^- = 35**
partially compensated respiratory acidemia

A. The pH of 7.32 is indicating acidemia.

B. Could a $PaCO_2$ of 70 be causing the acidemia? The answer is yes. A $PaCO_2$ this high would certainly cause an acidic pH.

C. Could a HCO_3^- of 35 be causing the acidemia? The answer is no. An HCO_3^- of 35 would cause the pH to go up – not down. The $PaCO_2$ of 70, therefore, is the offending value. It is the high $PaCO_2$ of 70 that is causing the respiratory acidemia.

D. Notice, however, that the HCO_3^- of 35 "followed" the high $PaCO_2$ so as to compensate for the high $PaCO_2$. It is the high $PaCO_2$ that is causing the low pH of 7.32 to begin with – an HCO_3^- of 35 doesn't cause a low pH. The pH is low because the $PaCO_2$ is too high, which is why the pH is reflecting respiratory acidemia. The response of the kidneys was to increase HCO_3^- so as to increase the amount of base in an effort to compensate for the high $PaCO_2$.

E. So what you have here is what is known as partially compensated respiratory acidemia. You could also state it as respiratory acidemia that is partially compensated by metabolic alkalemia.

F. This is a typical ABG for a chronic COPD patient. As you will learn in the mechanical ventilation chapter – your goal with these patients is to restore their acid/base balance to that which is "normal for them" – not textbook normal. For chronic COPDers, high CO_2 that is compensated with high bicarb is normal for them. You just have to find out what particular values are normal for them so you know what to work towards.

Example 10.   pH = 7.56   PaCO$_2$ = 50   HCO$_3$⁻ = 43
partially compensated metabolic alkalemia

A. The pH of 7.56 is indicating alkalemia.

B. Could a PaCO$_2$ of 50 be causing the alkalemia? The answer is no. A high PaCO$_2$ such as this would cause the pH to go down – not up.

C. Could a HCO$_3$⁻ of 43 be causing the alkalemia? The answer is yes. An HCO$_3$⁻ of 43 would certainly cause the pH to go up. The HCO$_3$⁻ of 43, therefore, is the offending value. It is the high HCO$_3$⁻ of 43 that is causing the metabolic alkalemia.

D. Notice, however, that the PaCO$_2$ of 50 "followed" the high HCO$_3$⁻ so as to compensate for the high HCO$_3$⁻. It is the high HCO$_3$⁻ that is causing the high pH of 7.56 to begin with – a PaCO$_2$ of 50 doesn't cause a high pH. The pH is high because HCO$_3$⁻ is too high, which is why the pH is reflecting metabolic alkalemia. The response of the lungs was to reduce ventilation so as to retain more CO$_2$, thus increasing the amount of acid in an effort to compensate for the high HCO$_3$⁻.

E. So what you have here is what is known as partially compensated metabolic alkalemia. You could also state it as metabolic alkalemia that is partially compensated by respiratory acidemia.

Example 11.   pH = 7.27   PaCO$_2$ = 38   HCO$_3$⁻ = 17
pure metabolic acidemia

A. The pH of 7.27 is indicating acidemia.

B. Could a PaCO$_2$ of 38 be causing the acidemia? The answer is no. A PaCO$_2$ of 38 is within normal range and would not cause an acidic pH.

C. Could a HCO$_3$⁻ of 17 be causing the acidemia? The answer is yes. A HCO$_3$⁻ of 17 is below normal and is the offending value that is causing the acidemia.

D. This therefore represents a pure metabolic acidemia.

G. Clinical Presentation of Acidemia and Alkalemia

Respiratory Acidosis

<u>Acute Respiratory Acidosis</u>

- pH < 7.35
- $PaCO_2$ > 45 mmHg
- HCO_3^- between 22 – 26

Causes of acute respiratory acidosis:

- Hypoventilation
- Cardiopulmonary arrest
- CNS trauma
- Chest trauma/pneumothorax
- Drug overdose
- Excessive sedation
- Restrictive lung disease

<u>Chronic Respiratory Acidosis (compensated)</u>

- pH between 7.35 – 7.40
- $PaCO_2$ > 45 mmHg
- HCO_3^- between 27 – 48

Causes of chronic respiratory acidosis:

- Hypoventilation
- COPD
- CNS Injury
- Chronic neuromuscular disease/muscle wasting

Signs & symptoms of respiratory acidosis:

- Rapid and shallow breathing
- Dyspnea
- Headache
- Diminished LOC
- Muscle weakness
- Hyperkalemia
- Cardiac dysrhythmias

Respiratory Alkalosis

Acute Respiratory Alkalosis

- pH > 7.45
- $PaCO_2$ < 35 mmHg
- HCO_3^- between 22 – 26

Causes of acute respiratory alkalosis:

- Increased alveolar ventilation (increased V_A)
- Severe infections/fever
- Pain and/or anxiety
- Pulmonary embolus
- Cirrhosis
- Encephalitis
- Hypoxemia

- Mechanical ventilation
- Salicylate intoxication (aspirin poisoning)

Chronic Respiratory Alkalosis (compensated)

- pH between 7.40 – 7.45
- $PaCO_2$ < 35 mmHg
- HCO_3^- between 12 – 21

Causes of chronic respiratory alkalosis:

- Increased alveolar ventilation that is often associated with long term mechanical ventilation

Signs & symptoms of respiratory alkalosis:

- Rapid and deep breathing
- Tachycardia
- Numbness and tingling in extremities
- Light headedness and lethargy and/or confusion
- Hypokalemia
- Nausea and vomiting
- Seizures

Metabolic Acidosis

Acute Metabolic Acidosis

- pH < 7.35
- $PaCO_2$ between 35 – 45 mmHg
- HCO_3^- between 12 – 21

Causes of acute metabolic acidosis:

- Ketoacidosis
  - alcoholic, starvation, diabetic
- Uremic acidosis (failure of renal acid excretion)
- Renal tubular acidosis
- Lactic acidosis (overproduction of acid)
- Loss of HCO_3^- (diarrhea)
- Renal loss of base (carbonic anhydrase inhibitors - Diamox)
- Conversion of toxins to acids (methanol, ethylene glycol, salicylate)

Chronic Metabolic Acidosis (compensated)

- pH between 7.35 – 7.40
- $PaCO_2$ < 35 mmHg
- HCO_3^- between 12 – 21

Signs & symptoms of metabolic acidosis:

- Kussmaul breathing
- Headache
- Diminished LOC (confusion, drowsiness)
- Nausea and vomiting
- Diarrhea
- Decreased blood pressure
- Hyperkalemia
- Warm, flushed skin
- Muscle twitching

Metabolic Alkalosis

Acute Metabolic Alkalosis

- pH > 7.45
- $PaCO_2$ between 35 – 45 mmHg
- HCO_3^- between 27 – 48

Causes of acute metabolic alkalosis:

- Ingestion of HCO_3^- (antacids), or administration of bicarb
- Licorice poisoning
- Diuretic induced hypokalemia or hypochloremia
- Prolonged vomiting
- Gastrointestinal suctioning
- Steroids (hypercortisolism)

Chronic Metabolic Alkalosis (compensated)

- pH between 7.40 – 7.45
- $PaCO_2$ > 45 mmHg
- HCO_3^- between 27 – 48

Causes of chronic metabolic alkalosis:

- Primary hypokalemic metabolic alkalosis with dehydration/ azotemia

Signs & symptoms of metabolic alkalosis:

- Compensatory hypoventilation
- Tachycardia and/or dysrhythmias
- Nausea and vomiting and diarrhea
- Altered LOC (confusion, dizziness, irritability)
- Muscle cramps, tremors, tingling in extremities

Chapter 6

Selected Topics in Hemodynamics

Hemodynamics essentially deals with the dynamics of blood flow. The *ultimate* goal of circulation is to ensure adequate delivery of oxygen to the tissues primarily through the manipulation of cardiac output. This chapter is presented with the presumption that you already have a functional understanding of the anatomy of the heart and blood vessels.

A. Pulmonary and Systemic Circulation

Pulmonary Circulation

Deoxygenated blood flows from the vena cava into the right atrium. The right atrium is the *pulmonary reservoir*. It then flows through the tricuspid valve into the right ventricle which is the pump. The right ventricle pumps the blood through the pulmonic valve into the pulmonary artery where the blood is ultimately distributed throughout the alveolar capillary bed.

The alveolar capillary bed is the capillary network that surrounds the alveoli. Within this capillary network is about 75 – 100 ml of blood spread over a surface area of approximately 70 square meters. The alveolar capillary bed thus has a very large surface area.

Systemic Circulation

From the alveolar capillary beds, blood then flows through venules and veins that ultimately lead into the four major pulmonary veins (2 left & 2 right) that return the oxygenated blood back to the left atrium. The left atrium is the *systemic reservoir*. From the left atrium, blood flows through the mitral valve into the left ventricle (the pump). The left ventricle then pumps the blood through the aortic valve where it enters into the systemic circulation.

Arteries & Arterioles – arteries carry oxygenated blood away from the heart. The exception to this rule is the pulmonary artery – although it is indeed carrying blood away from the heart, that blood however is still deoxygenated as it has not yet been oxygenated in the alveolar capillary beds.

Systemic Capillary Beds – are the capillary beds in the tissues. Oxygen is delivered to the tissues and carbon dioxide is removed from the tissues in the systemic capillary beds.

Venules and Veins – veins carry deoxygenated blood back to the heart. The exception to this rule is the pulmonary vein – although it is indeed carrying blood towards the heart, that blood is oxygenated as it has already passed through the alveolar capillary beds.

Pressure levels throughout the circulatory system

You need to know and remember these pressure levels. This is not just a bunch of data to fill up a page. In the ICU, you will often have patients that have invasive monitoring. In order for you to be able to understand what is going on you need to know the normal values. Nothing included in this book is something that you can forget. If it is in this book – it is essential.

Here are the normal values for the pressures throughout the
circulatory system.

Vena Cava (VC)	< 10 mmHg
Right Atrium (RA)	2 - 6 mmHg
Right Ventricle (RV)	25/0 mmHg
Pulmonary Artery (PA)	25/10 mmHg
Pulmonary Arterioles	12 mmHg
Pulmonary Capillary Bed	10 mmHg
Pulmonary Veins (PV)	9 mmHg
Left Atrium (LA)	6 - 8 mmHg
Left Ventricle (LV)	120/0 mmHg
Aorta	120/80 mmHg
Systemic Arterioles	30 mmHg
Systemic Capillaries	20 mmHg

B. Blood Volume of Pulmonary Circulation

At any given time, there is approximately 500 ml of blood
in the circulation between the pulmonary artery and the left atrium.
This is the "pulmonary circulation", and it accounts for about 10%
of the total circulation in the body. Of that 500 ml in the pulmonary
circulation, about 75 – 100 ml is in the pulmonary capillaries and the
other 400 – 425 ml is distributed between the pulmonary artery and
the pulmonary veins.

- The capillary volume is the volume ejected by the RV (right
  ventricle).
- The pulmonary capillary blood is almost completely replaced
  with each heartbeat.

- Blood remains in the capillary bed for ¾, or 0.75 seconds.
- The pulmonary vascular volume (the 500 ml) also serves as a backup reservoir that shields the left atrium from sudden changes in right ventricular output.
  - If venous return suddenly increased for example, the left ventricular filling does not change for 2 – 3 cardiac cycles.

C. The Cardiac Cycle

The cardiac cycle consists of contraction (systole) and relaxation (diastole) of both the atria and the ventricles.

- Average cycle time is 0.8 seconds.
- Diastole is normally twice as long as systole – this means that systole is about 0.27 seconds and diastole is about 0.53 seconds. The extra time for diastole is for the purpose of enabling adequate perfusion of the coronary arteries (perfusion of the heart itself). The opening of the aortic valve during systole somewhat blocks the coronary arteries, hence the prolonged diastole allows for adequate perfusion of the heart.
  - Extreme tachycardia however may shorten diastolic time so much that coronary blood flow becomes inadequate. (especially in patients whose coronary arteries are already narrowed).

The Actual Cycle

- The vena cava and the pulmonary veins fill the right atrium (RA) and the left atrium (LA) respectively.

- As the RA and LA fill, pressure builds so as to force open the tricuspid and mitral valves.

- Opening of the tricuspid and mitral valves results in blood flowing into the right ventricle (RV) and left ventricle (LV).
  - 78% of this flow is passive.
  - 22% of this flow is from atrial contraction.

- With the opening of these valves and blood flowing into the ventricles, the atrial pressure decreases and pressure begins to build in the ventricles as they begin to depolarize.

- As the RV and LV fill, enough pressure builds from ventricular contraction to close the tricuspid and mitral valves. THE CLOSURE OF THE TRICUSPID AND MITRAL VALVES IS WHAT YOU HEAR ON AUSCULATION AS S_1 – (the first heart sound).
  - note that although ventricular contraction has caused ventricular pressures to rise and has forced the closure of the tricuspid and mitral valves, this is known as *isovolumetric contraction* because there has been no change in ventricular volume during this time because the aortic and pulmonary semi-lunar valves are still closed at this time. This isovolumetric phase lasts for about 0.03 seconds, and what it does is allow for pressure to build in the RV and LV so that it becomes high enough to be able to overcome the opposing aortic and pulmonary artery pressure in order to force open the aortic and pulmonary semi-lunar valves.

- The continued pressure build-up from isovolumetric ventricular contraction then becomes sufficient enough to overcome the opposing aortic and pulmonary artery pressure and forces open the aortic and pulmonary semi-lunar valves such that blood then flows out of the RV and LV.

- Blood flows out of the RV and LV (ejection period) until the pressure in the RV and LV drops below the pressure in the aorta and the pulmonary artery. This leads to the closure of the aortic and pulmonary semi-lunar valves. THE CLOSURE OF THE AORTIC AND PULMONARY SEMI-LUNAR VALVES IS WHAT YOU HEAR ON AUSCULTATION AS S_2 – (the second heart sound).

- When the aortic and pulmonary semi-lunar valves close, flow in the aorta stops and the vessel itself recoils back to its original diameter. This can be seen on an EKG tracing and it is known as a ***dicrotic notch***. The absence of a dicrotic notch on the EKG may be indicative of arteriosclerosis.

End Diastolic Volume & End Systolic Volume

End diastolic volume (EDV) is the volume of blood in the ventricle at the end of diastole (or you can think of it as the amount of blood in the ventricle just before systole). It is the amount of blood that has filled the ventricle. To the extent that a greater EDV results in greater ventricular distension, EDV is thus a significant determinant of preload which will be discussed in a moment.

- EDV = 110 – 120 ml (the amount of blood in a filled ventricle at the end of diastole).

- Ventricular contraction (systole) then ejects about 70ml of blood. This is the *stroke volume*.

- Therefore, the difference between what was in the ventricle to begin with before contraction (EDV) and the amount that was ejected (70ml, the stroke volume) leaves you with 40 – 50 ml being left in the ventricle after systole. This is called the end systolic volume (ESV).

To summarize:

* At the end of diastole, EDV = 110 – 120 ml.
* The ventricle contracts (systole) and ejects 70ml (stroke volume).
* 40 – 50 ml remains in the ventricle (ESV).

The Ejection Fraction

The ejection fraction (E_f %) is simply the ratio between the stroke volume (SV) and the end diastolic volume (EDV). *It tells you percentage of the EDV that got ejected.*

$$E_f\% = \frac{SV}{EDV} \times 100$$

- A normal ejection fraction should be around 60%.
- Ejection fractions below 50% are not good. An ejection fraction below 50% is indicative of poor contractility and/or a failing pump.
- During exercise, the ejection fraction can get as high as 90% or more.

D. The Vascular System

- The main function of the systemic arterial system is to distribute oxygenated blood to the systemic capillary beds of the tissues throughout the body.

- Arteries become arterioles, and then arterioles become capillaries. Arterioles are considered the terminal component as they regulate the flow of blood through the arterial system by either constricting or dilating.

- By either constricting or dilating (under autonomic nervous system control), arterioles act as "gatekeepers" in the sense that they are able to allow blood to be diverted to an area of need.
    - e.g. – during a stress situation, arterioles in some areas can constrict so as to divert blood to other areas in greater need.

- Veins are responsible for returning blood to the heart.

- Veins have less smooth muscle than arteries and are more distensible. As such, veins contain about 65% of the overall blood volume.

- Large veins have one-way valves to help overcome gravity in allowing blood to return to the heart.

E. Cardiac Output

Cardiac output (CO) is the product of the heart rate and the stroke volume.

$$CO = HR \times SV$$

Cardiac output should equal venous return. The heart does not dictate the amount of blood to be pumped, but rather simply adjusts to what it is given. It automatically adjusts to incoming blood flow by pumping it out as fast as it enters.

- Normal CO is 5 LPM - (range of 4 – 8 LPM).
- Normal HR is 60 – 100 beats/min.

An increase in heart rate will increase cardiac output, but only to an extent. Once the HR reaches 170, there will no longer remain enough time for ventricular filling, so cardiac output will then drop. Conversely – a decrease in HR may not necessarily correspond to a decrease in cardiac output due to longer filling times.

The total cardiac output is pumped through both circulations (pulmonary & systemic) every minute.

The right and left ventricular outputs must equal over time, otherwise blood will start to accumulate.

Stroke Volume

The stroke volume (SV) is the amount of blood ejected during ventricular contraction (systole). SV = EDV – ESV, and it is around 70ml. Stroke volume is determined by 3 factors:

1) Preload
2) Afterload
3) Contractility

Preload

Preload is what you WANT. Preload is the stretching of the ventricle before contraction.   When you have increased preload, you have increased stroke volume which then results in better cardiac output. Preload is essentially EDV as it is the EDV that stretches the ventricle.

Factors that influence preload:

- Amount of venous return
- The compliance of the ventricle
- The duration of diastole
- Atrial contractions

Afterload

Afterload is what you DON'T WANT.   Afterload is the resistance that the ventricle must overcome in order to pump blood. When you have increased afterload, you have decreased stroke volume which results in less cardiac output.

Factors that increase afterload

- Hypertension
- Valve stenosis
- Polycythemia
- Vasoconstriction

Factors that decrease afterload

- Hypotension
- Anemia
- Vasodilation

Contractility

Contractility is the vigor of contraction of the heart. It's the strength of the contraction. Increased contractility leads to better stroke volume which in turn produces better cardiac output.

F.   Evaluation of Hemodynamic Status

Heart Rate & Rhythm

- An increase in HR could be indicative of a pending problem.
- You need to auscultate the quality of heart sounds.
- Check for murmurs and get an EKG for rhythm patterns.

Presence & Quality of Pulse

- You need to assess the strength of each pulse.
- Check the patient's upper and lower extremities.
- A shorter cardiac cycle will produce a weak pulse.
- Patients with hyperdynamic circulation (abnormally increased circulatory volume) will have increased pulse strength.
- Patients with significant tachycardia, arrhythmias, or hypo-dynamic circulation will have decreased pulse strength.

Capillary Refill

- Press the patient's nail bed between your fingers to squeeze blood from the underlying capillary bed.
- If tissue perfusion is normal – color will return to the nail bed ≤ 2 seconds.

Skin Color & Temperature

- Circulatory failure will cause compensatory vasoconstriction that diverts blood to the vital organs – hence the extremities will become cool to the touch.

LOC

- LOC is a sensitive indicator of tissue perfusion and hemodynamic status.
- Early signs of inadequate perfusion are:
  - Patient's inability to think or perform a complex mental task.
  - Restlessness and/or apprehension
  - Uncooperativeness or irritability
  - Short term memory loss

Urinary Output

- A decrease in urine output in an *adequately hydrated* patient is indicative of hypo-perfusion.

Neck Veins

- The jugular veins provide valuable information regarding the hemodynamic status of the right heart – assess for JVD.

Blood Pressure

- Blood pressure is directly related to cardiac output (CO) and systemic vascular resistance (SVR). BP = CO x SVR.

- An increase in blood pressure may be due to an increase in CO and/or SVR. Blood pressure gives you indirect information about a patient's cardiovascular status.

MAP (mean arterial pressure)

* MAP is the most useful parameter in assessing organ perfusion. MAP is the "profusion" pressure that is "seen" by the organs.

* MAP can be measured as follows:

1) MAP = DP + 1/3 (SP − DP)

or

2) MAP = $\dfrac{(2 \times DP) + SP}{3}$

where DP is the diastolic pressure, and SP is the systolic pressure

* Normal MAP is 70 − 105 mmHg.
* MAP < 65 mmHg is indicative of hypotension.
  - *the major concern with hypotension is adequacy of oxygen delivery to the tissues.*
* MAP > 110 mmHg is indicative of hypertension − this coincides roughly with a blood pressure of 140/90.

Arterial Compliance

* Decreased arterial compliance that occurs with age and/ or vascular disease causes aortic pressure to rise higher and more sharply during systole, and to fall more abruptly during diastole.

Determinants of Systolic & Diastolic Blood Pressure

* For a given volume of circulating blood, blood pressure is determined by:

- stroke volume
- arterial compliance
- arterial resistance

* For any given resistance and stroke volume, a stiffer aorta causes a higher systolic pressure.

* For any given compliance or resistance, an increased stroke volume will increase systolic pressure.

* Diastolic pressure is determined by SVR.

* Blood pressure is affected by:
  - fluid status
  - effects of medication
  - influence of the autonomic nervous system

Consequences of Hypertension

* Hypertension places excessive workload on the heart which will lead to heart failure if not treated.
* Hypertension can lead to the rupture of a major blood vessel in the brain (hemorrhagic stroke).
* Hypertension can lead to the rupture of blood vessels in the kidneys leading to extensive destruction of renal tissue and subsequent renal failure.

G. Central Venous Pressure Monitoring

Central venous pressure (CVP) is the blood pressure in the vena cava just as it enters the right atrium (RA).   Normal CVP is 2 – 6 mmHg and it is thought of as a good approximation for right atrial pressure. CVP is sometimes still used as a substitute for preload although the evidence suggests that it does not correlate with ventricular volume. Insofar as preload is the term used for ventricular stretching, we are speaking of CVP as a means of looking at the preload of the RV. Monitoring CVP is important because changes in CVP can be indicative of the following issues that may be of concern with your patient. If you look closely at the various causes for either increased or decreased CVP, you'll see that the CVP is enabling you to monitor fluid status and certain aspects of cardiac status. This is very important as fluid status is often a great concern in critically ill patients.

Causes of decreased CVP

- Hypovolemia
- Vasodilation
- Hemorrhage

Causes of increased CVP

- RV failure
- Hypervolemia
- Pulmonary valve stenosis
- Tricuspid valve stenosis

CVP is measured with a central venous catheter, otherwise known as a "central line", which is similar to an A-line in the sense that it is an invasive catheter. Whereas the A-line is placed into an artery, the central line is placed into a large vein – typically it could be the subclavian where it is then threaded through the vein until it rests in the superior vena cava just at the entrance of the RA.

The proper positioning of the pressure transducer is of the utmost importance in order to ensure an accurate reading of CVP. The transducer itself needs to be placed at the proper level of the heart. If the transducer is placed too high, you will get a false low reading of the CVP. If the transducer is placed too low, you will get a false high reading of the CVP. Ideally the transducer should be placed 5cm posterior to the left sternal border at the 4th intercostal space. This is the point that best represents the upper fluid level of the RA.

CVP Waveform

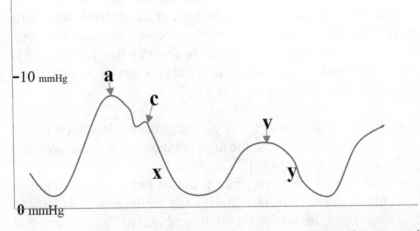

Interpreting the CVP waveform is something that you will gain experience with when you rotate through critical care. The CVP waveform is going to appear on the monitor. It will usually be right underneath the EKG waveform.

There are 3 upward waves (a, c, and v) and 2 downward waves (x & y)

wave	what it represents	when it is happening
a wave	atrial contraction	end of diastole
c wave	closing of tricuspid	early systole
x wave (descent)	ventricular contraction, atrial relaxation	mid systole
v wave	rapid, late systolic filling of atrium prior to the tricuspid opening	late systole
y wave (descent)	tricuspid opening – early ventricular filling	early diastole

The high point of the A wave (indicated by the arrow) is the atrial pressure at maximum atrial contraction. During the period of the A wave, the atrial pressure is greater than the ventricular diastolic pressure. At this point, the atrium is contracted and therefore the tricuspid is open. The high point of the A wave thus closely coincides with the right ventricular end diastolic pressure. *The key to visualizing all of this is to realize that when the tricuspid valve is open and the right ventricle is full - the ventricle, atrium and vena cava are all continuous.*

- To obtain the *mean* CVP, you can take the low point on the A curve and add it to the high point on the A curve and then divide that sum in half.
- Looking at the curve on the previous page – the low point on the A curve is about 1 mmHg and the high point is about 9 mmHg. The sum of that is 10, and half of 10 is 5 – and that is just about right since average CVP is 2 – 6 mmHg.

H. Pulmonary Artery Pressure (Swan Ganz)

The pressure in the pulmonary artery is often a parameter that is monitored. Pulmonary artery pressure is measured with a pulmonary artery catheter otherwise known as a Swan Ganz catheter. The Swan Ganz catheter is a thin flexible tube with a balloon located around the distal end of the catheter. The catheter is inserted through a large vein (often the subclavian vein) and threaded into the RA and then through the tricuspid valve into the RV. The catheter is then advanced through the pulmonary valve into the pulmonary artery. The balloon facilitates the threading of the catheter to its proper placement in the pulmonary artery by means of blood flow. When the balloon is inflated, it then "wedges" the catheter in the pulmonary artery where it is able to provide an indirect measurement of the pressure in the LA. The Swan Ganz catheter therefore enables measurement of pressures in the right atrium, right ventricle, pulmonary artery, and the pulmonary capillary wedge pressure (the filling pressure of the left atrium).

Insofar as the Swan Ganz provides a measurement of the **pulmonary capillary wedge pressure (PCWP)**, it is necessary for you to understand what this is telling you. When the balloon is inflated, it occludes the pulmonary artery at that point – so the pressure you are getting is very close to that of the LA. This is because from the point of where the pulmonary artery is occluded all the way through the rest of the pulmonary vasculature to the left atrium is basically acting as one long catheter that is able to "read" the pressure all the way to the LA. If the LA pressure is elevated – then the PCWP will reflect this by also being elevated. This is important to know because it is often *left ventricular failure* and/or *mitral valve stenosis* that causes an elevation in LA pressure – and thus an elevated PCWP. When the left ventricle is failing, or there is mitral valve stenosis, blood can get backed up in the LA and this will raise the pressure in the LA which is then seen as elevated PCWP. Elevated LA pressure is translated all the way back to the pulmonary capillaries where it raises the hydrostatic pressure in the pulmonary capillaries and can thus cause pulmonary edema. In fact, PCWP is considered the gold standard for determining pulmonary edema.

- Normal PCWP is 4 – 12mmHg
- PCWP > 18mmHg – early signs of pulmonary edema
- PCWP > 25mmHg – pulmonary edema

Causes of high PCWP
- Hypervolemia
- Left ventricular failure
- Mitral valve stenosis

Treatment could include administration of vasodilators and/or drugs that increase contractility of the heart.

Causes of low PCWP
- Low CO (cardiac output)

Treatment could include administration of IV fluids.

I. Cardiac Index

The cardiac index is the parameter that enables you to evaluate cardiac performance as a function of a patient's body size. The cardiac index is calculated as a ratio of the cardiac output to the body surface area over the course of one minute.

$$CI \text{ (cardiac index)} = \frac{CO \text{ (cardiac output)}}{BSA \text{ (body surface area)}}$$

$$or \quad CI = \frac{HR \times SV}{BSA}$$

- Normal range of cardiac index in rest is $2.6 - 4.2$ L/min/m^2.

- CI < 1.8 L/min/m^2 may be indicative of cardiogenic shock.

Chapter 7

Selected Topics in Oxygen Therapy (and Other Medical Gases)

A. The Dangers & Risks of Supplemental Oxygen

Great caution must be taken in the administration of oxygen as it has the potential to be quite toxic. At high oxygen concentrations, there is overproduction of oxygen free radicals that are very damaging to cells. The dangers of supplemental oxygen and oxygen toxicity (to include absorption atelectasis) will be given attention in this section.

Oxygen Toxicity

When it comes to oxygen toxicity, the degree of harmfulness is primarily determined by the PO_2 and the exposure time. Insofar as P_B is stable, it is going to be the FiO_2 that ultimately determines PO_2. Administering oxygen at an $FiO_2 > 50\%$ over a period of time > 24 hours can cause oxygen toxicity. Pulmonary toxicity can occur when administering a high FiO_2 at normal ambient pressures whereas CNS toxicity tends to occur when the patient is being given oxygen at a pressure above 1 ATM (hyperbaric pressure).

Therefore:

- Only give a patient an FiO_2 of 100% for 24 hrs. or less.
- High FiO_2's must be reduced to 70% within 48 hrs.
- And then further reduced to 50% within another 72 hrs.

Consider the following to understand the implications of exposing a patient to 100% oxygen:

<u>Effects of 100% O_2 < 6 hours</u>

1. Increased V_E (about a 5 – 20% increase)

- This happens due to an increase in CO_2 and local irritation. - 100% O_2 binds all the Hb leaving Hb unable to transport any CO_2 – hence the $PaCO_2$ rises and then V_E increases in an effort to get rid of the CO_2. Although CO_2 transport via Hb only accounts for about 21% of the total CO_2 transport (revisit chapter 3 if necessary to review CO_2 transport), that 21% is nonetheless significant enough that V_E will increase in an effort to get rid of the CO_2.

2. Absorption Atelectasis (N_2 washout atelectasis)

Realize that nitrogen is the gas that occupies the majority of the space in the respiratory tract. It is after all 78% of the air that you breathe. Nitrogen doesn't get absorbed across the A/C membrane; in fact you can just think of nitrogen as a place holder – it serves to help maintain the volume so as to keep the lungs open. But if you start breathing 100% oxygen, which is absorbed, and then consider that the CO_2 that is exchanged is exhaled – you have nothing left in the alveolar space to help keep it open. Whatever nitrogen that was in the lungs prior to the initiation of high FiO_2 oxygen therapy has now been "washed out" by the high concentration of oxygen and is no longer there to help maintain any alveolar volume – hence atelectasis will surely ensue.

- Absorption atelectasis can start to occur as soon as 30 minutes after initiation of O_2 therapy with 100% FiO_2.

- It occurs mostly with alveoli that are partially obstructed or in a dependent position.

- Atelectasis creates a V/Q imbalance because V becomes lower with respect to Q, hence you will have an increased physiologic shunt and worsened blood oxygenation.

- Absorption atelectasis is usually not a problem with patients that are awake and alert as periodic sighing and/or yawning will prevent alveolar collapse – but pay attention to them.

There is always an increased risk for absorption atelectasis when the FiO2 > 50%. And regardless of the FiO_2, pay particular attention to post-operative patients that are spontaneously breathing as they usually have lower V_T's due to pain and/or sedation.

Effects of 100% O_2 > 6 hours

1. Acute Tracheobronchitis – occurs after about 6 hours
   - Cough
   - Substernal chest pain
   - Depressed ciliary activity
   - Reduced mucus clearance

2. Pulmonary Function Measurements
   - Generally normal for 24 hours.
   - After 24 hours, VC (vital capacity) decreases.

3. Chest X-Ray (CXR)
   - Usually remains grossly normal for 1 – 4 days, except for decreasing VC.
   - *Decreased VC is the best objective index for pulmonary O_2 toxicity, and it is best observed on a CXR.*

4. After 1 – 4 days, the patient begins to have signs similar to bronchopneumonia.
   - Progressive dyspnea
   - Productive cough
   - Increased $P(A - a)O_2$

- Diffuse patchy infiltrates on CXR (more prominent in the lower lung fields)
- Basilar crackles

Pathophysiology of pulmonary oxygen toxicity

Pulmonary oxygen toxicity occurs in two phases – the early exudative phase, and the late proliferative phase.

Exudative Phase: this is the early phase – the phase where damage is done. The central issue is significant alveolar injury (damage to the alveolar epithelium). This phase occurs between 24 – 48 hours of exposure to an FiO_2 of 100%.

Signs of destruction and damage to the Type I Pneumocytes of the A/C membrane:

- Interstitial, perivascular, & intra-alveolar edema.
- Hemorrhage
- Influx of polymorphonuclear leukocytes (mainly neutrophils and macrophages).
- Pulmonary capillary endothelial necrosis.

These events cause build-up of fluid in the alveoli which then causes V/Q to be low (very low V with respect to Q) which results in physiologic shunting and hypoxemia.

Proliferative Phase: this is the late phase – the phase where the body makes an attempt to repair the damage. This phase occurs around day 4 of exposure to an FiO_2 of 100%.

- Type 2 pneumocytes increase until they virtually line the alveoli. (Remember that besides making surfactant, type 2 pneumocytes can make new type 1 pneumocytes – this is the attempt to repair the damage done to the type 1 cells.)
- Proliferation of fibroblasts in the pulmonary interstitium.
- Hyaline membranes form in alveolar region and pulmonary fibrosis and hypertension develop.

B. Oxygen Delivery Systems

Protocol Driven Oxygen Therapy – A therapist driven oxygen therapy protocol provides the following:

1) The patient receives an initial assessment.
2) The patient is evaluated for a *particular* protocol.
3) A treatment plan is implemented that is subject to modification as needed.
4) The O_2 therapy is D/C when no longer necessary.

When selecting an oxygen delivery approach, always remember the following: Purpose, Patient, & Performance.

Purpose: 1) Provide a sufficiently high enough FiO_2 to treat arterial hypoxemia.
2) Decrease the symptoms of hypoxia & decrease myocardial workload.

Patient: Consider the following with respect to your patient:
1) The underlying reason for their hypoxemia.
2) Their LOC
3) Their age
4) Are they predominately a nose or mouth breather?
5) Do they have a trach?
6) How stable is their V_E?

Performance: 1) If a patient is critically ill, they need a much more stable FiO_2 – use a fixed performance device. The goal is to maintain a $PaO_2 > 60$ mmHg with a $SaO_2 > 90\%$.
2) If the patient is less acute, there is less concern for the stability of the FiO_2 – you can use a variable performance device such as a nasal cannula or a simple mask.

With patients with chronic lung disease, the goal is to ensure adequate oxygenation without depressing ventilation. This is best met with a low flow nasal cannula or a low concentration air entrainment mask. Maintain PaO_2 at 50 – 70 mmHg for a SaO_2 between 85 – 92%.

Low Flow & High Flow – Variable vs. Fixed Performance

Before getting into the various oxygen delivery systems I want to take a moment to discuss the difference between low & high flow and variable vs. fixed performance. In clinical practice, low flow is often used interchangeably with variable performance and high flow is often used interchangeably with fixed performance. It is important however to understand the distinctions of what these terms imply so as to know what is most appropriate for the needs of your patient.

Low Flow / Variable Performance

A low flow device is a device that delivers O_2 at a flow rate that is generally < 8 - 10 LPM. It is not a sufficient enough flow rate to meet a patient's inspiratory demand. A low flow device provides a portion of the patient's V_E as pure oxygen, however the rest of the patient's V_E is entrained from the room air (the patient inspires it through their nose or mouth). Now the reason why the low flow device is considered to be of variable performance is because it is not able to *guarantee* a stable FiO_2. Variable performance by definition means that the FiO_2 will vary. Depending upon a patient's inspiratory effort (V_T, PIFR, and f), their PIFR often exceeds the flow rate of the device that is delivering the oxygen and there are fluctuations in V_T from breath to breath. Remember the discussion in chapter 1 on Bernoulli and air entrainment? Although Bernoulli's principle is not occurring in this case – air entrainment still is - the patient is doing the entraining themselves through their nose. Oxygen is being delivered at 100% from the wall source and the patient is mixing room air with that 100% oxygen with every breath that they take. The problem is that not every single breath that a patient takes is consistently always the same – so therefore the amount of air they entrain from breath to breath varies. This variation in the amount of entrained air causes variation in the FiO_2 – hence the reason why it is called a variable performance device.

Factors affecting the FiO_2 of a low flow system

V_T a decrease in the patient's V_T results in an increase in FiO_2.
because a decrease in V_T means less ambient air is being entrained, hence a higher FiO_2.
an increase in the patient's V_T results in a decrease in FiO_2.
because an increase in V_T means more ambient air is being entrained, hence a lower FiO_2.

PIFR   a decrease in the patient's PIFR results in an increase in FiO_2.
because a decreased PIFR means less ambient air is being entrained, hence a higher FiO_2.
an increase in the patient's PIFR results in a decrease in FiO_2.
because an increased PIFR means more ambient is air being entrained, hence a lower FiO_2.

RR   a decrease in the patient's RR results in an increase in FiO_2.
an increase in the patient's RR results in a decrease in FiO_2.

As long as the patient's breathing is stable, the variation in FiO_2 isn't that drastic, however it is still said to be variable insofar as it cannot guarantee a specific FiO_2 for every breath. We do have established FiO_2's for the various levels of flow for low flow devices, however it is with the understanding that it is variable. Those FiO_2's will be covered in the discussions of the various low flow devices that follow. The most *common* devices in this category are the nasal cannula and the simple mask.

High Flow / Fixed Performance

A high flow device is a device that delivers O_2 at a flow rate that is *generally* ≥ 60 LPM. Unlike low flow devices that only provide a portion of a patient's flow demand, a high flow device either meets or even exceeds a patient's inspiratory demands. As long as the device delivers a level of flow that meets or exceeds the patient's demand, the device can ensure fixed performance. The average PIFR during regular tidal breathing for a normal adult is *approximately* 3 x V_E. Since a V_E of 20 L/min. is generally considered to be the maximum level of ventilation that could be sustained by a patient that was sick, a flow rate of 60 LPM (3 x 20 L/min.) is usually sufficient to meet the flow demands of most patients. These devices are considered to be fixed performance because they are able to deliver a specific desired FiO_2. Fixed performance by definition means that the FiO_2 that is delivered is fixed. A fixed performance device is able to do this because there is no air entrainment by the patient through their nose that could alter the FiO_2 – 100% of the flow to the patient is being delivered by the high flow device. It doesn't matter if there is variation with a patient's V_T, PIFR, or RR because for any given breath – 100% of the flow for that breath is being given by the device, and hence the reason why it ensures a stable FiO_2. The most *common* devices in this category are the Venturi mask, the partial rebreather and non-rebreather mask, and the high flow nasal cannula.

Low Flow Systems

Nasal Cannula

The following chart gives you the approximate FiO_2 for the given flow rate when using a nasal cannula. Remember that the actual FiO_2 is influenced by the patient's V_T, PIFR, and RR, and whether they are breathing predominately through their nose or mouth. Notice that for each LPM of increased flow you increase the FiO_2 by 4%.

Flow Rate	FiO$_2$	
1 LPM	24%	*for neonates* – flow rates between
2 LPM	28%	0.25 – 2 LPM can produce FiO_2's
3 LPM	32%	between 35% - 70%
4 LPM	36%	
5 LPM	40%	
6 LPM	44%	

The nasal cannula should have a bubble humidifier attached if the flow rate is > 4 LPM in order to prevent patient discomfort. Flow rates higher than 6 LPM do not produce significantly higher FiO_2's and tend to cause nasal bleeding and/or drying of the nasal mucosa. Therefore – if you need a flow rate higher than 6 LPM, the nasal cannula is NOT the device of choice.

The nasal cannula is most suitable for patients who are in stable condition such that low flow oxygen with variable FiO_2 performance is sufficient enough to provide adequate oxygenation.

Simple Mask

The simple mask is one of the most commonly used low flow oxygen delivery devices. Just like the nasal cannula and the other low flow devices, the simple mask is also a variable performance device. The following little chart will give the FiO_2's that are associated with particular flow rates.

Flow Rate	FiO_2
5 – 6 LPM	40%
6 – 7 LPM	50%
7 – 8 LPM	60%

The simple mask utilizes flow rates between 5 – 10 LPM and generates FiO_2's from 40 – 60%. The FiO_2 varies because this is a variable performance device, so it is not a good choice if the patient needs a well-defined FiO_2. If more than 10 LPM is needed for the desired oxygenation, you need to use a different device. Realize that the mask itself is a 100 – 200ml reservoir – and it serves as an extension to the anatomic reservoir. This is why the simple mask can deliver a higher FiO_2 than a nasal cannula. But also realize that at flow rates < 5 LPM, the mask acts more like dead space and will then cause rebreathing of CO_2 because flow rates < 5LPM are not sufficient enough to wash out exhaled gas. Therefore, when using a simple mask, you always have to have the flow rate set to *at least* 5 LPM.

High Flow Systems

The first two devices to be discussed in this section are the partial rebreathing mask and the non-rebreather mask. These two devices don't exactly qualify as "high flow" as per the definition of high flow being $\geq$ 60 LPM, however they certainly are not low flow either - so they are being discussed here.

Partial Rebreathing Mask & Non-Rebreathing Mask

Both of these devices essentially look like a simple mask with a bag attached (typically a 1 liter bag). The bag acts as a gas reservoir and hence the reason why these devices can deliver much higher FiO_2's than a simple mask or a nasal cannula – although the non-rebreathing mask can deliver a higher FiO_2 than the partial rebreathing mask. Both of these devices must be run with a flow rate that is *at least* 10 LPM in order to prevent the bag from collapsing when the patient inhales. In most cases these devices are run with flow rates of 15 LPM or higher.

The fundamental difference between a partial rebreathing mask and a non-rebreathing mask is that a partial rebreathing mask has no valves whereas a non-rebreathing mask does. The ultimate implication of this is the level of FiO_2 that can be delivered.

Consider the following explanations:

With a partial rebreathing mask - when the patient inhales they are receiving gas from the bag, the O_2 source, and some entrained air as well as there are holes on the side of the mask. While the patient is exhaling, the bag is getting refilled from the source, however since there are no valves that separate the mask from the bag, the first 1/3 of the patient's exhalation (approximately 150ml) also goes into the bag as well – hence the reason for calling it a *partial* rebreathing mask. At about 1/3 of the way through the patient exhaling the bag is full again (from a combination of being filled by the source and the first 1/3 of the patient's exhalation) such that the remaining 2/3 of the patient's exhalation goes through the ports on the mask into the room. The important thing for you to realize is that the first 1/3 of the patient's exhalation that went into the bag came from the last portion of gas that they had inhaled on the previous breath. That last portion of gas that they inhaled on their previous breath never participated in gas exchange because it was all contained within the anatomic dead space where no gas exchange occurs (the conducting airways). There was therefore no depletion of O_2 nor any gain of CO_2 in that first 1/3 that they exhaled into the bag. As long as the flow rate is high enough to keep the bag from collapsing more than 1/3 during inhalation, there are usually no issues with rebreathing significant amounts of CO_2. The partial rebreathing mask is therefore what we might call a *moderate flow* device, but yet still variable performance insofar as the FiO_2 does vary as the partial rebreathing mask is still vulnerable to a considerable amount of gas dilution due to air entrainment because of the ports on the side of the mask and the fact that the mask itself does not maintain a perfect seal on the patient's face. Depending on the flow rate, partial rebreathing masks can generally achieve FiO_2's from 40 – 70%.

With a non-rebreathing mask - none of the patient's exhaled gas goes back into the bag. The mechanics of operation are essentially the same as a partial rebreathing mask except that a non-rebreathing mask has one way valves to prevent the patient's exhaled gas from entering the bag. The patient inhales 100% O_2 from the bag and the source, and during exhalation all of the exhaled gas exits the mask via a one-way valve and is prevented from entering the bag due to another one-way valve. (the one-way valve on the mask only allows gas to flow from the mask to the outside, and the one-way valve between the bag and the mask only allows gas flow from the bag into the mask). Because of there being 100% O_2 in the bag, the non-rebreathing mask offers a higher FiO_2 than the partial rebreathing mask. Depending on the flow rate, non-rebreathing masks can generally achieve FiO_2's from 60 – 80%. In theory, since the valves prevent any rebreathing and there is thus only 100% oxygen being delivered to the patient – you would think that the FiO_2 should be 100%. The reason why it isn't 100% and ranges instead from 60 – 80% (depending on flow rate) is as follows:

- There are 2 one-way valves on the mask – they both only allow gas flow from the mask to the outside. But for safety reasons, one of them is almost always removed. This is so that if there is a failure with the source gas that the patient can still breath air through the room. With the removal of that valve, air is now able to be entrained that will dilute the 100% gas from the bag.

- Most masks also do not provide a really good seal on the patient's face – so therefore you have leakage and thus air entrainment.

- The amount of air entrainment is going to depend upon the flow rate of the gas and the patient's PIFR.

The non-rebreathing mask is therefore what we would also call a *moderate flow* device, but yet still variable performance insofar as the FiO_2 does vary as the non-rebreathing mask is still vulnerable to gas dilution due to air entrainment because of the removal of one of the valves on mask and the fact that the mask itself does not maintain a perfect seal on the patient's face. Yes – in theory you could say it was fixed performance if both valves were on the mask and the mask had a perfect airtight seal – but such is not the case in clinical reality, so therefore the non-rebreather is variable performance device. But because it is able to achieve FiO_2's in the 60 – 80% range, the non-rebreather is very often the device of choice in the case of emergencies where a high FiO_2 is needed.

Blending Systems

A blending system is a system where you have 2 separate flowmeters – one flowmeter that is specifically for oxygen and another flowmeter that is for regular air. The blending system takes the flow from each of these flowmeters and combines them so as to give you an FiO_2 and a total flow rate. This is true high flow as the flow rates are usually ≥ 60 LPM, and they are fixed performance as they deliver a controlled FiO_2. A blending system is often useful for a patient with a high V_E that needs a high FiO_2 as well, but the problem is that these systems are prone to inaccuracy and failure. But when they do work they are quite good. If you are using a blending system on a neonate, always keep an O_2 analyzer in line at all times.

The following 2 tables will give you the FiO_2 and total flow rate you will get as a function of blending oxygen and air. Table 1 has O_2 as the primary gas with you blending air into the O_2, and table 2 has air as the primary gas with you blending O_2 into the air. As you will see from the two tables below, you have a lot of flexibility in your selection depending upon the FiO_2 needs and flow demands of your patient.

Table 1
Primary gas source: OXYGEN
Secondary gas source: AIR

Primary	Secondary	Total flow	FiO_2
(O_2 flowrate - LPM)	(Air flowrate - LPM)		
40	0	40 LPM	100 %
40	5	45 LPM	91.2 %
40	10	50 LPM	84.2 %
40	15	55 LPM	78.4 %
40	20	60 LPM	73.6%
40	25	65 LPM	69.6%
40	30	70 LPM	66.1%
40	35	75 LPM	63.1%
40	40	80 LPM	60.5%
40	45	85 LPM	58.1%
40	50	90 LPM	56.1%
40	55	95 LPM	54.2%
40	60	100 LPM	52.6%
40	65	105 LPM	51.1%
40	70	110 LPM	49.7%

Table 2
Primary gas source: AIR
Secondary gas source: OXYGEN

Primary (Air flowrate - LPM)	Secondary (O$_2$ flowrate - LPM)	Total flow	FiO$_2$
40	0	40 LPM	20.9%
40	1	41 LPM	22.9%
40	2	42 LPM	24.8%
40	3	43 LPM	26.5%
40	4	44 LPM	28.2%
40	5	45 LPM	29.8%
40	6	46 LPM	31.3%
40	7	47 LPM	32.8%
40	8	48 LPM	34.2%
40	9	49 LPM	35.5%
40	10	50 LPM	36.8%
40	15	55 LPM	42.5%
40	20	60 LPM	47.3%
40	25	65 LPM	51.4%
40	30	70 LPM	54.9%
40	35	75 LPM	57.9%
40	40	80 LPM	60.5%
40	45	85 LPM	62.8%
40	50	90 LPM	64.9%
40	55	95 LPM	66.7%
40	60	100 LPM	68.4%
40	65	105 LPM	69.9%
40	70	110 LPM	71.3%

Air Entrainment Mask (note that venturi, or venti mask is a misnomer)

An air entrainment mask is a device that operates on the principle air entrainment. In section G of chapter 1, the physics of air entrainment was discussed in detail. Understanding the physics of air entrainment is important enough that I will reiterate some of that material now. If necessary, you can return to that section in chapter 1 for the complete discussion.

To reiterate from chapter 1 - when a fluid (gas flowing from the wall source) encounters a very narrow passageway (the jet that is part of the air entrainment mask), the velocity of the gas increases and the lateral pressure decreases (Bernoulli's Principle). Remember that the increase in velocity can be so great that it will cause the lateral pressure to drop below ambient. That lateral pressure is the pressure that the gas is exerting inside the tube. Remember also that there is not only gas flowing through the tube that is feeding into the adapter (where the jet is contained), but there is also gas (air) in the room surrounding the adapter. If the gas that is flowing through the tube is forced into a jet of much smaller diameter such that its velocity increases to the point where that causes the lateral pressure to drop below ambient (and thus become negative with respect to the pressure in the room), then the air in the room surrounding the adapter is going to flow into the opening on the adapter (the entrainment port) and thus be entrained into the overall flow of gas going to the patient. This happens because gases will naturally flow from areas of higher pressure to lower pressure. If the pressure has dropped to below ambient within the adapter, then the air in the room which is at higher pressure is going to flow into the entrainment port on the adapter. Thus you have room air at 21% O_2 flowing into the entrainment port that is now being combined with the 100% O_2 that is coming from the wall – and that mixing will result in the 100% O_2 from the wall being reduced down to the FiO_2 desired.

The air entrainment device therefore serves 2 overall purposes:

1) You already have flow coming from the wall according to however many LPM you have the flow meter set at. Now that you are also entraining room air as well, you have effectively increased

the total flow of gas to the patient. This is important as you always want to be able to deliver enough flow to meet a patient's inspiratory flow demand.

2) As already discussed, it is a way to be able to deliver a specific percentage of gas (FiO_2). To reiterate – Oxygen comes out of the wall at 100%. If you only want 60%, then you attach an adapter that has an entrainment port of appropriate size so as to mix enough room air with the 100% oxygen coming from the wall in order to bring the percentage of oxygen down to 60%.

The amount of air entrained depends on 2 things.

1) The size of the jet
   - Making the jet smaller increases the amount of air entrained and thus increases total flow.

2) The size of the air entrainment ports
   - For a fixed jet size – increasing the size of the air entrainment ports will increase the volume of air that is entrained and thus increase total flow.

Now that the physics of how the air entrainment mask works has been reviewed, let us return to discussing the actual use of an air entrainment mask. The air entrainment mask can be considered true high flow at FiO_2's $\leq 35\%$. This is because at an $FiO_2 \leq 35\%$ you can achieve a total flow rate ≥ 60 LPM. This makes the air entrainment mask particularly useful with hypoxemic COPD patients because these patients usually only get an FiO_2 between 24 – 35%, and at that FiO_2, the flow will always be adequate to meet their flow demands. *But you have to be mindful and remember that in order to have true high flow, you have to keep the $FiO_2 \leq 35\%$.*
The central issue involved with using an air entrainment mask is in determining the amount of total flow you are going to get. And that is dependent on the FiO_2 that you set. Most physicians that are experienced with this are going to know that if they want to achieve high flow that they have to order an FiO_2 that is $\leq 35\%$. Having said that, let me show you the two ways that will enable you

to determine the amount of flow you will achieve as a function of the FiO_2.

The first way is to use what one of my professors referred to as the magic box. In my opinion it is not only more time consuming and requires calculations, but it also only provides a rough estimate of the air:O_2 ratio – and it is not even a good estimate when the FiO_2 is < 40%. The second way is to memorize the chart that I have made for you because not only is it exact, but it has everything in it that you need to know. But I will cover the magic box since you may see it on an exam.

The magic box

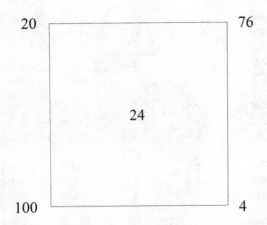

Here is how it works:

100 ALWAYS goes at the bottom left
20 ALWAYS goes at the top left
The FiO_2 you desire ALWAYS goes in the middle of the box

The 76 comes from subtracting 100 – 24. (*76 is the air part of the ratio*)
The 4 comes from subtracting 20 – 24 (don't worry about the negative sign – everything is positive). (*4 is the O₂ part of the ratio*)

Now you look at the 76 and the 4 as a quotient – 76/4, which is 19, and you set that 19 as a ratio to 1 - which is 19:1. And this is why I say that it's not even a good rough estimate because the air:O_2 ratio at an FiO_2 of 24% is 25:1 – NOT 19:1. The magic box doesn't start to become reasonably accurate until you get up to an FiO_2 of 40%. From 40% on up the magic box is pretty accurate, but realize that in order to achieve high flow you cannot exceed an FiO_2 of 35% - so since you are mostly concerned with the flow you are getting at FiO_2's at or below 35%, my advice to you is to memorize the chart below – and copy it and keep it in the pocket of your lab coat.

100% O2	Entrained Air	Air:O2 ratio	Total Parts	Total Flow	FiO2
1 LPM	25 LPM	25 to 1	26	26 LPM	24% (.24)
4 LPM	100 LPM	25 to 1	26	104 LPM	24% (.24)
1 LPM	10 LPM	10 to 1	11	11 LPM	28% (.28)
4 LPM	40 LPM	10 to 1	11	44 LPM	28% (.28)
1 LPM	8 LPM	8 to 1	9	9 LPM	30% (.30)
4 LPM	32 LPM	8 to 1	9	36 LPM	30% (.30)
1 LPM	5 LPM	5 to 1	6	6 LPM	35% (.35)
4 LPM	20 LPM	5 to 1	6	24 LPM	35% (.35)
8 LPM	40 LPM	5 to 1	6	48 LPM	35% (.35)
1 LPM	3 LPM	3 to 1	4	4 LPM	40% (.40)
4 LPM	12 LPM	3 to 1	4	16 LPM	40% (.40)
8 LPM	24 LPM	3 to 1	4	32 LPM	40% (.40)
1 LPM	1.7 LPM	1.7 to 1	2.7	2.7 LPM	50% (.50)
4 LPM	6.8 LPM	1.7 to 1	2.7	10.8 LPM	50% (.50)
8 LPM	13.6 LPM	1.7 to 1	2.7	21.6 LPM	50% (.50)
1 LPM	1 LPM	1 to 1	2	2 LPM	60% (.60)
4 LPM	4 LPM	1 to 1	2	8 LPM	60% (.60)
8 LPM	8 LPM	1 to 1	2	16 LPM	60% (.60)
1 LPM	0.6 LPM	0.6 to 1	1.6	1.6 LPM	70% (.70)
4 LPM	2.4 LPM	0.6 to 1	1.6	6.4 LPM	70% (.70)
8 LPM	4.8 LPM	0.6 to 1	1.6	12.8 LPM	70% (.70)
1 LPM	0.3 LPM	0.3 to 1	1.3	1.3 LPM	80% (.80)
1 LPM	0 LPM	0 to 1	1	1 LPM	100% (1)
4 LPM	0 LPM	0 to 1	1	4 LPM	100% (1)
8 LPM	0 LPM	0 to 1	1	8 LPM	100% (1)

When it comes to knowing what total flow will be (which is what you are concerned with), it is the air:O_2 ratio that will tell you what this is going to be. *The air:O_2 ratio tells you the factor by which you multiply the liter flow of oxygen in order to know the liter flow of air that is entrained.* Understand what this means: Go the first line of the chart – the air:O_2 ratio is 25:1. This is the air:O_2 ratio for when the FiO$_2$ is 24%. What this means is that when the FiO$_2$ is 24%, for every LPM of flow you have for O_2, you are going to have 25 times that amount of air being entrained into the device. So if your flow of O_2 from the wall source is at 1 LPM, you will entrain 25 LPM of air and have a total flow of 26 LPM at an FiO$_2$ of 24%. Now 26 LPM isn't "high flow", but look what happens when you raise the flow of the O_2 flowmeter to 4 LPM. We're on the second line of the chart now – still 24% FiO$_2$ which is still a 25:1 air:O_2 ratio. By having raised the flow of the O_2 to 4 LPM, the flow of the air is now 100 LPM because 25 x 4 = 100. And that results in a total flow of 104 LPM which totally high flow. At an FiO$_2$ of 24%, the amount of air entrained is always going to be 25 times the flow of the oxygen.

Let's skip down now to the part of the chart where the FiO$_2$ is 35%. At an FiO$_2$ of 35%, the air:O_2 ratio is 5:1. This means that for every LPM of flow from the O_2 flowmeter, there will be 5 times as much air entrained. Look at the line where the O_2 flow is 8 LPM. The flow of the air entrained is 40 LPM because 8 x 5 = 40. Therefore the total flow is 8 + 40 = 48 LPM. Now that isn't exactly high flow, but look what happens when you raise the O_2 flow to 10 LPM – 10 LPM of O_2 flow with an air:O_2 ratio of 5:1 will give you 50 LPM of entrained air – and 50 LPM of entrained air added to 10 LPM of O_2 gives you a total of 60 LPM – and that's high flow. The example with 10 LPM of O_2 that I just gave you isn't on the chart – but it doesn't have to be. I purposely picked an example that wasn't on the chart to show you that you can always figure it out very easily.

You will obviously always know the FiO$_2$ that is desired – and by knowing that, you will always know the air:O_2 ratio. The key here is to MEMORIZE the air:O_2 ratios for the respective FiO$_2$'s. If you do that, then no matter what the FiO$_2$ is – by knowing the air:O_2 ratio you will always be able to know the LPM of entrained air as a factor of the LPM of the O_2. And by then knowing both the LPM of the O_2 and the entrained air – you will know your total flow and thus know if it is high enough to be high flow. You already know that the way you select the FiO_2 is to either select the particular FiO_2 you want on the dial on the adapter, or you use a color-coded adapter that is for the particular FiO_2 that you want. Now since you understand air:O_2 ratios, you know how to set the flow on the O_2 flowmeter in order to know how much air will be entrained so as to achieve the total amount of flow you desire.

A few things to keep in mind:

- In order for the air entrainment mask to remain a fixed performance device, the total flow has to exceed the patient's inspiratory demand. As shown already – when you keep the FiO_2 at 35% or less – which results in an air:O_2 ratio of 5:1 or greater – it is very easy to get a total flow $\geq$ 60 LPM which should always be more than enough flow.

- Note also that as you get higher up on the chart ($FiO_2 > 40\%$) that the air:O_2 ratios start to get much smaller which means that you will be entraining significantly less air. At these higher FiO_2's you won't be able to entrain enough air to achieve a total flow sufficient enough to exceed the patient's flow demand. When the flow from the air entrainment device becomes less than the patient's inspiratory demand, then air dilution occurs and the FiO_2 becomes variable.

- The take home message therefore is that when you are using an air entrainment mask and you want to keep it at fixed performance – Keep the $FiO_2 \leq 35\%$.

High Flow Nasal Cannula

Depending upon the needs of the patient, the high flow nasal cannula can often be an excellent choice in oxygen therapy. A high flow nasal cannula can often be used instead of CPAP or NIPPV because the high flow delivered from a high flow nasal cannula is capable of improving issues with hypoxemia and hypercapnia, as well as effectively reducing the patient's WOB. Because of the high flow rates, a high flow nasal cannula is able to keep the upper airway (anatomical dead space) flushed of end expiratory gas that is high in CO_2 which in turn helps with hypercapnia. Not only does the high flow flush the upper airway of CO_2, but this high flow is also simultaneously keeping the anatomic reservoir full of oxygen.

The high flow rate of a high flow nasal cannula also creates the effect of mild pressure that is very similar to the way that PEEP exerts its effects. Although it is not quite exactly the same thing as PEEP, when the patient exhales against an incoming flow that is at such a high flow rate, it has a similar effect as PEEP in that it helps with keeping the alveoli distended. This effect decreases atelectasis, improves V/Q, and thus helps with improving oxygenation. This "PEEP" effect also decreases a patient's WOB and can counteract intrinsic PEEP (autoPEEP) in the same way that applied (extrinsic) PEEP does. A rough estimate is that for every 10 LPM of flow from the high flow nasal cannula, approximately 1 cmH_2O of positive pressure (or "PEEP") is generated.

- A nasal cannula is typically the means of delivery for a high flow nasal cannula system, however it can be adapted to be delivered via a tracheal adapter when needed.

- With a high flow nasal cannula system, the delivered gas is completely humidified (44mg/L) and heated (37°C).

- A high flow nasal cannula is a fixed performance device because the FiO_2 delivered can be considered to be precise. The constant flushing of the upper airway due to the high flow rate essentially maintains an oxygen rich reservoir that reduces the amount of entrained ambient air to such a minimum that the FiO_2 being delivered by the device is truly what is being inspired by the patient.

- The high flow nasal cannula is generally well tolerated by patients because of the gas being humidified and heated. It is much more comfortable than a CPAP or BiPAP, and since it is a nasal cannula, patients can still eat and talk. There is also virtually no need for the sedation that is often needed with more invasive means of therapy.

- Utilizing the high flow nasal cannula is becoming the new trend in oxygen therapy choice post-extubation. Typically when a patient is extubated they are placed on an aerosol mask. Although that is certainly still done, there is a trend now to use the high flow nasal cannula rather than an aerosol mask.

There are several versions of high flow nasal cannula delivery systems available today. The Vapotherm® high flow nasal cannula is capable of delivering flow rates up to 40 LPM with 95 – 100% relative humidity at temperatures ranging from 33°C to 43°C. The Optiflow® high flow nasal cannula can deliver flow rates up to 60 LPM with precise control of humidity and temperature at 44mg/L and 37°C respectively.

With high flow oxygen therapy being utilized more and more often as an oxygen delivery strategy, I cannot urge you enough to become well acquainted with these devices as you do your clinical rotations. They are very effective devices that very often can enable a patient to avoid non-invasive or invasive mechanical ventilation.

Enclosure Systems

Oxygen Tents

The oxygen tent, otherwise known as a Croupette® or a cool mist tent, is essentially a canopy or tent that can be used to treat hypoxemia and help liquefy secretions - mainly with toddlers or small children in cases of croup or cystic fibrosis. It is rarely ever used with adults or older children. It provides an oxygen enriched and humidified environment at temperatures that are often 10 – 12 degrees lower than room temperature. It can provide FiO_2's from 40 – 50% at flows of 12 – 15 LPM, but it is a variable performance device as the FiO_2 will vary due to frequent leaking. Because of the fact that nowadays there are other more efficient and effective ways to deliver oxygen therapy and humidification, the oxygen tent really isn't used all that much.

Oxygen Hoods (oxyhood)

The oxyhood is generally a solid, clear plastic structure that fits over the head of the patient. It is a fixed performance device that is used to deliver controlled FiO_2's up to 100% to neonates. It is therefore considered one of the best methods for O_2 therapy with neonates when fixed performance is needed. The oxyhood is indicated for:

- Hypoxemia (as indicated by decreased SpO_2 or PaO_2)

- Increased WOB

- Respiratory distress

- Cold stress

- Persistent pulmonary hypertension of the newborn (PPHN)

When using the oxyhood with a neonate, there are several things that you need to keep in mind.

- Make sure that the gas temperature is set at NTE (neutral thermal environment). The neutral thermal environment refers to the narrow range of environmental temperatures whereby the neonate is able to maintain its normal body temperature with the least expenditure of energy. The baby's basal metabolic rate and oxygen consumption are at a minimum when you properly maintain a NTE. The idea behind this is to enable the neonate to utilize their energy for growth and other vital functions rather than having to spend energy to keep themselves warm. A precise NTE is a function of the baby's weight and age, however the following are rough guidelines for NTE:

Newborns < 1500 grams   NTE = 35°C

Older infants > 2500 grams   NTE = 32°C

- Make sure the flow rate of gas going into the oxyhood is at least 5 – 10 LPM. It needs to be high enough to flush out exhaled CO_2.

- Be ever so mindful of the consequences of hyperoxia. Oxygen toxicity can cause retinopathy of prematurity.

- Use an O_2 analyzer to monitor the FiO_2 in the hood and regularly check the PaO_2 of the baby. A baby in a NICU is going to have a line in place so nursing will be able to get an ABG for you easily.

Incubators (also known as an Isolette®)

The incubator provides convection heating along with supplemental O_2. It is therefore the best device to provide neonates and infants with a stable NTE. Besides providing strict thermal and humidity control of the environment, the incubator also serves to shield the baby from the noise of the room. If supplemental oxygen therapy if being provided via the environment of the incubator, it is going to be variable performance. Very often, due to the issues related to their pre-maturity and/or condition, the baby is intubated and receiving mechanical ventilation while they are in the incubator. Depending on the situation, the baby could be on high flow, or it is even possible that they could be using an oxyhood. The point of using the incubator is for its ability to provide a very stable and controlled environment. Providing ventilation and/or oxygen therapy can be always delivered via other means while the baby is in the incubator if their needs are beyond the variable performance oxygen therapy that is available through the incubator.

C. Other Medical Gases

<u>NO (Nitric Oxide)</u>

Nitric oxide is a non-flammable gas that has a slight metallic odor at room temperature. Although it is non-flammable, it does support combustion. It has a density of 1.245 kg/m^3 and a specific gravity of 1.04 at 21.1°C at 760mmHg. Nitric oxide is highly unstable in the atmosphere. Nitric oxide exists in 3 biologically active forms in tissue. Those 3 forms are:

- Nitrosonium (NO+)
- Nitroxyl anion (NO-)
- Free radical (NO)

In the presence of air, NO combines with O_2 to form NO_2 (nitrogen dioxide) which is a strong oxidizing agent. In the presence of moisture, NO can form nitrous and nitric acids, both of which can cause corrosion.

Both NO_2 and nitric acid are very toxic and can cause chemical pneumonitis, pulmonary edema, and death.

However – although NO is toxic in high concentrations, experimental data suggest that low doses act as a powerful pulmonary vasodilator. NO acts as a potent pulmonary vasodilator by inducing smooth muscle relaxation through its activation of cGMP. Very low concentrations (2 – 80 ppm) have been used to for the following situations:

- To treat persistent pulmonary hypertension of the newborn (PPHN).
- To reverse pulmonary vasoconstriction in ARDS (acute respiratory distress syndrome).
- It is used as an adjunct to treatment of congenital cardiac defects.
- It is also used to possibly reverse bronchoconstriction caused by histamine and/or methacholine.

As a potent pulmonary vasodilator, the use of NO will help:

- Decrease resistance in the pulmonary vasculature
- Decrease pulmonary arterial pressure

which will then

- Improve shunting
- Improve the PaO_2

N$_2$O (Nitrous Oxide)

Nitrous oxide is a colorless, non-flammable gas with a slightly sweet odor and taste that is slightly soluble in water, alcohol, and oils. It is an oxidizing agent and it supports combustion. Nitrous oxide is used primarily as a CNS depressant.

- Consistent with its CNS depressing effects, N_2O can be used as an anesthetic.

- However, insofar as N_2O is a weak general anesthetic, N_2O must be used in conjunction with other drugs to achieve effective anesthesia.

- Adequate O_2 must always be given along with N_2O – failure to provide sufficient O_2 may cause brain damage or even be fatal.

Heliox

Heliox is used on a limited basis with patients with large airway obstruction. Heliox is a combination gas consisting of helium and oxygen. Whereas the density of oxygen is 1.326 kg/m^3 at 21.1°C and 760mmHg, the density of helium is only 0.165 kg/m^3 at 21.1°C and 760mmHg. The lower density of heliox promotes laminar flow, thus there is much less resistance as it passes through the airway and this translates to a reduction in the patient's work of breathing. It is therefore quite useful as a means to deliver oxygen therapy to patients with severe airway obstruction in cases such as:

- Asthmatic patients with acute respiratory failure
- Post-extubation stridor

Heliox can also be used in the ventilatory support of patients with severe COPD, as well as in the delivery of anesthetic agents, particularly in cases when having to use a very small diameter endotracheal tube.

Heliox comes in 3 forms (or mixtures):

He : O_2

80 : 20	This mixture is 1.8 times less dense than 100% O_2.
70 : 30	This mixture is 1.6 times less dense than 100% O_2.
60 : 40	This mixture is 1.4 times less dense than 100% O_2.

The first two – 80:20 and 70:30 are what you are going to see being used most often in clinical practice.

Now – realize that as a result of not being as dense as oxygen, the actual flow of heliox is greater than the set flow. The factor of the increased amount of flow is consistent with the factor of decreased density just indicated. What this means is as follows:

- If you are using 80:20 heliox – the actual flow is 1.8 times the liter flow of the set flow.

- If you are using 70:30 heliox – the actual flow is 1.6 times the liter flow of the set flow.

- If you are using 60:40 heliox – the actual flow is 1.4 times the liter flow of the set flow.

Example:

You are using 80:20 heliox. The set flow on the flowmeter is 10 LPM.

10 LPM x 1.8 = 18 LPM

18 LPM is the actual flow.

Conversely – you can take the flow rate you *want* and divide that by 1.8 – and then set the flow meter accordingly:

Example: you *want* a flow rate of 10 LPM. Take 10 LPM and divide by 1.8 (10 ÷ 1.8 ≈ 5.5). Set the flow meter at 5.5 LPM – because you know that since the actual flow is 1.8 times greater than the set flow – your actual flow will be 5.5 x 1.8 ≈ 10 LPM.

When giving heliox to a patient that is intubated, the heliox is introduced directly into the ventilator. When giving heliox to a non-intubated patient, administer it via a non-rebreather mask. Do not give heliox via a nasal cannula as there is just too much leakage, and do not give heliox via a hood as the helium collects at the top of the hood.

CO_2/O_2 (Carbogen)

The gas mixture of CO_2/O_2, otherwise known as Carbogen, is used for the following:

- To stimulate ventilation when there is depression of ventilation
    * Inspiration of carbogen is perceived by the body as if it were not receiving adequate O_2. Therefore, the rate and depth of breathing increase, and cardiac output is increased due to an increase in heart rate.

- Treatment of central retinal artery occlusion

- Also used as an adjunct to radiation therapy in the treatment of certain cancers

- Carbogen was used in psychiatric research.

- Although rare, there are some individuals who use carbogen recreationally for its psychedelic effects.

Carbogen is available as:

$CO_2 : O_2$

    5 : 95
    7 : 93

Carbogen is typically administered via a non-rebreather.

Clinical signs of CO_2 toxicity to watch for when administering carbogen:

- Hypoxemia

- Extra systole (pre-mature ventricular contractions)

- Flushed skin

- Full and bounding pulse

- Hypertension

- Muscle twitching

- $PaCO_2 > 70mmHg$

Chapter 8

Selected Topics in Mechanical Ventilation

Whether or not you have intubation privileges will depend entirely on the institutional policies of where you work. The degree of independence and autonomy you will have in ventilator management will also depend on policy as well as the level of trust you have earned from the physicians that you work with. Whether you happen to be in a setting that enables you to exercise independent clinical judgment, or you are in a setting that limits you to following orders or protocols – it is absolutely essential in either case that you understand the basics of mechanical ventilation as you will be one of the main clinicians involved with the care of patients that are being mechanically ventilated. Having said that – it is incumbent upon you to know as much as you possibly can because caring for someone who is being mechanically ventilated is serious business and not to be taken lightly.

The presentation of material in this chapter is going to be succinct and to the point, but yet with enough detail to enable you to understand the rationale behind what is being said. There are volumes of texts and journals on the subject of mechanical ventilation, and as you grow in your understanding of the subtleties of respiratory physiology and gain experience in the clinical nuances of managing patients, those texts will offer many insights into different strategies that can be employed in your attempt to help your patients. But for now, it is essential that you get grounded in basic fundamentals – the bedrock of knowledge on mechanical ventilation upon which everything else you will ever learn about this topic is built.

A. Introduction

Understand that mechanical ventilation is *strictly supportive* – it cannot cure anything. Mechanical ventilation provides a patient with the support they need by sustaining ventilation until the underlying issues which got them on the ventilator in the first place are resolved.

Recall that the two aspects of normal breathing are ventilation and respiration.

Ventilation (spontaneous breathing) – this is the bulk movement of air in and out of the lungs. Of the two aspects of breathing that we are discussing here, when it comes to mechanical ventilation, this is the one that we can *guarantee*. In other words - mechanical ventilation is able to guarantee the bulk movement of air into the lungs. Remember that exhalation is passive.

Respiration – this is gas exchange, and this CANNOT be guaranteed by mechanical ventilation.

External Respiration is gas exchange between the lungs and the blood.

Internal Respiration is gas exchange between the blood and the tissues.

Why can mechanical ventilation guarantee ventilation but not respiration? The ventilator can guarantee ventilation because that is simply a matter of forcing air into the lungs. The ventilator is just an air pump – a rather sophisticated one indeed, but at the end of the day it is fundamentally just acting as a pump to force air into the lungs. Whereas ventilation is just a matter of moving air and can thus be guaranteed by a mechanical ventilator, respiration (gas exchange) is much more complex and involves many other factors that are beyond the scope of what could be guaranteed by a ventilator. There could be problems with the A/C membrane. There could be lung consolidation due to disease. There are any number of other pathological issues that could compromise either external or internal respiration, and although the ventilator is certainly able to help *improve* issues with respiration – it can never guarantee respiration in the same manner as it is able to guarantee ventilation.

As a side note – also realize that your patient's lungs may be perfectly fine and they are receiving mechanical ventilation for reasons other than lung issues. Perhaps they have suffered a traumatic brain injury or maybe they have neuromuscular disease. In either of those cases their lungs are fine but yet they still require mechanical ventilation because they are unable to adequately ventilate on their own due to their condition. But even in cases where we are providing mechanical ventilation to a patient who otherwise has normal healthy lungs, the ventilator can still only guarantee ventilation and can never guarantee respiration. Always keep in mind that mechanical ventilation is supportive – it is providing ventilation until the underlying issues (respiratory or otherwise) are resolved.

B. Indications for an Artificial Airway

1. TO MAINTAIN A PATENT AIRWAY

It is essential to always have a patent (open) airway.

For example - a patient with an edematous airway - airway edema for example that is secondary to smoke inhalation (like a burn patient that was in a fire). You treat this prophylactically with steroids and intubation in order to maintain a patent airway. Airway edema is serious regardless of the cause. The edema itself causes significant narrowing of the airway and therefore it is an "obstruction" to adequate flow of air into the lungs. You cannot risk the edema worsening such that you lose the airway.

2. TO PROTECT THE AIRWAY

It is essential to protect the airway from aspiration.

For example - when a patient has lost their gag reflex due to a drug or alcohol overdose. If a patient lacks an adequate gag reflex for whatever reason such that they cannot protect their airway from aspiration – then you have to intubate.

3. TO FACILLITATE SUCTIONING

It is essential to be able to adequately clear secretions.

For example - a patient whose condition is causing excessive secretions, but yet that patient has an inadequate cough mechanism. Uncleared secretions are obstructions to air flow – so if a patient has excessive secretions but does not have an adequate cough – you'll need to intubate in order that you can suction them.

4. SUPPORT OF VENTILATION

For example - when the patient is under anesthesia, or in the case of when the patient has suffered a traumatic brain injury – or any other reason which would require invasive mechanical ventilation.

The indications for an artificial airway that have just been discussed are different from the indications for mechanical ventilation that we are about to discuss (with the exception of #4 which is common to both categories.) One may ask themselves – *would you ever intubate a patient and then not put them on the ventilator?* – well sometimes maybe, but rarely. Having a patient breath spontaneously through an ETT (endotrachael tube) is going to be challenging as their WOB (work of breathing) will increase because of the additional resistance being imposed by the ETT itself. Look back at the first indication – to maintain a patent airway. In the example given, the patient is breathing on their own and our reason for intubating is to ensure patency of the airway in the event that the edema worsens. Could this patient continue to breath on their own through the ETT? Maybe - but it would certainly require much more effort, and considering the condition they are in already, we are not going to want to add to that burden by causing them to have to work even harder to breath. In a situation like this we would connect them to the ventilator and possibly utilize a partial support mode like pressure support for example that would enable them to continue to spontaneously breath on their own since they are able to anyway, but yet the ventilator will give them some help. The different modes of ventilation will be discussed in detail later in this chapter. Almost all the time - if you're going to intubate, then that means you are going to put the patient on the ventilator. As we turn our attention now to discussing the indications for mechanical ventilation, remember that although mechanical ventilation cannot guarantee respiration, when a patient is unable to achieve appropriate ventilation to maintain adequate gas exchange and/or acid-base balance on their own, then mechanical ventilation is initiated in order give them the best chance at being able to improve and maintain homeostasis.

C. Indications for Mechanical Ventilation

General Indications

1. ACUTE VENTILATORY FAILURE

Acute ventilatory failure is when:

*   pH < 7.30 (acidosis)

these numbers come from the ABG

* $PaCO_2$ > 50mmHg

BUT – use good clinical judgment and KNOW your patient. A chronic COPD patient will often have a "walking & talking" $PaCO_2$ at this level – this means that these numbers may be normal for them and they might not be in any distress. This is why it is important for you to know the history of your patient.

2. IMPENDING VENTILATORY FAILURE

Impending ventilatory failure is when you have progressive hypoventilation and acidosis. You will know if this is happening by looking at the *trends* in the blood gas (ABG). Progressive acidosis is indicated when you start seeing the pH drop over time. Progressive hypoventilation is when you start seeing the $PaCO_2$ rise over time. It is the patient's inability to adequately ventilate that is causing the $PaCO_2$ to rise. The patient isn't moving enough air and thus they are not exhaling enough CO_2 such that it is now starting to build up in the blood – and this is being indicated by the progressive rise in $PaCO_2$ and the simultaneous drop in the pH. Remember that CO_2 acts as an acid - if it builds up in the blood, that is going to be indicated by a drop in the pH.

Trending example:

T_1	pH = 7.39	$PaCO_2$ = 40 mmHg	PaO_2 = 90 mmHg
T_2	pH = 7.32	$PaCO_2$ = 48 mmHg	PaO_2 = 80 mmHg

T_1 for example is the first time you drew a blood gas and saw that all the values indicated are within normal range. Then say two hours later you draw another blood gas (T_2) and you see that the pH has dropped and the $PaCO_2$ is elevated. This is showing a trend of progressive acidosis and hypoventilation. It is indicating impending ventilatory failure. If this trend continues, your numbers are going to reach those of acute ventilatory failure that were just discussed in #1. The idea is to not reach the point of acute failure. By being observant of the trends in the ABG you can see where your patient is headed and thus get them intubated and on mechanical ventilation so as to begin supporting them before they get to the point where they are in full blown acute ventilatory failure.

NOW – don't forget that despite everything that was just said about impending ventilatory failure, you must still observe the clinical manifestation of your patient. You always have to look at your patient to see how they are doing – clinical practice is always about more than just the numbers.

Consider this as an example:

Asthma patients tend to hyperventilate when they are having an asthmatic episode. Now with hyperventilation your numbers are going to be the opposite of what was just discussed. With hyperventilation, they are going to be blowing off even more CO_2 than usual so the blood gas you just got from this patient is going to reflect a pH on the alkaline side (say 7.48) and a $PaCO_2$ of 32 mmHg for example. Now let's say two hours later you get another blood gas on this patient and all their numbers are within perfect normal range and you think to yourself that now they are fine. But are they really? Are their numbers really "normal" - or have they become normal because this patient is now exhausted? All that hyperventilation from their asthmatic episode has made them so tired that their rate and depth of breathing has now slowed down – and it's the slowing down of their rate and depth that has made their ABG numbers seemingly return to normal. But that which now appears as normal with the numbers could in fact be on its way to being impending ventilatory failure because this patient's WOB has been so severe and they have become so tired that they may no longer have enough energy to enable themselves to maintain adequate ventilation. This is why you have to closely observe your patient. Obviously you would consider getting another ABG to see if they were indeed trending towards impending ventilatory failure, but the point of having said all of this is to make you understand that your ability to properly care for your patient involves not only your understanding of numbers and trends, but also being able to make sound clinical judgment based on your observation of them. If this patient has indeed become exhausted and is heading towards not being able to have enough energy to sustain their own ventilation – you're going to know this by your observation of them long before you get that next ABG.

3. SEVERE REFRACTORY HYPOXEMIA

Refractory essentially means "not responding to". In this case, it means that you are giving a patient oxygen therapy with the highest possible FiO_2 (100%), but yet they are not improving. In other words, no matter how much oxygen therapy you give the patient – they do not respond with any improvement.

Severe refractory hypoxemia is when:

$PaO_2 < 40$ mmHg

$SaO_2 < 75\%$

There are a number of issues that could be causing this to happen. There could be atelectasis that is compromising adequate gas exchange. There could be issues with the A/C membrane that are inhibiting gas exchange. The patient could have pneumonia or pulmonary edema, in which case the lung consolidation from either of those would cause shunting that will result in hypoxemia. Lung consolidation is when fluid is in the alveolar space rather than air, and consolidation causes shunting. Shunting is when you have adequate blood perfusion to the alveoli but yet there is no gas in the alveoli to be exchanged. The alveoli aren't ventilated with gas because they're consolidated due to the pneumonia for example. Blood therefore perfuses the alveoli but yet doesn't get to pick up any oxygen because the alveoli are filled up with fluid rather than gas. And that will definitely lead to hypoxemia. Regardless of the cause, when oxygen levels reach the point of indicating hypoxemia to this degree – it is time to intubate and initiate mechanical ventilation.

4. PROPHYLACTIC VENTILATORY SUPPORT

If needed: post – anesthesia
               post - surgery

Specific Indications

1. Apnea or imminent respiratory arrest

2. Hypoxemic respiratory failure that is refractory to a high FiO_2 with high flow OR if accompanied with: patient is unable to to protect their airway, CV instability. altered LOC

3. Ventilatory insufficiency secondary to neuromuscular disease, AND one of the following:

   - VC (vital capacity) < 10 – 15 ml/kg
   - MIP (max inspiratory pressure) > -20 to -30 cmH$_2$O
   - Respiratory acidosis

4. Acute exacerbation of COPD with SOB, tachypnea, respiratory acidosis, AND one of the following:

   - Unable to protect their airway
   - Copious secretions
   - Altered LOC
   - Unable to do NIPPV due to facial problems
   - CV(cardiovascular) instability

D. Contraindications for Mechanical Ventilation

1. UNTREATED TENSION PNEUMOTHORAX

The pneumothorax MUST be treated first before you can put a patient on mechanical ventilation. You cannot introduce positive pressure mechanical ventilation until the integrity of the lung has been re-established by having treated the pneumothorax.

2. PATIENT'S INFORMED CONSENT

Again – you must know who your patients are and be well informed regarding any advance directives they may have.

DNR – Do Not Resuscitate – This means you don't intubate, etc. This is a no code. You do nothing.

DNI – Do Not Intubate – This means that you don't intubate, but you do everything else.

3. MEDICAL FUTILITY

This is a decision made by the physician when you are in a medically hopeless situation. Clinically you have arrived at the point where it has been determined that mechanical ventilation would be of no benefit.

E. Goals & Objectives of Mechanical Ventilation

General Goals & Objectives

1. MAINTAIN PHYSIOLOGIC VENTILATION

To maintain physiologic ventilation means to maintain adequate alveolar ventilation so as to support pulmonary gas exchange. *BUT remember that maintaining normal physiologic ventilation for your patient is in accordance with what is normal for them.* The numbers from the ABG are one thing, but you need to interpret those ABG numbers in light of what you know is going on with your patient. With respect to the fact that mechanical ventilation is a means by which you are able to help a patient to restore and/or maintain arterial and systemic acid/base balance – realize this does not necessarily mean that you are going to manipulate the ventilator in order to achieve textbook normal ABG values for every single patient. As already previously stated – it is incumbent upon you to know what is going on with your patient. Your patient may be a chronic COPDer whose "normal" $PaCO_2$ is say 60 – 65 mmHg. *If this is the case, then your job is to maintain that.* Once you understand more about the complexities of the pathophysiology of COPD, you will understand why you absolutely cannot "over-ventilate" a COPD patient in an effort to bring their $PaCO_2$ down to within normal textbook range. The problem with a chronic COPD patient is not so much with getting air in, but rather with being able to exhale fully. Remember that exhalation is always passive – even when a patient is on a mechanical ventilator. These patients often experience dynamic airway collapse upon exhalation which in and of itself is an obstruction to airflow and this prolongs the time needed to exhale. This reduced ability to exhale is further complicated by the fact that an obstructed airway also causes air trapping at the end of exhalation which in turn causes the pressure in the alveoli to be greater than atmospheric pressure - this is what is known as autoPEEP (positive end-expiratory pressure), and it is self-induced due to their inability to adequately empty their lungs. If you over-ventilate them in an attempt to get their ABG numbers to within textbook normal you are actually going to worsen their condition. You'll end up making them even more acidotic because by over-ventilating them you will have added to the amount they need to exhale which is already more than what they can handle. Over-ventilation is also going to increase the autoPEEP which can cause barotrauma to the lung as well as impede venous return to the heart which will then reduce their cardiac output.

Furthermore, chronic COPDers compensate for their CO_2 retention by having elevated bicarbonate (HCO_3-) levels – this is what enables their pH to remain stable. If you did somehow succeed in normalizing their $PaCO_2$ to textbook normal, then the elevated bicarb that is present due to their natural COPD status will in all likelihood put them in a state of metabolic alkalemia and this is not what you want. Even though the kidneys will excrete the bicarb in a few days and your "numbers" will look good to you and you'll think that you have restored acid-base balance – when you then attempt to wean this patient off the ventilator they will in all likelihood go into acute respiratory acidosis or even respiratory failure because that initial issue of air trapping due to airway collapse that causes them to retain CO_2 is still present. The last few days that you have been monkeying around with the ventilator trying to make their $PaCO_2$ textbook normal and thinking you were giving the kidneys time to enable the bicarbonate levels to go back to normal was actually removing the compensation that their body had adjusted to in order to handle their chronically elevated CO_2 due to their COPD. CO_2 levels can change in a matter of minutes to hours whereas changes in bicarbonate levels take a few days. As soon as you remove them from the ventilator their $PaCO_2$ is going to go back up and their pH is going to drop (all within a matter of minutes to an hour or so) because there will not be enough bicarb to compensate because it'll take another few days for the kidneys to catch up with this and you'll end up with a patient in acute ventilatory failure. Much more will be said of this later in this chapter and also in the pathology chapter when COPD is discussed at length. But hopefully what was covered just now drove home the point of just how critically important it is to *know your patient and to understand that your goal in maintaining physiologic ventilation is to maintain that which is normal for them.*

With it being understood that you are to maintain ventilation in accordance with what is "physiologically normal" for your patient, realize that very often this will indeed just be a matter of you maintaining ventilation so as to maintain textbook normal values for $PaCO_2$. This is called *eucapnic ventilation.*

Eucapnic Ventilation – this is maintaining alveolar ventilation so as to maintain $PaCO_2$ levels within the normal range of 35 – 45 mmHg (40 mmHg). This is the "regular normal" that would be for a patient that did not have obstructive lung disease or other issues that would otherwise require you to have to take into account everything that was just discussed with regards to you maintaining "what is normal for them". In other words, eucapnic ventilation is when your goal is to maintain textbook normal values for $PaCO_2$.

There will be times however, because of the particulars of a patient's condition, that you will need to maintain ventilation that results in having elevated $PaCO_2$ (hypercapnia or hypercarbia). This is referred to as *permissive hypercapnia* because your ventilation strategy is purposely allowing for the elevated $PaCO_2$.

Permissive Hypercapnia – although this is still obviously supporting a patient's alveolar ventilation, it is manipulative in the sense that it is purposely allowing for elevated $PaCO_2$ levels. There are times when it is necessary to implement ventilator strategies that are specifically aimed at protecting the lung, and these strategies involve using low tidal volumes and/or frequencies that will ultimately result in elevated $PaCO_2$ levels. Clinical evidence has shown that the benefit of protecting the lung outweighs the elevated $PaCO_2$ insofar as in most cases elevated $PaCO_2$ is well tolerated.

Examples of this are as follows:

A. COPD – Reducing the tidal volume and/or respiratory rate in order to minimize intrinsic positive end-expiratory pressure (auto-PEEP) in patients with COPD greatly enhances the ability to protect the lung from barotrauma (injury to the lung due to the increased pressure from the autoPEEP). Lower tidal volumes and / or respiratory rates will result in an elevation of $PaCO_2$, however this is permitted for the benefit of protecting the lung.

B. ALI (acute lung injury) – This is a low tidal volume ventilation strategy to protect the lung from ventilator-associated lung injury in patients with acute lung injury. Again, lower tidal volumes will result in an elevation of $PaCO_2$, however this is permitted for the benefit of protecting the lung.

C. ARDS (acute respiratory distress syndrome) – Evidence has clearly shown that low tidal volume ventilation strategies improve outcomes in patients with ARDS. Although the respiratory rate is routinely increased during this low tidal volume ventilation strategy in an effort to maintain adequate minute ventilation, the increases in the respiratory rate may not be sufficient enough to compensate for the low tidal volumes such that hypercapnia may develop. As with the previous two examples, the elevation of $PaCO_2$ is permitted for the benefit conferred by the low volume ventilation strategy.

2. IMPROVE EFFICIENCY OF EXTERNAL RESPIRATION

The key word here is improve – not guarantee. Remember from our earlier discussion that mechanical ventilation can never guarantee respiration – it can only help improve respiration. *But recognize that the usual natural consequence of improving ventilation is to also improve external respiration (gas exchange between the alveoli and the blood).* Once we get into learning about modes and other features of the ventilator, you'll learn about the ways that you can have control over the volume and /or pressure of the breath that you deliver to the patient. In certain instances this enables you to have control over the extent to which you increase the lung volume. Lung expansion therapy can be a very useful *ventilatory strategy* that enables you to treat atelectasis which in turn does wonders to improve external respiration. Extrinsic PEEP (to be discussed in detail later in this chapter) is another feature of mechanical ventilation that is used to help improve oxygenation, and oxygenation *essentially implies* the same thing as external respiration. *(Oxygenation reflects the quality of external respiration)*

Improvement in external respiration, or oxygenation, will result in the patient having a better PaO_2. And if the patient's hemoglobin (Hb), cardiac output (Q_t) and oxygen saturation (SaO_2) are otherwise normal – then improving or optimizing the PaO_2 will then help enhance oxygen delivery to the tissues. Remember oxygen delivery (DO_2) is given by:

$$\dot{D}O_2 \quad = \quad \underbrace{CaO_2}_{\substack{\text{dissolved } O_2 \quad | \quad \text{bound } O_2}} \quad x \quad \dot{Q}_t$$

$$\dot{D}O_2 \quad = \quad [(0.003 \text{ x } \mathbf{PaO_2}) + (Hb \text{ x } 1.34 \text{ x } SaO_2)] \quad x \quad \dot{Q}_t$$

*Improving the efficiency of **external respiration** (i.e. oxygenation – PaO_2) always helps improve DO_2 (as long as Q_t, Hb, and SaO_2 are normal). By improving DO_2 you have enhanced oxygen delivery to the tissues and thus you have helped to optimize **internal respiration** as well. Hopefully this illustration of throwing DO_2 into the picture has started to help you see how things work together.*

3. DECREASE THE WORK OF BREATHING

There are several issues that could cause an increase in a patient's work of breathing (WOB) – an acute asthmatic episode, an exacerbation of COPD, etc. Pretty much anything that is going to cause an increase in resistance in the airway and/or a decrease in lung compliance is going to cause a patient to have to work harder to breathe. When a patient can no longer keep up with the work of breathing, you need to decrease their work of breathing by actually taking over the work of breathing for them by putting them on the ventilator. WOB = $\Delta P \times \Delta V$, and the normal value is 0.5 ± 0.2 joules/L.

4. DECREASE MYOCARDIAL WORK

Whenever a patient's condition is such that it forces them to have to work harder to breath, it places increased demands on the heart. When tissues (respiratory muscles in this case) are having to work harder (from increased WOB), they demand more oxygen. The heart then has to work harder in order for the cardiac output to be sufficient enough to keep up with the oxygen demand of those muscles. So number 3 and number 4 go hand in hand in that the way you decrease the myocardial work is to decrease the work of breathing – and you do that by putting the patient on the ventilator.

Specific goals & objectives for mechanical ventilation:

1. To correct respiratory failure
2. To correct acute respiratory distress
3. To correct hypoxemia
4. To treat atelectasis and maintain FRC
5. To alleviate respiratory muscle fatigue
6. To facilitate sedation and/or paralysis
7. To minimize systemic oxygen consumption
8. To minimize myocardial oxygen consumption

F. Clinical Signs to Recognize Acute Respiratory Failure

When speaking of acute respiratory failure, there are generally 2 types:

1) <u>Hypoxemic Respiratory Failure</u> (this is analogous to what was introduced previously in section C of this chapter under the heading of severe refractory hypoxemia.

2) <u>Hypercapnic Respiratory Failure</u> (this is analogous to what was introduced previously in section C under the heading of acute ventilatory failure.

In some ways, this material could have been covered in section C – Indications For Mechanical Ventilation, but I have chosen to give this its own section in order that you will be able to see the comprehensive nature of what is involved when making determinations as to whether or not you are going to need to intubate and place your patient on mechanical ventilation.   Throughout this chapter I have mentioned several times how important it is to know what is going on with your patient and to have been carefully observing them.   The earlier you are able to determine that your patient is in distress, the better off you will be in being able to help them. This section is going to highlight what that entails.

<u>Determining if your patient is in distress</u>:

- Assess their LOC

- Assess their vital signs
    - Oxygenation – *is it adequate?*
    - Respiratory Rate – *are they tachypneic?*
    - Heart Rate – *are they tachycardic?*
    - Blood Pressure – *are they hyper or hypotensive?*
    - Temperature – *are they febrile?*

- Look at their skin
  - are they cyanotic?
  - are they diaphoretic?

- Are they experiencing dyspnea?

- Are they exhibiting any outward signs of distress?

- Are they tripoding or using accessory muscles?

Now let us consider the 2 types of acute respiratory failure. Acute respiratory failure is the inability of the patient to maintain $PaCO_2$, PaO_2, and/or pH at acceptable levels.

1) Hypoxemic Respiratory Failure
   This is life threatening because the patient's inability to maintain an adequate PaO_2 will lead to organ failure due to tissue hypoxia.

Hypoxemic respiratory failure is *generally* caused by:

- Severe $\dot{V} / \dot{Q}$ mismatch (R – L shunting)
- Diffusion defect
- Hypoventilation (alveolar)
- High altitudes (inadequate inspired O_2)

2) Hypercapnic Respiratory Failure
   This is when the patient is unable to maintain a normal $PaCO_2$.

Hypercapnic respiratory failure results when the ventilatory pump is not working correctly. What is meant by this is that the respiratory muscles could be fatigued and are thus not able to keep up with the demands of ventilation (this will be seen as increased WOB). On the other hand, the inability to maintain adequate ventilation could be due to neurological issues with the CNS or neuromuscular disease. In either case, you are going to be seeing diminished ventilation which will be evidenced by an elevated $PaCO_2$ and a drop in the pH (acidosis).

You're going to treat acute respiratory failure with:

- O_2 therapy (although this often doesn't work when you are dealing with severe shunting).
- CPAP
- Intubation with mechanical ventilation (including PEEP).

It is very important that you recognize either of these quickly and commence treatment immediately. Untreated hypoxemia or hypercapnia (with its resultant acidosis) will lead to cardiac dysrhythmias, ventricular fibrillation, and cardiac arrest. Also note that in the case of when a patient is hypoventilating, you may very well end up with a mixture of both hypoxemia and hypercapnia. The fact that they are not moving enough air means that they will not only retain CO_2 (hypercapnia) and develop acidosis, but in all likelihood are also not inspiring sufficient O_2 such that they will be experiencing hypoxemia as well.

Physiologic Parameters to Assess the Status of Your Patient

1. **MIP** (Maximum Inspiratory Pressure) – MIP measures respiratory muscle strength. It indicates maximum inspiratory pressure effort against an occluded airway. You may also see it referred to as NIF (Negative Inspiratory Force).

   - Normal value is -80 cmH_2O.
   - Acceptable values are between -20 and -80 cmH_2O.
   - Above -20 cmH_2O is not acceptable – this is because at least -20 cmH_2O is needed in order to produce a sufficient enough tidal volume to enable an adequate cough.

2.   VC (Vital Capacity)

- Normal value is 65 – 75 ml/kg of IBW (Ideal Body Weight).
- Acceptable value is greater than/equal to 10 ml/kg IBW.
- Below 10 ml/kg IBW is not acceptable because a VC less than this is not enough to maintain normal ventilation or to enable a productive cough.

NOTE: These first 2 assessments (MIP & VC) are particularly important when assessing a patient with neuromuscular disease because these patients typically have issues with being able to maintain sufficient respiratory muscle strength.

3.   PEFR (Peak Expiratory Flow Rate) – this is one of the main assessments you will use with *asthma patients*. The PEFR is a reliable indicator of R_{AW} and is therefore indicative of the risk of not being able to maintain a patent airway.

It is important to know your patient's baseline PEFR (their normal PEFR when they are not having an acute asthmatic episode) in order that you have something to compare to when evaluating their current status. This will enable you to know how much progress they are making.

Generally speaking though, normal PEFR's are around 10L/sec or 600 L/min, but note that gender and height must be accounted for when doing a precise calculation. You must also take into consideration what is "normal for your patient".

Normal R_{AW} is 0.6 – 2.4 cmH$_2$O/L/sec. Anything beyond this is indicating excessive airway resistance. Some material may say it is 0.5 – 1.5 cmH$_2$O/L/sec. When a patient is being mechanically ventilated it will be 5 – 9 cmH$_2$O/L/sec because the ventilator adds 4 – 6 cmH$_2$O/L/sec.

4. **Respiratory Rate** (or respiratory frequency) – this is the number of breaths per minute the patient is taking.

   - Normal values are between 12 – 20 breaths/min.
   - Acceptable values are between 8 – 20 breaths/min, but be mindful to be observing your patient for other signs if they are at either extreme of this range.
   - Above 20 breaths/min & below 8 breaths/min are not acceptable. If the patient's rate is either above 20 or below 8 you need to determine what is going on and take appropriate action. At respiratory rates above 35 breaths/min, alveolar ventilation will not be adequate.

5. V_E (minute volume or minute ventilation or expired volume per minute).

   - Normal values are 5 – 6 L/min.
   - Acceptable values are those under 10 L/min.
   - If minute ventilation falls below 5 L/min, they are not adequately ventilating. If minute ventilation is above 10 L/min, the patient's WOB is going to be too high and they are going to become exhausted.

6. **$PaCO_2$** (partial pressure of carbon dioxide) – _$PaCO_2$ is the best indicator of adequate ventilation._

   - Normal values are 35 – 45 mmHg.
   - Below 35 mmHg indicates hyperventilation and you'll also see a pH indicating alkalemia _(unless it is compensated)._
   - Above 45 mmHg indicates hypoventilation and you'll also see a pH indicating acidosis _(unless it is compensated)._

   Since $PaCO_2$ is indeed the best indicator of adequate ventilation, I want to take a moment to expand upon this. Some of the ideas that I am going to expand upon were introduced in chapter 3 on gas exchange, so please refer back to that material if needed.

Failure to bring in enough fresh air to adequately eliminate carbon dioxide is essentially what is causing hypercapnic respiratory failure – regardless of the reason. So then appreciate that it is hypercapnia, or elevated $PaCO_2$, that is the hallmark of ventilatory failure. In essence you have diminished alveolar ventilation (V_A) with respect to carbon dioxide production by the body's cells. Your cells are continuously producing CO_2 as a byproduct of metabolism, but yet there is not sufficient alveolar ventilation to ensure its removal. Decreased alveolar ventilation can occur from anything that decreases V_E – and V_E is decreased by things that will decrease either the V_T or the f (frequency or respiratory rate). Recall that V_E = V_T x f, and when either the V_T or the f is decreased, V_E is decreased and thus V_A is decreased. Remember that V_A = (V_T – V_D) x f – so for a *constant* V_D, lowering V_T or f is going to have the same net effect of lowering V_A as it did on lowering V_E. A drug overdose that depressed the respiratory drive, or respiratory muscles that are weak are examples of things that could decrease the V_T or f. Whatever the actual clinical cause, V_E is reduced enough such that V_A is decreased and thus $PaCO_2$ becomes elevated.

But also remember that when V_D *increases*, it will affect V_A. Recall that increased dead space ventilation (V_D) will cause a decrease in alveolar ventilation (V_A). An increase in dead space is actually more often the cause of hypercapnia than decreased minute ventilation. Later when we get into the pathology of obstructive and restrictive lung disease, you will come to appreciate that increased dead space ventilation is often the underlying issue that leads to CO_2 retention and thus increased $PaCO_2$ levels. In fact, when you see elevated $PaCO_2$ levels, it is suggestive that V_D is increased relative to V_T.

An increase in V_D affects the V/Q relationship as it leads to V/Q mismatching. In other words, an increase in the V_D/V_T ratio leads to an imbalance in the ventilation/perfusion (V/Q) relationship. In obstructive lung disease (COPD) there is often significant V/Q mismatching because of a relative increase in V_D with respect to V_T which then lowers V_A which then causes hypercapnia and acidosis. This is because COPDers often resort to a rapid, shallow breathing pattern that increases the V_D/V_T ratio with each breath. They do this to minimize the muscle fatigue and the feeling of breathlessness, but it doesn't ultimately solve their problem. When you see V/Q mismatching as it pertains to increased dead space, it is usually being caused by either an increase in the V_D/V_T ratio (too much of the V_T remains in the conducting airways) that was just discussed as it pertains to COPD, or it can also be caused by a pulmonary embolus, a pulmonary vascular injury, or regional pulmonary hypotension.

Increased V_D relative to V_T can also be seen in patients with restrictive lung disease (e.g. pulmonary fibrosis). In similar fashion to the COPD patient, these patients also exhibit a rapid, shallow breathing pattern that increases the V_D/V_T ratio which then ultimately decreases V_A that results in hypercapnia.

Realize that in either of these cases (obstructive disease or restrictive disease), even if the V_E is normal, the distribution of V_E is abnormal. In other words, the ratio of dead space to tidal volume (V_D/V_T) is abnormally high and that is going to decrease V_A and thus you are going to have elevated $PaCO_2$ (hypercapnia).

7. PaO₂

- Normal range is 85 – 100 mmHg.

PaO_2 is one of the indicators of how well a patient is oxygenating. A low PaO_2 on room air is indicative that the patient is having problems with oxygenation and is hypoxemic. Note that a patient could have a normal PaO_2 and still be experiencing hypoxia due to other reasons that are compromising oxygen delivery to the cells.

8. SpO₂ (oxygen saturation measured by a pulse oximeter)

- Normal range is 94 – 100%.
- Below 90% is indicating hypoxemia.
- Below 80% there is risk of compromised organ function – especially the heart and brain.
- Continued low oxygen can also lead to cardiac or respiratory arrest.

9. CaO_2

- Normal range is $16 - 20$ ml/dl.
- Remember that oxygen content is determined by the following equation:

$$(PaO_2 \times 0.003) + (Hb \times 1.34 \times SaO_2)$$
Dissolved O_2   *Bound O_2*

10. PaO_2/PAO_2

- This is your "a / A" ratio. This is telling you the proportion of oxygen that is getting from the alveoli into the blood.
- It should be as close to 1 as possible – at least 0.9 or 90%.
- If it is less than 0.15, you have a critical situation.

11. PaO_2/FiO_2

- This ratio is showing you the comparison between the oxygen level in the blood and the fractional concentration of the oxygen that is being inspired.
- Acceptable values for this ratio are $350 - 450$ mmHg.
- Values below 300 mmHg indicate ALI (acute lung injury).
- Values below 200 mmHg indicate ARDS (acute respiratory distress syndrome).

G. Pathological Conditions that Increase the Risk for Mechanical Ventilation

There are three particular conditions that put a patient at increased risk for needing mechanical ventilation. They are:

1. Central nervous system (CNS) issues
2. Neuromuscular disease
3. Increased work of breathing (WOB)

1.   Central Nervous System (CNS) Issues

   A. Drugs
      - (particularly depressants)
   B. Tumors
   C. Stroke
   D. Head Trauma
      - Cerebral hemorrhage
      - Increased intracranial pressure (ICP)

   Injuries and/or other issues that affect the brain have the potential to depress the respiratory drive (the neural regulation of breathing). Although $PaCO_2$ is the principle drive for ventilation, it requires a properly functioning brain that is able to interpret $PaCO_2$ (remember it's actually H^+ and not CO_2 directly) in order to ensure the proper regulation of breathing. When there is injury or trauma to the brain, or a drug overdose, the neural mechanisms responsible for regulating and maintaining the drive to breath can be adversely affected such that mechanical ventilation becomes a necessity.

   When the respiratory drive is diminished due to a brain injury, you end up with a decreased V_E and thus a decreased V_A which in turn results in hypoxemia, hypercapnia, and acidosis. Furthermore, Cheyne-Stokes or Biot's respiration patterns can also be present with brain injuries, and this further destabilizes the patient's ability to maintain proper ventilation. Thorough assessment and close monitoring of the ventilatory and oxygenation status of these patients is absolutely necessary in order to determine if mechanical ventilation will be necessary.

A word about ICP

   Intracranial pressure is the pressure inside the skull, and thus the brain and the CSF (cerebrospinal fluid). Normal values for ICP are 5 – 10 mmHg, although some literature indicates it being 7 – 15 mmHg for an adult in the supine position. In either case, any type of head trauma as well as several other pathologies can cause the ICP to increase. If the ICP reaches 20 mmHg or more, it has to be treated. When you have a patient with elevated ICP due to an acute brain injury, it is important that you ensure a patent airway, adequate ventilation, and adequate oxygenation. Low PaO_2 (hypoxemia) and/or high $PaCO_2$ (hypercapnia) will cause the cerebral blood vessels to dilate and this causes increased blood flow to the brain that will elevate the ICP. Furthermore, hypoxemia forces the brain to resort to making ATP via anaerobic metabolism which produces lactic acid that lowers the pH even more and that contributes to more vasodilation that just ends up making the problem even worse. On the other hand, vasoconstriction occurs when carbon dioxide levels are below normal – so hyperventilating a patient with ICP can temporarily reduce the ICP. By hyperventilating the patient, you are effectively increasing their V_E, and remember that increasing V_E also increases V_A – and when you increase V_A you decrease $PaCO_2$. By decreasing $PaCO_2$ you decrease the ICP because decreasing carbon dioxide raises the pH which then causes cerebral vasoconstriction that lowers cerebral perfusion which lowers ICP.

Let me clarify something here: When we are talking about ICP – we are not talking about the pressure inside the blood vessels of the brain. In your normal sense of understanding you think of vasoconstriction as something that increases the blood pressure and vasodilation as something that lowers the blood pressure – and that is correct as far as the pressure inside the blood vessel itself is concerned. But this is not what we are talking about when it comes to ICP. As it pertains to ICP, we are not talking about the pressure inside the vessels themselves, but rather we are talking about the "spaces" in the brain though which those vessels course along. ICP is the pressure being exerted on the brain itself. Blood vessels in the brain course along pathways within the brain, and those blood vessels are right next to the brain tissue itself. If you dilate that vessel and thus make it bigger, even though the blood pressure inside that vessel will have been reduced by becoming bigger – by now being bigger it is exerting more pressure on the brain tissue that is immediately next to it. Conversely, if you constrict those vessels and thus cause them to become smaller, what you have done is created more space between the vessel itself and the brain tissue that surrounds the vessel. And by doing this you have effectively given the brain more room so to speak, and this enables the pressure within the brain tissue itself to be reduced.

Realize though that this strategy is not without a cost. The hyperventilation strategy that results in the vasoconstriction that can lower the ICP can also limit the amount of blood flow to the brain – and this could be problematic especially if you are dealing with a patient that already has some degree of brain ischemia. Cases like this are not cut and dry and this is why you will need to work closely with the attending physician regarding the strategies that are going to be employed in the management of these types of patients. Depending upon the situation, the physician may decide to try to reduce the ICP by administering IV mannitol. By using mannitol, you will create a hypertonic solution within the blood that will draw water out of the neurons and this will help reduce the fluid within the intracranial space and thus reduce the ICP. Just be cognizant that managing patients with these types of issues is far from simple and pay close attention to your attending physician.

2. Neuromuscular Disease

- Disease of muscle tissue itself
  - e.g. muscular dystrophy

- Disease that affects the neuromuscular junction
  - faulty transmission of nerve impulses
    - e.g. Myasthenia Gravis

- Motor neuron disease
  - e.g. ALS, paralytic poliomyelitis

- Polyneuropathy
  - e.g. Guillain-Barré Syndrome

When dealing with patients with neuromuscular disease, it is important to monitor the progression of muscle weakness. This means that you are going to need to monitor their MIP and VC every 2 – 4 hours. Refer back to the discussion of MIP and VC in the last section.   You will also want to monitor their ventilatory and oxygenation status.

3. Increased work of breathing (WOB)

When considering the work of breathing, we are looking at both the rate and depth of the patient's breathing. Under normal circumstances, the work of breathing usually only amounts to about 1 – 4 % of a patient's total oxygen consumption. But when a patient is in distress, the increased oxygen demand from their respiratory muscles due to their increased work of breathing can then account for up to 40% of that patient's total oxygen consumption.

There are several things that can lead to an increase in a patient's WOB:

- Exacerbation of COPD
- Increased R_{AW} from secretions, airway inflammation, mucosal edema, bronchoconstriction, or foreign body aspiration
- Thoracic trauma - pneumothorax
- Pulmonary edema
- Pleural effusion & hemothorax
- Pulmonary fibrosis
- Air trapping

Increased WOB, especially if severe, is going to lead to significant fatigue which is going to result in hypoventilation and impending ventilatory failure. Go back to the discussion on impending ventilatory failure in section C and revisit the example given with the asthmatic patient. This is a case of severely increased WOB. The hypoventilation that results from their fatigue causes their V_A to decrease and they end up having hypoxemia, hypercapnia, and acidosis. In cases of severe WOB, intubation and placement on mechanical ventilation will likely be necessary due to the fact that their respiratory muscles have become so tired that they no longer have the muscle strength to maintain adequate ventilation on their own.

H. Triggering & Cycling

TRIGGERING – triggering is the mechanism used to BEGIN INSPIRATION. There is the time trigger, and then there are two types of patient controlled triggers – pressure & flow:

1. TIME TRIGGER

Inspiration begins according to a set interval of time. When you set the frequency on the ventilator – this establishes the time trigger.

2. PATIENT CONTROLLED TRIGGERS

Think of patient controlled triggers as sensitivity controls. Pressure and/or flow are two variables that we can enable the ventilator to be sensitive to insofar as enabling the patient to trigger a breath. We can make the ventilator sensitive to either pressure or flow, but not both at the same time.

- You will always set a sensitivity.
- Although you can set either a flow or a pressure sensitivity, flow is the default setting on most new ventilators.

Pressure Trigger

- The pressure trigger is set at **-2 cmH$_2$O (this is the sensitivity).**
- What this means is that you are going to set the ventilator so that it will detect a slight negative pressure coming from a slight inspiratory effort from the patient.
- If/when the patient attempts to take a breath (so long as their effort is at least -2 cmH$_2$O), then the ventilator will sense this effort from the patient and deliver them a breath.

Flow Trigger

- The flow trigger is set at **2 LPM (this is the sensitivity).**
- There is a constant flow of gas through the ventilator circuit – this is known as bias flow.
- If/when the patient attempts to take a breath, it will cause the flow rate of the bias flow to decrease. As long as the patient's effort is at least 2 LPM, that will sufficiently reduce the bias flow such that the ventilator will detect that drop in bias flow and thus deliver a breath.

CYCLING – cycling is the mechanism used to END INSPIRATION. There are four types of cycling mechanisms: (volume cycling, pressure cycling, flow cycling, and time cycling).

1. Volume Cycling

- Sometimes this is also referred to as volume – targeted.
- Inspiration ends when a pre-set V_T has been delivered.
- The pressure will vary during the delivery of the V_T.
  - Hence you need to set a pressure limit (high pressure alarm) because volume cycling carries the risk of barotrauma.
- Since you are controlling V_T, and you also control RR or f, volume cycling enables you to control V_E.

Therefore: the V_T is controlled and guaranteed so long as the pressure does not exceed the pressure limit. The pressure needed to deliver that V_T is going to vary according to resistance (both the elastic resistance of the lung and R_{AW}) and lung compliance. But pressure cannot be allowed to get too high because then it becomes unsafe for the patient. $30 - 35$ cmH$_2$O is generally considered the upper limit for pressure – beyond this is the risk for barotrauma. Hence the need for the pressure limit or pressure alarm.

A word about the pressure limit:

A limit mechanism is simply defining the maximum value that a variable can attain. In volume cycling, a pressure limit is set (via setting a pressure alarm) such that if/when that pressure limit is reached, inspiration will end. If the pressure limit is reached, it causes a premature ending of inspiration. It has to be this way in order to protect the lung from barotrauma as already mentioned.

Example:

Say you want to deliver a V_T of 600 ml and you set a pressure limit (alarm) at 50 cmH_2O.

The ventilator begins to deliver the breath, and let's say at the point where the ventilator has delivered 100 ml, the pressure is 20 cmH_2O.

and at 200 ml, the pressure is up to 30 cmH_2O

and at 300 ml, the pressure is up to 50 cmH_2O

At the point of 300 ml, the pressure limit of 50 cmH_2O has been reached – inspiration will be prematurely terminated and the patient will only get a V_T of 300 ml rather than 600 ml. This is to protect them from the damage that could be done from letting the pressure get too high.

Now – every ventilator has a built in internal manometer that measures **PIP (peak inspiratory pressure).**

- PIP is measured at the end of inspiration.
- PIP tells us how hard the ventilator is working – in other words it is telling you the amount of effort/work that it is taking in order to overcome the elastic and frictional resistance in order to deliver the V_T.

Although PIP is piece of data that tells you the amount of pressure that it is taking to deliver the breath – consider the following example as something you can do in volume cycling in order to gain more information about what is going on when pressures change. This will enable you to determine what is going on with your patient.

At 8am your patient's PIP is 20 cmH_2O. But then when you measure it again at 10am it has risen to 50 cmH_2O. Now we're not talking about limits or alarms here, or whether the breath is going to be prematurely ended – what we're talking about here is trying to figure out what is going on with your patient with regards to *why* the pressure went up so much. This is how you start thinking like a discerning clinician.

Obviously this change in PIP is indicating a rather drastic increase in the amount of pressure, but at this point you can't tell if it is due to an increase in R_{AW}, or if it is due to the changes in the compliance of the lung. In order to narrow it down and pinpoint the cause of this pressure increase - you have to do the following:

Every ventilator has a button on it that is called the **inspiratory pause (or inspiratory hold)** *button.* When you press the inspiratory pause button it is going to give you a number called the **plateau pressure (P_{PLT}).**

When you hit the inspiratory pause button at the end of inspiration, flow is halted and exhalation is prevented so that you get a static measurement of P_{PLT}. P_{PLT} is the pressure inside the lung – it's telling you the pressure that is needed to keep the lung inflated.

Now let's look at two possible scenarios:

A. Let's say your P_{PLT} was 15 cmH_2O. That is telling you that it is taking 15 cmH_2O in order to keep the lung inflated. You have a total PIP of 50 cmH_2O from the example given for this scenario, but yet only 15 cmH_2O of that 50 cmH_2O is being used to keep the lung inflated. That tells you that the other 35 cmH_2O is in the airway – so this is telling you that you have a R_{AW} issue. Something has increased the resistance in the airway, and one of the first things you should consider is if they have developed a mucus plug or excessive secretions that need to be suctioned to relieve the problem. Other things for you to consider is if they are having a bronchospasm or if perhaps the endotrachael tube has become occluded.

B. Let's say your P_{PLT} was 40 cmH$_2$O. That is telling you that it is taking 40 cmH$_2$O in order to keep the lung inflated. You have a total PIP of 50 cmH$_2$O from the example given for this scenario, and 40 cmH$_2$O of that 50 cmH$_2$O is needed to keep the lung inflated, and the other 10 cmH$_2$O is in the airway. This is telling you that you have a compliance issue. Something has changed with the dynamics of their lungs and you'll need to investigate further to see what is going on. Issues of lung compliance don't usually change that drastically over the course of just 2 hours, but you will nonetheless need to do further clinical evaluation to determine what is going on with them because high P_{PLT} is seen with pulmonary edema, pneumonia, ARDS, or if they have developed a pneumothorax.

Therefore:

Low P_{PLT} with respect to a high PIP is indicating a R_{AW} issue. High P_{PLT} with respect to a high PIP is indicating a lung compliance issue. Anything that causes a decrease in the compliance of the lung such as pulmonary edema, pneumonia, ARDS, or a pneumothorax for example, is going to cause the P_{PLT} to be high. At a minimum, you should always check the P_{PLT} during the first ventilator check of your shift because the P_{PLT} is going to give you information about lung compliance and R_{AW}.

* In mechanically ventilated patients, $R_{AW} = \dfrac{PIP - P_{PLT}}{PIFR}$

2. Pressure Cycling

- Sometimes this is also referred to as pressure – targeted.
- Inspiration ends when a pre-set pressure has been reached.

- There are no modes that "pressure cycle" directly. Pressure cycling essentially amounts to what happens when you reach a set pressure limit (alarm). You could be in a mode for example that is utilizing volume cycling – but if you have a pressure limit (alarm) set, and that pressure is reached – then it's going to pressure cycle and inspiration will be ended.

Students often confuse pressure cycling with pressure control ventilation. They are not the same thing. Pressure control ventilation is a mode that is time cycled and we will cover that later. Think of pressure cycling as a safety feature that protects the patient from high inspiratory pressures. When a certain set pressure limit (alarm) is reached, inspiration is cycled into exhalation.

As a preview though to the pressure control mode that will be discussed shortly, one of the drawbacks with pressure control is that you can't do an inspiratory pause like you can do in volume control (which is volume cycled) because pressure is constant – therefore, if the V_T does drop, you won't be able to tell if it's from increased R_{AW} or a decrease in lung compliance. But when you start to see V_T rise – that is telling you that something is improving. Oftentimes when you have a patient in volume control ventilation and their pressures are consistently too high – you'll switch them over to pressure control ventilation so that you can control the pressure – but then you have to concern yourself with whether they are getting a sufficient enough V_T.

3. Flow Cycling

- In flow cycling, inspiration ends when the inspiratory flow reaches a pre-determined minimum.
- Flow cycling is used in modes that allow for *spontaneous breathing* – like pressure support for example.

Flow is always highest at the beginning of the breath – it starts out at 100%. Inspiration ends at a set point where flow is at its lowest – say 10 – 15%, because the flow rate is lowest at the end of the breath.

4. Time Cycling

- In time cycling, inspiration ends when a pre-set T_I (inspiratory time) is reached.

You will see time cycling being used when you are in the pressure control mode for example:

- you would set an inspiratory pressure – say 20 cmH$_2$O
- you would set a T_I – say 3 seconds

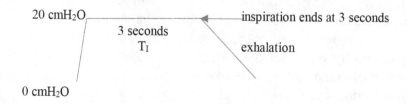

20 cmH$_2$O ———————————————◄———inspiration ends at 3 seconds

3 seconds
T_I exhalation

0 cmH$_2$O

I. Initiation of Mechanical Ventilation

This section is going to introduce the initial settings for the various different parameters of the ventilator. The Mode you are in will determine which of these parameters you actually set. Modes in be addressed in depth in the next section (section J).

Select the mode – as just mentioned, modes will be covered extensively in the next section, however I list it here as the mode is the first thing you have to decide upon. Although volume control is commonly used as an initial mode, any mode can be used initially. Here are some of the basic modes for you to become familiar with.

- AC, VC, CMV, PCV – these modes are full support modes.
- SIMV, PSV – these modes are partial support modes.

AC, VC, CMV, and SIMV are volume cycled.
PCV is time cycled.
PSV is flow cycled.

Minute Ventilation (V_E) – provide a minute ventilation that matches the patient's needs and provides adequate gas exchange.

- Normal values are 5 – 6 L/min.
- Acceptable values are those under 10 L/min.
- If minute ventilation falls below 5 L/min, they are not adequately ventilating. If minute ventilation is above 10 L/min, the patient's WOB is going to be too high and they are going to become exhausted.

You don't directly set V_E – there is no button or knob for V_E. In volume ventilation, you determine V_E by setting the V_T and f because $V_E = V_T$ x f. Note though that in the pressure control mode V_T is variable (you don't set a V_T in pressure control mode) – so you'll need to pay attention to make sure that V_E is appropriate.

Set the Initial Tidal Volume (V_T) – *in volume ventilation modes*

- 5 – 8 ml/kg of Ideal Body Weight (IBW)
- Some texts will say 5 – 10 ml/kg IBW

You must determine IBW in kg in order to set V_T – it is not an option – you must do this with every patient.

Determining IBW in kg:

Males   50 + 2.3(height in inches – 60)

Females   45.5 + 2.3(height in inches – 60)

Example: you have a male patient that is 6'2" that weighs 230 lbs.

50 + 2.3(74 inches - 60 inches)
50 + 2.3(14)
50 + 32.2
82.2 kg is their IBW

If V_T is 5 – 8 ml/kg IBW, then 5 x 82.2 = 411, and 8 x 82.2 = 657.6

Therefore, you can set their V_T between 410 – 650 ml.

Note: Their IBW of 82.2 kg is the same as 181 lbs. (82.2 kg x 2.2 lbs./kg = 181 lbs.), which is 49 lbs. less than their actual weight of 230 lbs. But it is the IBW of 82.2 kg – not their actual weight that you must use when determining the range for tidal volume. IBW always has to be used because larger or heavier patients may have bigger bodies, but they don't have bigger lungs just because their bodies are bigger. Always be aware of this.

Set the Initial Frequency (f)

- The normal frequency range for a spontaneously breathing patient is 12 – 20 breaths/min. – so you want to stay within this range when they are being mechanically ventilated.

Realize that the only time that a patient will *only* be getting breaths according the to the frequency that you have set is when they are sedated. If the patient is not sedated, they will always be able to trigger the ventilator themselves – so you want to try to set the rate on the ventilator to be in synch with how the patient is breathing. The way you do this is as follows: Immediately after intubating them, bag them with a BVM, and though the process of giving them manual breaths via the BVM you figure out what their rate is so that you can then set the frequency on the ventilator accordingly. By doing this you can help avoid issues of having the patient being out of synch with the ventilator. You always want the patient to be in synch with the ventilator. It can become very uncomfortable for them if they are out of synch (out of synch means for example that while they are exhaling the ventilator is trying to give them another breath – and this becomes quite uncomfortable for them). Unless they are sedated, the patient always controls the frequency. Even though you set a frequency – the patient can always trigger the ventilator and thus you can end up having a frequency higher than what you set. In fact – when you see the actual frequency being consistently higher than the set frequency – that is telling you that they are either out of synch with the ventilator or they are having other problems which you will need to address.

Setting the Sensitivity

This means setting the patient controlled trigger. Remember that the time trigger is a function of the frequency that is set. This breath (time triggered) happens automatically as per the set frequency. What we're talking about here is the trigger (sensitivity) that enables the patient to trigger a breath. And as previously discussed – there is a flow trigger and a pressure trigger. Refer back to the beginning of section H for the details if necessary. You're going to set either a flow trigger or a pressure trigger, but not both. It's one or the other, and flow is usually the default trigger.

Setting the Initial FiO$_2$

There is some variation regarding the initial FiO$_2$ setting, so I am going to give you three possible scenarios. The policies and practice standards of the institution where you work, and ultimately the orders of the attending physician will determine the FiO$_2$, however these are the possibilities that you will likely encounter.

Scenario 1 - Prior to being intubated and being placed on mechanical ventilation, the patient was either breathing room air, or you have no information regarding this patient. Place this patient on an FiO$_2$ of 40 – 60%.

Scenario 2 - Prior to being intubated and being place on mechanical ventilation, the patient was receiving oxygen therapy. In this case, you set the FiO$_2$ on the ventilator to be at the same level as it was for the oxygen therapy they were previously receiving prior to being intubated.

Scenario 3 – Set the initial FiO$_2$ on the ventilator at 100%.

- Then gradually decrease the FiO$_2$ so as to maintain a PaO$_2$ between 80 – 100 mmHg.
- Maintain FiO$_2$ < 50% with a SpO$_2$ > 90%.
- The goal is to maintain adequate oxygenation at the lowest possible FiO$_2$.

<u>Rationale for starting out with an FiO_2 of 100%</u>

By starting out with an FiO_2 of 100%, you can look at the $P(A - a)O_2$ gradient in order to determine O_2 transfer efficiency and to know if there is shunting going on.

Remember the $P(A - a)O_2$ gradient from chapter 3? You get the PaO_2 from the ABG, and calculate the PAO_2 using the alveolar air equation. Once you have both the PaO_2 and the PAO_2, then you can look at the difference between them; $(PAO_2 - PaO_2)$.

- When breathing room air ($FiO_2 = 21\%$), you know that the (A - a) gradient should be no more than $5 - 10$ mmHg, although it does increase with age and that was discussed in chapter 3.
- At 100% FiO_2, however, the (A – a) gradient should be no more than 65 mmHg.
- Furthermore, when using an FiO_2 of 100% - you know that for every 50 mmHg difference in (A - a) that you have a 2% shunt.
  - e.g.: your (A – a) = 350. That is indicating a 14 % shunt.
- If the (A - a) gradient on a FiO_2 of 100% is greater than 450 mmHg, then that is indicating severe refractory hypoxemia or intrapulmonary shunting – just look at the math again, if the (A – a) is 450, that is indicating an 18% shunt. If it was even higher than 450, it would be even worse.

The PaO_2/FiO_2 ratio (P/F ratio) can also be looked at. This was discussed in section F; however, it is being mentioned again here as it is relevant to the current discussion. Although the P/F ratio can be calculated at any FiO_2, *it nonetheless provides a rough estimate of whether or not there is a significant (A -a) gradient present as just discussed above.* Whereas the (A - a) gradient requires more calculations to obtain, the P/F ratio can be figured out quickly. The interpretation of the P/F ratio is according to how it was already discussed in section F.

(P/F ratio) – reiterated from section F:

- This ratio is showing you the comparison between the oxygen level in the blood and the fractional concentration of the oxygen that is being breathed.
- Acceptable values for this ratio are 350 – 450 mmHg.
- Values below 300 mmHg indicate ALI (acute lung injury)
- Values below 200 mmHg indicate ARDS (acute respiratory distress syndrome)

Note however that even though the P/F ratio is easier to calculate than the (A - a) gradient, it cannot distinguish hypoxemia due to hypoventilation from other causes such as V/Q mismatching, whereas the (A – a) gradient can. So, in actual clinical practice, the P/F ratio should only be used to give a rough estimate for detecting an (A - a) gradient when the $PaCO_2$ is normal and shunting is not suspected. Many clinicians however consider a P/F < 200 to be generally indicative of a shunt > 20%.

Setting the Initial PIFR

- The peak inspiratory flow rate is determined by the following equation. This equation enables you to determine the PIFR that is needed for a desired I:E ratio.

PIFR = V_E x Σ I:E ratio
Which is to say that PIFR = minute ventilation x the sum of the I:E ratio.

Example: V_T = 600ml, f = 12, and the desired I:E ratio is 1:3

Therefore, V_E = V_T x f, 600ml x 12/min. = 7200ml/min. and the sum of the I:E ratio is 1+3 = 4

So PIFR = 7200ml/min x 4 = 28,800ml/min or 29 LPM.

* And in the clinical setting we would add an additional 15-20 LPM.

Let us revisit some concepts from chapter 2 to review and better understand PIFR and the I:E ratio. If necessary, return to the section in chapter 2 where I:E ratios are discussed as it is absolutely relevant with respect to mechanical ventilation. The I:E ratio is simply the ratio of the inspiratory time and the expiratory time. Basic math enables us to calculate total cycle time (TCT), inspiratory time (T_I), and expiratory time (T_E) during delivery of an assisted breath. The total cycle time always equals inspiratory time plus expiratory time (TCT = T_I + T_E). It is determined by the frequency (or RR) because TCT is also 60/f. For example, if the frequency is 12 breaths per minute and the patient is not breathing above the set rate, then the total cycle time is 5 seconds (60/12 = 5). By way of another example, if the frequency is 20 breaths per minute, then the total cycle time is 3 seconds (60/20 = 3). Inspiratory time is determined by V_T and the inspiratory flow rate. For example, if V_T is 1000 milliliters (1L) and inspiratory flow is 60 liters per minute (1 liter per second), then inspiratory time is 1 second. In the second example above, the patient is breathing 20 times per minute. Thus, the TCT is 3 seconds. A 1-liter tidal volume (1000ml) delivered at 60 liters per minute (1 liter per second) takes 1 second to deliver. Since the TCT is 3 seconds, that leaves 2 seconds available for exhalation. The ventilator inspiratory-to-expiratory time ratio (I:E) is thus 1:2.

I did this to reinforce how you can figure out different things depending upon what variables you know. In the initial discussion of this section you were shown how to determine PIFR given that you knew V_E and the I:E ratio. In the subsequent discussion you reviewed how you are able to determine the I:E ratio when you know the frequency (and thus TCT), V_T, and the flow rate. Getting comfortable with being able to either determine the PIFR needed to establish a desired I:E ratio, or determining the I:E ratio from knowing the VT, TCT and flow rate is simply a matter of working with these ideas and illustrating the math to yourself until it becomes second nature to you – and it will.

One last thing I want to leave you with in this section is the idea of "meeting you patient's inspiratory demand" so that you can make sure that they never feel as though they are not getting enough flow. The following formula is what you use to determine a patient's inspiratory demand:

$$\frac{V_T}{T_I} = \frac{X \text{ ml}}{60 \text{ sec}}$$

Solving for X gives you the flow needed to meet the patient's demand:

Let us solve this equation using the same numbers as in the original PIFR problem at the beginning of this section:

$$\frac{600 \text{ml}}{1 \text{ sec}} = \frac{X \text{ ml}}{60 \text{ sec}}$$

X ml/sec = 36,000ml/sec, or 36 LPM

I was never taught this formula for determining a patient's flow demand in any of my lectures and I never read it in a book. It was taught to me by my department chair one day while I was in his office talking to him about a few things. Since the last thing I wrote in the initial part of this PIFR section was to tell you that you need to add an additional 15 – 20 LPM to the flow that you calculated from PIFR = V_E x (sum of I:E), it stood to reason that the results of the equation I just showed you for determining a patient's flow demand was the reason why. Although 36 LPM is only 7 LPM more than 29 LPM, adding an additional 15 – 20 LPM to the calculated PIFR is sufficient enough to always ensure that the patient has more than enough flow to satisfy any demand they may have.

Setting Initial PEEP

PEEP is going to be discussed in much more detail in section K of this chapter, but here is the information for initial ventilator settings for PEEP.

- Set initial PEEP at 3 – 5 cmH$_2$O (some sources will say to set it at 2 – 6 cmH$_2$O).
- If the patient was on CPAP prior to being intubated, then you could set the PEEP at the same level the CPAP was set.

Note that this initial PEEP setting is not therapeutic. Its purpose is to restore FRC and the physiological PEEP that existed prior to intubation. Subsequent changes to PEEP will be based on ABG results.

PEEP is used to treat refractory hypoxemia. It is contraindicated when the patient is hypotensive, has elevated ICP, or has an untreated pneumothorax.

Setting Alarms

High Minute Ventilation Alarm

Set at 2 LPM above the patient's baseline V_E (the patient's *actual* V_E).
- This alarm is to alert you when patient is becoming tachypneic (respiratory distress).
- Or the ventilator is self-triggering – sensitivity may need to be adjusted.

High Respiratory Rate Alarm

Set at 10 – 15 breaths/minute above the *observed* respiratory rate.
- This alarm is also to alert you when patient is becoming tachypneic (respiratory distress).
- Or the ventilator is self-triggering – sensitivity may need to be adjusted.

Low Exhaled Tidal Volume Alarm

Set at 100 ml lower than the set V_T.
- This alarm is usually due to a circuit disconnection, a system leak, or an ET tube cuff leak.

Low Exhaled Minute Ventilation Alarm

Set at 2 LPM below the average V_E (the patient's actual).
- This alarm is also usually due to a circuit disconnection, a system leak, or an ET tube cuff leak.

High Inspiratory Pressure Alarm

Set at $10 - 15$ cmH$_2$O above the peak inspiratory pressure (PIP).
- This alarm is usually caused by:
  - water in the circuit
  - kinking in the ET tube
  - secretions in the airway
  - bronchospasm
  - tension pneumothorax
  - decrease in lung compliance
  - increase in R$_{AW}$
  - coughing
  - too much flow

Low Inspiratory Pressure Alarm

Set at $10 - 15$ cmH$_2$O below the observed PIP.
- This alarm is usually due to a circuit disconnection, a system leak, an ET tube cuff leak, or insufficient flow.

High PEEP/CPAP Alarm

Set at $3 - 5$ cmH$_2$O above PEEP.
- This alarm is usually due to a circuit or exhalation manifold obstruction, or patient autoPEEP.

Low PEEP/CPAP Alarm

Set at $2 - 5$ cmH$_2$O below PEEP.
- This alarm is usually due to a circuit disconnect.

Apnea Alarm

The apnea alarm is set when you are using a mode that allows for spontaneous breathing – e.g. SIMV or PSV.

Set with a $15 - 20$ second time delay. With most, if not all ventilators, this will trigger an apnea ventilation mode. Set the ventilator to provide full ventilatory support at 100% FiO_2 while in the apnea mode.

<u>Alarms usually set only with infants</u>

<u>High FiO_2 Alarm</u>

Set at 5% above the analyzed FiO_2.

<u>Low FiO_2 Alarm</u>

Set at 5% below the analyzed FiO_2.

<u>High / Low Temperature Alarm</u>

As it pertains to heated humidification

High Temperature Alarm – Set at 37° C. You don't want the temperature going above this.
Low Temperature Alarm – Set at 30°C. You don't want the temperature going below this.

Setting Humidification

- Normal humidification is to provide 100% relative humidity at body temperature (37°C).
- This contains 44 mg/L H_2O.
- With humidifiers – set a minimum of 30 mg/L H_2O at 31°C - 35°C.
- Usually set the temperature at 35°C - 37°C.

Flow Patterns

The two flow patterns I am going to discuss are the two patterns that you will encounter most often in clinical practice – they are the constant flow pattern and the descending flow pattern.

<u>Constant</u>

Constant flow is shown with a square wave.

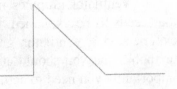

- Constant flow gives the shortest T_I.
- You set a PIFR: the PIFR initiates at the set rate and stays at that rate continuously until the V_T is delivered and the breath ends – hence the square wave.
- Constant flow gives you higher peak pressures, but lower mean airway pressures – this is because T_I is quick in this case.

<u>Descending</u>

Descending flow is shown with the following wave: *Descending flow is what you usually start out with.*

- With descending flow, flow is greatest at the beginning of inspiration and it decreases to baseline by the end of inspiration.
- Descending flow gives you lower peak pressures, but higher mean pressures because T_I is longer.

<u>Some advantages to descending flow</u>

If your patient has low lung compliance – a descending flow pattern may be beneficial by keeping PIP lower and mean airway pressure higher so as to improve gas distribution.

If your patient has high R_{AW} – a descending flow pattern is more likely to deliver a set V_T at lower pressure and provide better distribution of gas throughout the lung.

Say for example that you start out with a descending flow pattern but you have I:E problems such that you want to gain T_E. You could see this with a COPDer who is trapping air and needs more time to exhale.

To gain T_E, you could switch to constant flow. In so doing, you will decrease T_I and gain the T_E you desire.

But going to constant flow will increase the PIP – so you may then need to decrease your PIFR.

Therefore – be aware that changing the flow pattern changes the I:E ratio and it changes the PIP.

Flow Graphics

Ventilator graphics in general are not so much something that needs to be explained, but rather something that needs to be experienced. Ventilator graphics are covered in your primary textbook, and you should also receive lectures as well - but more importantly you need to actually spend time with the ventilator and become comfortable with the way the ventilator graphically depicts a breath, pressures, resistance & compliance, flow, etc., and all the nuances that pertain to all these parameters. Most students usually have no issues with this area in their lectures or textbook reading, and since it is really learned by actually experiencing it on a real ventilator, no further coverage will be given in this book.

But I do want to include a flow graphic to illustrate one of the important points that was made in the previous section on PIFR – and that is the idea of making sure that your flow is always meeting your patient's inspiratory demand. A typical, and often desired I:E ratio is 1:2 - 1:3. This can usually be achieved with a PIFR around 60 LPM (range of 40 – 80 LPM). But since no two patients are the same, you always need to be observing them, and watching the ventilator and the monitors to make sure everything is ok.

Consider the following two graphical representations of flow that will enable you to know whether the flow to the patient is sufficient.

Adequate Flow During Volume Ventilation

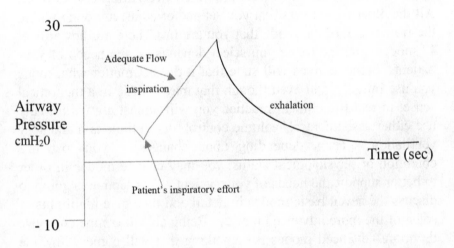

Patient Outbreathing the Set Flow

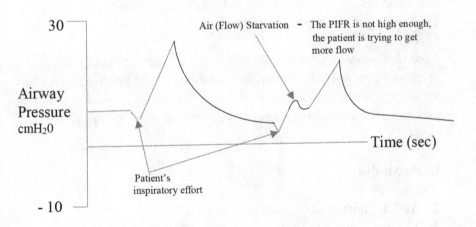

J. Modes of Ventilation

In the last section - Initiation of Mechanical Ventilation, selecting the mode was indicated as the first thing that you do when putting a patient on a mechanical ventilator. Think of the mode as the overall framework through which everything else is done. All the other parameters that you set and/or adjust are done within the framework of the mode that you are in. There are upwards of 17 modes, and the mode you select depends on the needs of your patient. Some sources will state that it doesn't matter what mode you use initially, and even though that may be true in a theoretical sense, in real life clinical practice you will almost always initially use either assist control, volume control, or continuous mandatory ventilation.   Then, depending upon changes in your patient's condition or physiological status, you may change modes in order to better support the needs of your patient. This section is going to discuss the seven basic modes in detail and then give highlights of some of the more advanced modes. Being able to competently use the more advanced modes is something that will come with time as you gain clinical experience. As the features and capabilities of ventilators continue to evolve, it will always be necessary for you to stay current in this area as you will be the main clinician that everyone else will look to for understanding when it comes to the functioning of the mechanical ventilator.

Note that as we now begin to discuss the particular modes, the settings I give you for the various parameters are uniquely specific for the mode being discussed. Refer to the previous section for the settings of other parameters and alarms that may be applicable.

Basic Modes

1. **Assist Control (AC)**
2. **Volume Control (VC)**
3. **Continuous Mandatory Ventilation (CMV)**

These first three modes are being discussed collectively because they all mean essentially the same thing – volume ventilation, and volume ventilation is what we usually start with. These are full support modes which means that they are giving full ventilatory support. They are also referred to as control modes in that the ventilator controls the various ventilatory parameters, including T_I and the set baseline respiratory rate. Remember though that the rate can exceed the set rate if the patient initiates (triggers) extra breaths.

Full support is indicated:

- When the patient needs complete rest.
- When you need controlled hyperventilation to help reduce elevated intracranial pressure (ICP).
- When using paralytics to induce paralysis in the patient. *Remember that when this is done – **the patient is always sedated first, then paralyzed.***

When you want total ventilatory control over the patient – rather than fooling around with sensitivity settings, you will sedate and paralyze them. You will however, always set a sensitivity setting regardless.

In giving full support, you are essentially enabling the ventilator to take over the WOB for the patient. It is by eliminating the WOB from the patient that the ventilator enables them to have complete rest. The only work for the patient would be the slight effort they would make to initiate a breath (as per the sensitivity setting), but even if they don't make this slight effort the ventilator will still deliver regular breaths based upon the time trigger which is a function of the set frequency.

Remember these modes are TIME or PATIENT TRIGGERED and VOLUME CYCLED (Refer back to the previous discussion on triggering and cycling to reinforce these concepts if necessary).

<u>Parameters you set with AC, VC, or CMV</u>

- Set V_T ⟶ this controls V_E – remember that changes in either of these
- Set f ⟋ will change V_E.
- Set sensitivity
- Set PIFR
- Set pressure limit (alarm)

* In volume ventilation, pressure varies according to lung dynamics.

<u>Important things to keep in mind with volume ventilation.</u>

Since you are setting the frequency (f), and PIFR in volume ventilation, you need to have a firm understanding of how these two things interact with each other.

<u>For a constant PIFR (i.e. - PIFR is held constant)</u>

If you increase the frequency – you thus decrease the TCT. But only the T_E is affected, so you effectively decrease T_E.

If you decrease the frequency – you thus increase the TCT. But again, only the T_E is affected, so you effectively increase T_E.

<u>For a constant f (i.e. – f is held constant)</u>

When f is held constant, TCT does not change.

Therefore:

If you increase the PIFR, you decrease T_I and thus increase T_E accordingly.

If you decrease the PIFR, you increase T_I and thus decrease T_E accordingly.

Consider the following for an application of what was just discussed:

For a "normal patient", I:E ratios are usually around 1:2 - 1:3. But let's say you have a COPD patient who is air trapping and you want to be able to increase T_E in order to give them more time to exhale. In this case that could mean for example that you want to change the I:E ratio to 1:4. You can do this one of two ways. As discussed above, one of the ways you can do this is by increasing the PIFR (f remaining the same). When you increase the PIFR you are increasing the speed at which the breath is delivered. If the breath is getting delivered faster that means it's taking less time to be delivered, hence T_I is less. But remember that since the frequency has not been changed that means that TCT has remained unchanged – and in that scenario that means that a reduction in T_I will result in having a longer T_E, and therefore you have given your patient more time to exhale. The other way you can accomplish extending T_E is by decreasing the frequency (in this case PIFR remains constant). When you decrease the frequency you increase the TCT, but remember that only the T_E is affected. T_I remains the same because the PIFR has remained constant. In this scenario, by decreasing the frequency you have increased T_E by virtue of increasing the TCT, and thus you have given your patient more time to exhale.

Another thing to note – if you raise the V_T while keeping the PIFR and the frequency the same (meaning no change in the TCT), then you will have increased the T_I because for the same PIFR it is going to take longer to deliver a larger volume of gas. In this case T_E will have been shortened. Therefore, if you want to raise the V_T but yet keep the I:E ratio the same – then you are going to have to increase the PIFR, because the only way you're going to deliver more gas without altering T_I (and thus maintaining the same I:E ratio) is to deliver it faster – hence the rationale behind having to raise the PIFR in this scenario.

4. Synchronized Intermittent Mandatory Ventilation (SIMV)

SIMV is one of those modes that you will either love or hate. Some old-school physicians still love SIMV for reasons I won't get into, but among respiratory therapists, SIMV is fading from popularity. There are good points and bad points about SIMV, and once you become more experienced with mechanical ventilation you can make up your own mind on how you feel about this mode. But for now let's get into what SIMV is all about.

- SIMV is a *partial support mode* which means that in order to use this mode your patient must have an intact respiratory drive and thus have the ability to breathe spontaneously.

As with volume ventilation (AC, VC, CMV), SIMV is also TIME or PATIENT TRIGGERED and VOLUME CYCLED.

Parameters you set with SIMV

Just as it was with volume ventilation, with SIMV you set the same parameters.

- Set V_T
- Set f
- Set sensitivity
- Set PIFR
- Set pressure limit (alarm)

With everything being the same as volume ventilation so far, you may now be asking what makes SIMV different? As just mentioned – SIMV is mode that provides *partial support* rather than full ventilatory support, and as this discussion continues you will come to appreciate what that means. Another aspect unique to SIMV is that is can be used as a weaning mode – and SIMV can be used in this way by virtue of the fact that it is a partial support mode.

Therefore, SIMV is indicated:

- When you only want partial support. This means that the patient has an intact respiratory drive and can breathe on their own, *but they need help.*

- As a means to wean the patient off the ventilator. Since SIMV enables the patient to have time to breathe on their own, it is a mode that enables you to start transferring the WOB back to the patient gradually.

How SIMV works and what makes it so similar to, but yet different from volume ventilation.

Insofar as SIMV is triggered and cycled the same way as volume ventilation, and you set the same parameters as volume ventilation, the fundamental thing that makes SIMV different is the way in which you set the frequency. *In SIMV the frequency is purposely set so as to enable a long enough TCT to enable the patient to be able to breathe spontaneously in between the mechanical breaths.*

Consider the following as a generic example:

You set the frequency (f) at 6. Your TCT is then 60/f or $60/6 = 10$ seconds. Now you set your PIFR so that you get a T_I of 2 seconds. Since the TCT is 10 seconds, if T_I is 2 seconds, then T_E has to be 8 seconds because $TCT = T_I + T_E$. Now a T_E of 8 seconds is a ridiculously long T_E, but we are doing this on purpose because it is during this long T_E that we are giving the patient a chance to take a breath on their own.

If during this long T_E the patient triggers (they attempt to take a breath on their own), their effort opens a demand valve that gives them access to the gas so that they can draw a breath on their own. They only get access to the gas – they don't get any flow from the ventilator – the flow of gas during this patient triggered breath is controlled by the patient. One of the things you should be realizing by now is that during the times that the ventilator is delivering the breath, the WOB is being done by the ventilator. During the times when the patient is triggering a breath, the WOB is being done by the patient. It is through this process of being able to temporarily transfer the WOB back to the patient during the times that they trigger that this mode is able to be useful in weaning. One of the issues with weaning is whether or not the patient has sufficient respiratory muscle strength to sustain adequate ventilation on their own. By transferring the WOB back to the patient during the times that they trigger enables a way to help them start building back up their muscle strength. This mode is designed such that if the patient triggers a breath, the ventilator will reset so as to stay in synch with the patient.

Realize however, that experience from clinical practice has shown that utilizing T piece trials (spontaneous breathing trial - SBT) and/or gradual reductions in pressure support results in much shorter weaning times than using SIMV. This is one of the reasons why SIMV has fallen out of favor with many respiratory therapists. Patient discomfort that can be caused by the potential variation that can occur with flow patterns and inspiratory time frames when using SIMV is another reason that many RT's no longer favor SIMV. But as it was indicated at the beginning of this section, there are still enough physicians that like to use this mode such that you'll need to become comfortable with using it. Once you gain experience as a therapist and earn the trust of the physicians that you work with, you can then share your expertise regarding mode selection and/or strategy options that are perhaps better suited than SIMV.

Some very important things to keep in mind with SIMV.

One of the recurring themes of this book is to always be paying attention to your patient – as a licensed medical practitioner that needs to become second nature to you. If it doesn't, you won't last very long. Look at how this pertains to monitoring someone on SIMV.

Since there are times when they are breathing on their own in this mode – you need to pay close attention to the tidal volumes they are achieving during the times they are spontaneously breathing. You will be able to look directly at the ventilator and it will indicate to you the V_T they are achieving during a spontaneous breath. Remember you have purposely set a low f in order to establish a longer TCT in order to give them time to breathe on their own. But it is essential that they are achieving a good enough V_T because they still need to maintain an adequate V_E.

So you need to be paying attention to the *trends* in the V_T they achieve during the times they take a spontaneous breath. The mechanical breaths delivered by the ventilator are always going to be consistent with what you have set – it's the spontaneous breaths that they take in between where you have to pay attention and make sure they are getting enough V_T.

Example: You observe the following pattern in the V_T the patient is achieving during their spontaneous breathing.

Spontaneous breath 1 – V_T = 275 ml

Spontaneous breath 2 – V_T = 225 ml

Spontaneous breath 3 – V_T = 250 ml

Spontaneous breath 4 – V_T = 225 ml

Spontaneous breath 5 – V_T = 200 ml

This is a trend that is showing an overall decline in achieved V_T. Even without the downward trend, these are not great spontaneous tidal volumes anyway. In fact they are rather poor, and furthermore it's mostly dead space ventilation anyway so they probably won't have a good $PaCO_2$ from the ABG. This trend is telling you that this patient does not yet have adequate muscle strength to achieve a proper V_T. They can't handle the WOB required of them to achieve a proper V_T. Some of the burden of the WOB that is obviously still too much for them has to be relieved.

You handle this one of two ways:

1) Increase the frequency – increasing the frequency will make the TCT shorter. Remember that only T_E is affected – T_I remains consistent because we are not altering the PIFR. Although T_E does get shortened, it is the shortening of the whole TCT that will make the next time triggered breath (machine breath) happen sooner. The patient ends up getting more machine delivered breaths because the time given to them to breathe on their own has been reduced. The ventilator has assumed more of the WOB and this gives the respiratory muscles a chance to

rest - thus the V_E and the ABG will improve. *Note that the more you increase the frequency, the more you make SIMV become like volume ventilation (AC, VC, CMV) – just food for thought.*

2) Add pressure support – rather than increasing the frequency, you can add pressure support. You keep all the parameters as they are and the patient continues to have the same intervals of spontaneous breathing, but you add pressure support to the spontaneous breaths. This way they still have the same time frame through which to be able to breath on their own, but they get some assistance with the WOB from the pressure support you have added to their spontaneous breaths. Although pressure support is its own mode – it can also be added to some of the other modes in order to help reduce the patient's WOB. This enables the patient to rest while yet maintaining an adequate V_T and V_E, and helps improve their ability to successfully wean.

5. Pressure Control Ventilation (PCV)

Just like AC, VC, and CMV – pressure *control* ventilation (PCV) is a full support mode. DO NOT get this confused with the pressure support mode that was just mentioned at the end of the SIMV discussion. They are completely different things and pressure support will be discussed right after this section on pressure control.

Pressure control is a mode that is often used when pressures get too high while in volume ventilation. Remember that pressure is variable in volume ventilation, and if there are issues with R_{AW} or lung compliance, you may end up with pressures that are not safe for the patient. When this happens, switching over to pressure control is an option because in pressure control the pressure is set and thus fixed. Being able to fix the pressure at a set level is what enables us to protect the lung from barotrauma, therefore PCV is considered one of the lung protection strategies. When you are in PCV it will be volume that varies, so you will need to pay attention to the V_T in order to make sure that the patient is maintaining an adequate V_E.

PCV is TIME or PATIENT TRIGGERED, and it is TIME CYCLED.

Parameters you set with PCV

- Set inspiratory pressure level
- Set frequency (f)
- Set T_I (T_I defines the length of time for the time cycling)
- Set sensitivity

When you are in PCV, if you need to increase the V_T, there are two things you can do:

1) Increase the inspiratory pressure – this is an option as long as the pressure isn't getting too high. Remember that $30 - 35$ cmH$_2$O is about as far as you want to go – beyond that you will have to start concerning yourself with barotrauma.

2) Increase T_I – When you increase T_I, you are allowing more time for inspiration, and therefore you will achieve a higher V_T. But be aware – you have only increased T_I - you did not alter the frequency. Therefore the TCT has remained the same which means that when you increase the T_I, the T_E is going to decrease. Pay attention to your patient and make sure they are getting enough time to exhale.

With PCV:

V_T varies *directly* with the set inspiratory pressure, T_I, and lung compliance.

V_T varies *inversely* with R_{AW}.

6. Pressure Support Ventilation (PSV)

Pressure support was previously mentioned as an adjunct that could be used along with SIMV. Here we are going to discuss how it is used as its own unique mode.

- PSV is a totally *spontaneous* mode of ventilation. This means that the patient must have an intact and stable ventilatory drive.
- If the patient does not make an inspiratory effort – they get nothing.
- The aim of PSV is to help decrease the WOB – therefore it is useful as a weaning mode.

PSV is PATIENT TRIGGERED, and it is FLOW CYCLED.

Parameters you set with PSV

- Set inspiratory pressure level (the level of pressure support).
  * *Even though in PSV you are only setting a small amount of pressure just to provide support, you are nonetheless still setting a pressure.*

- Set sensitivity

Parameters controlled by the *patient* with PSV

- The patient controls the V_T.
- The patient controls the inspiratory flow.
- The patient controls the frequency (f).
- The patient controls T_I.

Realize that this mode is simply augmenting the spontaneous V_T of the patient. V_T is going to vary in this mode.

A) V_T will vary with the level of pressure support being given.

B) V_T will also vary according to lung dynamics.

- V_T will vary directly with lung compliance.
- V_T will vary inversely with R_{AW}.

Since V_T varies in this mode – you have to pay attention to the V_T the patient is achieving. You also have to pay attention to the frequency because that is also under the patient's control, and their spontaneous V_T and f are going to determine their V_E.

PSV$_{MAX}$

With PSV, the amount of pressure support you are going to give is largely dependent upon how much help they need in order to achieve an adequate enough V_T so as to ensure an adequate V_E. In general you will use the least amount of pressure necessary to sustain an adequate V_T because the idea here is to enable the patient to carry as much of the WOB as they can handle. If you are changing over to PSV from the patient having been in volume ventilation, you could determine the initial pressure support by taking the difference between the PIP and P_{PLT} that they had when they were in volume ventilation (pressure support setting in PSV = PIP – P_{PLT} from previous volume ventilation).

PSV$_{MAX}$ is a level of pressure support that is high enough to totally support the patient. Theoretically speaking, you could provide so much pressure support that it would essentially provide total support for the patient and the only work being done by the patient would be to trigger the ventilator. So depending upon the circumstances of your patient, you could start the level of pressure support at PSV$_{MAX}$. By starting out this way, as you then start to lower the inspiratory pressure support over time – you are gradually transferring the WOB to the patient. And this is one of the ways that is successful in weaning patients off the ventilator. If along the way during the weaning process your patient starts to exhibit difficulty

– you can increase the amount of pressure support. This will shift some of the WOB from the patient back to the ventilator.

7. Continuous Positive Airway Pressure (CPAP)

CPAP and PEEP are extremely similar. Whereas CPAP is a mode on the ventilator as well as a stand-alone device, PEEP is only a setting on the ventilator. Setting PEEP within the various modes was not discussed in this section on modes because PEEP is going to be discussed in depth right after we are finished with modes. Along with being discussed here, CPAP will also appear later in the section on non-invasive ventilation as CPAP is used to treat pulmonary edema and obstructive sleep apnea.

- CPAP is a totally spontaneous mode – the patient is breathing fully on their own – therefore they must have an intact ventilatory drive.
- CPAP helps with oxygenation – NOT ventilation. It helps to maintain FRC, improves V/Q, and helps with refractory hypoxemia.
- CPAP essentially changes the baseline pressure of the lung. The slight continuous positive pressure from CPAP helps keep the alveoli open – which in turn is effective in preventing atelectasis and thus improving oxygenation and preventing/treating hypoxemia.
- CPAP helps decrease the WOB in patient's whose lung compliance is low.
- CPAP can be used in weaning.
- Even though it is a totally spontaneous mode, you can set alarms to know if your patient is in distress.
- Depending on what it is being used for, CPAP settings can vary. CPAP of $3 - 5$ cmH$_2$O is typically sufficient to maintain physiological PEEP and prevent/treat atelectasis, and $7 - 12$ cmH$_2$O is typically sufficient to address obstructive sleep apnea. CPAP can go higher if needed.

Advanced Modes

8. Airway Pressure Release Ventilation (APRV)

APRV is considered to be an "open lung" approach to ventilation. The patient is being ventilated at the top of the compliance (volume – pressure) curve. What you have in this mode is essentially 2 levels of CPAP that are occurring at alternating time limits. This allows for unrestricted spontaneous breathing throughout the ventilatory cycle. The continuous CPAP with regular, short releases in airway pressure facilitates alveolar ventilation and CO_2 removal.

In the APRV mode you have the following:

P_{high} – this is the upper level of CPAP – it is set to the previous P_{PLT} pressure (generally between 15 – 30 cmH$_2$O), although some clinicians will use the mP$_{AW}$ (mean airway pressure) from the conventional mode when setting P_{high} in APRV. In APRV, P_{high} is considered baseline.

T_{high} – this is the length of time that P_{high} is maintained. It is set between 4.5 – 5.5 seconds (but never less than 4 seconds). You can go as high as 12 – 15 seconds, but this must be done gradually in small (0.5 – 2 second) intervals.

P_{low} – this is the lower level of CPAP – it is set between 0 – 15 cmH$_2$O, however the trend with more protocols these days is to set it at 0.

T_{low} – this is the length of time that P_{low} is maintained. It is set between 0.6 – 1 second.

P_{high} and P_{low} are thus TIME TRIGGERED AND TIME CYCLED.

P_{high} facilitates alveolar recruitment and therefore enhances gas exchange. The extended time (T_{high}) that occurs during P_{high} allows alveolar units with slower time constants to open. The timed releases in pressure (P_{low}) allows the alveolar gas to be exhaled via natural lung recoil. The short T_{low} prevents the loss of FRC, and this is important as we do not want de-recruitment of the lung to occur. The optimal duration of T_{low} and the setting of P_{low} are functions of the time constant, and the V_T during T_{low} is dependent upon the compliance of the lung, R_{AW}, the duration of T_{low}, and ΔP. Complete exhalation of V_T would be about 4 time constants. The higher the pressure gradient (ΔP), which is the difference between P_{high} and P_{low}, the greater the expiratory flow and thus a better V_T. V_T is attempted to be maintained at 4 – 6 ml/kg IBW. Pressure support may also be added to either P_{high} or P_{low}, or both.

Indications for using APRV

- With low compliance lung disorders.
- Refractory hypoxemia (ARDS/ALI).
- When P_{PLT} is exceeding 30 – 35 cmH$_2$O.
- In cases of acute lung injury.
- With atelectasis after major surgery.

Contraindications for APRV

- Unmanaged increases in ICP.
- A large bronchopleural fistula.
- Asthma
- COPD

Advantages to using APRV

- Lower pressures needed to maintain ventilation and oxygenation in patients with ALI.
- Requires a lower V_E suggesting decreased dead space ventilation.
- Avoids shear stress and stretch injury.
- Decreased hemodynamic compromise.
- Allows for spontaneous breathing at all points in the respiratory cycle.

- Spontaneous breathing tends to improve V/Q matching.
  - because spontaneous breathing provides better ventilation to dependent lung regions.
  - spontaneous breathing retains diaphragmatic function which helps offset any atelectasis that would occur at the lung bases.
- Spontaneous breathing prevents ventilatory muscle atrophy.
- With APRV there is less need for sedation and nearly no need for neuromuscular blocking agents.

Disadvantages to using APRV

- Volumes are affected by changes in compliance and R_{AW} – therefore close monitoring is required.
- Fear of integrating new technology.
- Limited research and clinical experience.
- Asynchrony can occur when spontaneous breaths are out of synch with release time.

Management of APRV

1) To increase PaO_2

- Increase P_{high} in 2 cmH_2O increments (increase mP_{AW}).
- Increase FiO_2
- Increase T_{high} *(this will also probably increase $PaCO_2$)*.
- Decrease T_{low} to increase intrinsic PEEP *(this will also probably increase $PaCO_2$)*.
- Put patient in prone position if needed.

2) To decrease $PaCO_2$ (if $PaCO_2$ is too high resulting in acidosis)

- Decrease T_{high} – this will result in more releases per minute, thus it will increase V_E.
  - but be careful – the P_{high} - T_{high} combo is what is providing the mP_{AW} and thus oxygenation. If T_{high} is decreased to the point where the breath releases exceed 12 per minute, this will affect oxygenation.

- Increase P_{high} – this will increase V_T, but don't increase P_{high} to any more than $30 - 35$ cmH$_2$O.
- V_T may be augmented by using pressure support (+5), but the PIP cannot exceed 35 cmH$_2$O.

3) To increase PaCO$_2$ (if PaCO$_2$ is too low resulting in alkalemia)

- Increase T_{high} - this will result in less releases per minute and thus lower V_E.
- Decrease T_{low}
- Many consider T_{low} to be the key variable. It must be short enough to prevent lung de-recruitment, but long enough to maintain a V_T that is $4 - 6$ ml/kg IBW. Utilize the flow/time graphics on the ventilator – never let the expiratory flow reach baseline as this helps to avoid lung de-recruitment.

Weaning from APRV

- The first priority should be to reduce the FiO$_2$.
- There are many different protocols to discontinue APRV.

    1) Maintain oxygenation with FiO$_2 \leq 45\%$.

    2) Decrease P_{high} by 2 cmH$_2$O increments, and increase T_{high} by 1 second increments.

    3) When a P_{high} of 12 cmH$_2$O is reached – change to PSV with a PEEP of 5.

9. Pressure Regulated Volume Control (PRVC)

Think of PRVC as a hybrid mode that combines volume and pressure control ventilation. In this mode you are able to deliver a guaranteed V_T by using PCV in the sense that the ventilator adjusts the inspiratory pressure to provide the V_T at the lowest possible pressure. This is accomplished by means of continuous feedback of the measured V_T.

PRVC is PATIENT or TIME TRIGGERED, and TIME CYCLED.

Parameters you set with PRVC

- Set target V_T
- Set T_I
- Set f
- Set sensitivity
- Set pressure limit (alarm)

How PRVC works:

As a breath is being delivered, the ventilator measures the V_T that is being delivered and compares it to the set (targeted) V_T – this is a closed loop (feedback) system.

As this is a volume targeted, pressure controlled means of delivering a breath,

- If the delivered V_T < set (targeted) V_T
  - then the ventilator will increase the pressure in small increments over the next several breaths until the delivered V_T is equivalent to the target V_T.

- If the delivered V_T > set (targeted) V_T
  - then the ventilator will decrease the pressure accordingly so as to equate to the target V_T.

Note:

When using PRVC, some ventilators will *initially* do a test breath in order to do an inspiratory pause. The P_{PLT} obtained from the inspiratory pause during this test breath will then be the pressure control level for the next breath. The pressure level of subsequent breaths will either increase or decrease by a maximum of 3 cmH_2O in order to achieve the set (targeted) V_T.

In the PRVC mode, the ventilator will not permit the pressure to exceed 5 cmH_2O below the upper pressure limit setting. This means that if the upper pressure limit is 30 cmH_2O and the ventilator needs to apply more than 25 cmH_2O to deliver the V_T, then the alarm is going to go off and the pressure is going to be limited to 25 cmH_2O. This means that in a case such as this, you may end up not achieving the target V_T.

Conversely, as the patient's condition improves (better lung compliance and/or less R_{AW}) – the amount of pressure needed to deliver the V_T will decrease in response to the improvements in lung mechanics. But regardless of the amount of improvement and less need of pressure to deliver a breath - the baseline pressure, which is PEEP, will always be maintained.

Advantages of PRVC

- The pressure adjusts for changes in C_L and R_{AW}.
- It uses the lowest possible pressure to deliver the set (targeted) V_T.
- It decreases the risk of barotrauma and volutrauma.
- It decreases the risk of hypoventilation.
- The inspiratory pressure automatically decreases as the patient improves.
  - but realize that what this means is that the patient is assuming more of the WOB. If you are observing that the patient is able to reach, or even exceed the target V_T at much lower pressures – it is indeed an indication that they are improving, but monitor them closely because the reduced pressure from the ventilator is because the patient is doing more of the WOB on their own, and you want to watch them for any signs of fatigue.

Disadvantages of PRVC

- Intermittent patient effort will result in variable V_T's.
- Potential asynchrony with variable patient effort.
- PRVC is not suitable for patients with asthma or COPD.
- PRVC is not well tolerated by patients that are awake or non-sedated.

- A *sudden increase* in ventilatory demand may result in a temporary decrease in ventilatory support because changes in the pressure are made progressively - not immediately. *This is the one you really have to pay attention to with PRVC as it is one of its major downfalls.*

10. Volume Support (VS) - "Volume Targeted PSV"

As you are about to see, this mode is somewhat similar to PRVC. Whereas in PRVC you are delivering a targeted V_T via *pressure control*, in the volume support mode (VS) you are doing the same thing except that you are delivering the targeted V_T by using *pressure support*. This hybrid mode basically boils down to being pressure support with a targeted volume.

Volume support can be used as a weaning mode, although its value in weaning is not clearly established. Volume support is a partial support mode that can only be used with a patient that has an intact respiratory drive that is able to breathe spontaneously.

Volume Support (VS) is PATIENT TRIGGERED, and it is FLOW CYCLED (just like PSV).

Parameters you set with VS

- Set the target V_T
- Set sensitivity
- Set pressure limit

Since this is a support mode – the patient is controlling the other parameters (T_I, f, and flow).

You don't set an inspiratory pressure level like you do in PSV - because in VS, the level of pressure support needed to achieve the target V_T is going to vary according to lung dynamics. In regular PSV, the amount of pressure support that is given for each breath is always the same – it's whatever you set it at. But in VS, the amount of pressure support given for each breath in order to reach the target

V_T is going to vary in accordance with lung dynamics (lung compliance and R_{AW}) – and this is the aspect of VS that makes it very similar to PRVC.

In VS, just as in PRVC, you have a closed (feedback) loop whereby the ventilator is measuring the V_T of each breath and comparing it to the targeted V_T. And just like it was in PRVC, the ventilator adjusts the pressure accordingly for each subsequent breath in order to meet the targeted V_T. It will either increase the level of pressure support (not to exceed the pressure limit) to meet the targeted V_T if needed, or it will decrease the amount of pressure support in the event that not as much pressure is needed to reach the targeted V_T. A reduction in pressure is what you would see when the patient is improving.

So you may ask – if volume support (VS) and PRVC are so similar, why have both? The subtlety lies herein: PRVC delivers a targeted V_T via *pressure control* - and even though the pressure delivering each breath varies with respect to lung dynamics – it is still a FULL SUPPORT mode which means that the ventilator is controlling everything. With VS you still have a targeted V_T, but it is being delivered via *pressure support*. Of course the amount of pressure support that is delivering each breath varies with respect to lung dynamics just like it did with PRVC, but VS is a PARTIAL SUPPORT mode which means that the patient is controlling most of the parameters of breathing. Flow is controlled by the patient, inspiratory time is controlled by the patient, & frequency is controlled by the patient.

Both PRVC and VS, like PCV, are considered modes that are consistent with lung protection strategies by virtue of the fact that they impose pressure limits. Protection of the lung is further enhanced in that both of these modes are also volume targeted which if you think about it also means that they are volume limited as well, and that is also consistent with protecting the lung.

Just as it was with PRVC, when your patient is in VS mode - if you start observing that the patient is able to reach, or even exceed the target V_T at much lower levels of pressure support – it is indeed an indication that they are improving, but monitor them closely because the reduced pressure support coming from the ventilator is indicating that the patient is doing more of the WOB on their own, and you want to watch them for any signs of fatigue.

11. Mandatory Minute Ventilation (MMV)

This is a mode that is designed to maintain a minimum V_E. Although research on the effectiveness of this mode is still lacking, it can still be used to support being able to maintain a minimum V_E. This mode is used mostly in conjunction with SIMV – so you are basically adding MMV to SIMV. Note though that you can use MMV with the control modes as well (e.g. CMV).

The basic idea of how this works is as follows: Say for example that you have your patient in SIMV – remember that in SIMV there are going to be periods of time when the ventilator is going to be giving mandatory breaths, but then there will also be times when the patient is breathing spontaneously.

You are going to have a V_E as a result of the mandatory mechanical breaths – that is your "mechanical" V_E, which is just V_T x f as per however you have the ventilator set for the mandatory breaths.

But since the patient is also spontaneously breathing in between the mechanical breaths – you then also have a spontaneous V_E that is determined by the patient's own effort.

You need to look at both of these in order to determine their total V_E, which is going to be the mechanical V_E + their spontaneous V_E. It's only after you see what their total V_E is that you can then determine where you want to set the MMV.

You determine the amount of MMV as follows:

Let's say your patient is on SIMV and their total V_E is 10 LPM. Now that's a little high since "normal" is 5 – 6 LPM, but a V_E that is ≤ 10 LPM is still acceptable – and for the purpose of this example it is fine. For a patient that is on SIMV, you set the MMV at 90% of the mechanical (mandatory) V_E.

For this patient that is on SIMV with a total V_E of 10 LPM, let us say hypothetically that 8 LPM of that total is coming from the mandatory (mechanical) V_E. From what I just told you with regards to how to set the MMV, you would set the MMV at 90% of 8 LPM – or 7 LPM.

Now MMV is a closed (feedback) system that has the ability to tell when the V_E has dropped such that it can then react accordingly – and here is how it does that:

Let's say that the total V_E of the patient drops to 6 LPM. Because of the feedback mechanism, the ventilator is going to recognize this and take action to bring it back up to 7 LPM. It will do this by increasing the mechanical (mandatory) V_T and/or frequency in order to get the V_E back to at least 7 LPM.

The drawback with MMV is that MMV is not able to distinguish between "good" ventilation and "bad" dead space ventilation. Referring back to the example above – you've set the MMV at 7 LPM (that's the minimum V_E) – and let's say that this minimum V_E is either being met or exceeded. The problem is that the MMV mode doesn't know *how* it's being met. If the V_T x f = V_E is say 585 x 12 $\approx$ 7 LPM, then all is well. But what if the V_T x f = V_E is from 350 x 20 = 7 LPM. This is not good because it is mostly dead space ventilation that is happening as a result of a rapid and shallow breathing pattern. The mandatory machine breaths are always going to be at the V_T and f that you set. But since in SIMV the patient is also able to breath spontaneously on their own, it is necessary to access the *quality* of those spontaneous breaths that are contributing to the MMV. All the ventilator sees is a number (the V_E) – it cannot discern the quality of the breaths that are making up the V_E. Because of this mode's inability to distinguish the quality of the ventilation that is producing the V_E, it will be necessary for you to set a high frequency alarm and a low V_T alarm so that *you* will be able to discern the quality of the ventilation.

If MMV is being used with CMV, the MMV can be set at 80% of their V_E so long as there is no remarkable hypocapnia or alkalemia. If there is minor hypocapnia or alkalemia, then set the MMV at 75% of their V_E. *(in CMV there is no spontaneous V_E - there is only a mechanical V_E because CMV is a full support control mode).*

----

12. Automode (Variable PSV)

Automode, also known as variable PSV, is an interactive mode of ventilation that facilitates weaning. This mode can alternate from a time triggered mandatory breath in a control mode (e.g. CMV) to a patient triggered support breath in a support mode (e.g. VS).

If the patient makes no spontaneous effort, then all the breaths are mandatory (mechanical) as per the set V_T, etc. If the patient does make an inspiratory effort, then they would take a spontaneous breath with support. Automode is usually set up so that if no patient trigger is sensed within a time frame of 7 – 12 seconds then the control mode takes over until such time that the patient triggers.

Earlier weaning is made possible due to the elimination of annoying apnea alarms. Observing your patient over 24 hour periods enables the assessment of breathing activity and patterns. As such, this mode may be good for patients who have periods of apnea, neuromuscular disease, or who have exhibited Biot's or Cheyne-Stokes breathing patterns.

Examples of interaction in Automode:

Control Mode	Support Mode	
VC	VS	----- provides equal set V_T's
PRVC	VS	----- provides equal set V_T's
PCV	PSV	----- enables the clinician to select different set pressure levels to vary patient/ ventilator workloads (this is a replacement to conventional SIMV.)

K. PEEP

General Points

- PEEP is not a mode – it's a setting on a ventilator.

- PEEP, otherwise known as positive end expiratory pressure, is a means by which positive pressure is applied at the end of expiration. Instead of the pressure being 0 at the end of exhalation, PEEP enables us to keep it just slightly positive.

- PEEP takes the place of a sigh or a yawn that occurs with a normal individual. A normal person yawns or sighs to keep lower alveoli open – but a patient on a mechanical ventilator can't yawn, so PEEP offsets this incapacity. PEEP is a way of keeping the alveoli open without having to use excessive volumes or pressures. $3 - 5$ cmH$_2$O PEEP from the ventilator is about what it takes to replace the physiologic PEEP (the sigh or yawn). Every patient that is intubated and being mechanically ventilated is going to get at least this minimal amount of PEEP to keep their alveoli open because they are not able to sigh or yawn on their own.

- PEEP and CPAP are cousins in the sense that they both provide positive airway pressure. CPAP provides it continuously whereas PEEP provides it at the end of exhalation, but nonetheless remember that CPAP is a MODE that requires a spontaneously breathing patient whereas PEEP is a SETTING within a mode. Most mechanically ventilated patients (regardless of the mode being used) get a small amount of PEEP $(3 - 5$ cmH$_2$O) to prevent end-expiratory alveolar collapse.

- Besides replacing the sigh or yawn and thus enabling the alveoli to remain open, the main indication for PEEP is to treat refractory hypoxemia - in other words PEEP is used to treat a shunt. PEEP improves oxygenation.

- PEEP restores FRC and helps improve lung compliance.

- PEEP is also used to reduce ventilator-associated lung injury in patients with ALI (acute lung injury), and ARDS (acute respiratory distress syndrome).

Optimal PEEP

Optimal PEEP is that which provides for the best static compliance with the best O_2 delivery at the lowest FiO_2. The idea is to recruit recruitable alveoli without over distending normal alveoli while keeping the $P_{PLT} \leq 30 - 35$ cmH$_2$O. Some alveoli are recruitable and will respond to PEEP whereas other alveoli will never respond and just won't open no matter how much pressure is applied. Remember also that PEEP contributes to the overall amount of pressure in the lung – so if you are in PCV for example and delivering the V_T with a pressure of 25 cmH$_2$O – realize that you won't want to set the PEEP more than $5 - 10$ cmH$_2$O because you don't want to exceed a total pressure of $30 - 35$ cmH$_2$O.

You must always be aware of the patient's hemodynamic status when using PEEP as the use of PEEP has hemodynamic consequences. Since PEEP by definition is applying positive pressure into the lung (and the thorax by extension), a natural consequence of this is the potential to reduce venous return and thus reduce cardiac output. This is why it is always imperative that you continuously monitor your patient's hemodynamic status.

There are several charts and algorithms, etc. that are available to tell you how to figure out the best PEEP to give your patient. And in cases of ARDS these charts may have slightly more applicability, but the reality of determining the right amount of PEEP comes down to applying common sense through the lens of a few variables as follows:

- The ideal (optimal) PEEP level is that which is enabling the best oxygenation at the lowest FiO_2 without causing any hemodynamic instability. The simplest and most clinically relevant way to figure this out is to do a PEEP study.

The PEEP Study

When trying to optimize the level of PEEP – especially with a patient with ALI or ARDS, consider the following as this will enable you to be very effective at finding the optimal PEEP with just a few pieces of data you are able to quickly ascertain at the bedside.

1) Obtain baseline values for static compliance, P/F ratio, and SpO$_2$. (you need baseline values as a reference for comparison)

2) Start increasing the PEEP by about 2 – 3 cmH$_2$O every 20 minutes.

3) At the end of each 20 minute interval – look at the following:

- **Static Compliance** $C_{stat} = \dfrac{V_T}{P_{PLT} - PEEP}$

This is easy to figure out: You get the P_{PLT} by doing an inspiratory hold. The PEEP you'll know because you set it, and then you'll look at the ventilator to see their exhaled V_T. Do the calculation to determine their static compliance. Normal range is 60 – 100 ml/cmH$_2$O.

- **P/F Ratio** (PaO$_2$/FiO$_2$)

You'll get the PaO$_2$ from the ABG. They should have an A-line so that you're not sticking them every 20 minutes. The FiO$_2$ will be whatever you have it set at. Do the calculation and refer to the information below to determine the status of your patient.

- Normal values for this ratio are 350 – 450 mmHg.
- Values below 300 mmHg indicate ALI (acute lung injury)
- Values below 200 mmHg indicate ARDS (acute respiratory distress syndrome)

- SpO$_2$

  This is derived from simple pulse oximetry. The goal is to maintain an SpO$_2 \geq 92\%$, or at the level specified by the physician.

4) At the end of each 20 minute interval, if you find the C$_{stat}$, P/F ratio, and SpO$_2$ increasing – then you know that your strategy of raising the PEEP 2 – 3 cmH$_2$O every 20 minutes is working. Continue the strategy of raising the PEEP in 2 – 3 cmH$_2$O increments every 20 minutes until the data dictates otherwise. And what is meant by that is as follows:

   - At the point when the P/F ratio becomes $\geq$ 200, or if the static compliance decreases – THEN STOP - and set the PEEP at the setting where it was just prior.

   Realize also that as you are doing this protocol that you have to remain aware of, and take into consideration, other parameters of hemodynamic stability. You're going to have to continue to monitor their vitals to include their heart rate and blood pressure. Knowing whether or not the PEEP is compromising cardiac output is going to be more difficult to calculate because you don't know the stroke volume. Cardiac output (Q$_t$) is easy to figure out when you know the stroke volume because it's simply the heart rate x stroke volume. You can get the pulse easily, but not having the stroke volume means that you would have to figure out Q$_t$ using the Fick equation and that is a bit more involved. However – if your patient is oxygenating well and there are no other signs to indicate a reduction in cardiac output, then Q$_t$ is probably not being adversely affected by PEEP. Clinical signs though that would prompt you to suspect that Q$_t$ is being compromised would be a decrease in blood pressure, changes in the EKG (arrhythmias), rapid breathing, decreased urine output, anxiety, or decreased LOC. Remember to also monitor their end tidal CO$_2$ (EtCO$_2$) as this will give you a close approximation to their PaCO$_2$ which will enable you to tell how well they are ventilating.

Also:

If the systolic BP is less than 90, DO NOT increase the PEEP.

Try to keep the mean airway pressure (mP_{AW}) $\leq$ 15 cmH2O. If mP_{AW} rises above this, it can lead to a decrease in Q_t.

AutoPEEP (Intrinsic PEEP)

When a patient receives a mechanical breath, or takes a spontaneous breath (in partial support modes) - the lung volume at the end of exhalation *should* be FRC and the pressure *should* be ambient. However, when exhalation is incomplete (does not reach FRC), you develop an issue of progressively trapping air. This progressive hyperinflation of the lung due to incomplete exhalation that is increasing the alveolar pressure at the end of expiration is what is known as autoPEEP.

This unintentional PEEP can be due to several things, but most often it is a consequence of the expiratory flow limitations that arise from the obstructed and/or narrowed airways that are characteristic of COPD. Mucus plugs that obstruct the airways will inhibit expiratory airflow and thus cause air trapping. An asthma patient in status asthmaticus is going to have severely narrowed airways that will inhibit expiratory airflow and thus cause air trapping. When expiratory flow limitations are imposed due to obstructed and/or narrowed airways, not only is lung emptying incomplete, but the interruption of the expiratory phase by a new phase of inspiration further contributes to worsening the problem of hyperinflation. A time triggered ventilator delivers breaths according to the set frequency – it is not aware of these air trapping and incomplete exhalation issues going on with the patient. Expiratory flow limitations aren't the only problem that can cause autoPEEP. Another issue that will cause autoPEEP to develop is when a patient hyperventilates and thus has a high V_E.

Roughly 30% of patients on mechanical ventilation have dynamic hyperinflation and autoPEEP. For whatever the reason (some just mentioned), their lungs are not adequately emptying and autoPEEP is occurring. AutoPEEP has to be addressed because it has adverse effects such as causing diminished venous return to the heart which then leads to reduced cardiac output.

One way to determine if the patient is indeed experiencing autoPEEP is to do an expiratory hold. By doing an expiratory hold you will be able to get a measurement of the static PEEP in the lung, and if it is higher than the set PEEP, then you'll know that you have true autoPEEP occurring. A problem with this though, is that when you're measuring autoPEEP via the expiratory hold maneuver, you're only getting data for the lung units that are open and accessible. At the end of expiration, however, many of the small airways are closed and therefore the pressure in the alveolar units that are distal to these closed airways is not being accounted for. The measurement you derive from the expiratory hold is therefore underestimating the true value of the actual amount of autoPEEP.

In any case, the way you prevent and/or treat autoPEEP is to provide an adequate enough I:E ratio so as to give them enough time to exhale – and when they are in volume ventilation (VC, AC, CMV) for example, that means you need to increase T_E. You already know from the discussion on volume ventilation in the last section on modes that you can manipulate T_E a couple of different ways. If you need to – now would be a good time to review the nuances of how you adjust PIFR, frequency, and V_T as a means to manipulate the T_E.

During the course of your efforts to alter the V_T or f or PIFR in order to maximize T_E in an effort to reduce autoPEEP, you may find yourself in a situation of not being able to establish an adequate V_E. Your patient may then start to trigger excessively and this is just going to defeat the whole purpose and make things worse. In cases like this you may ultimately need to have the patient sedated and paralyzed in order for you to be able to control the V_E.

Another situation you may encounter is when you have a patient that is making inspiratory efforts, but those efforts are not able to trigger the vent. Your first instinct may be to think that it is a sensitivity setting issue. But when you're dealing with a patient with autoPEEP issues, the problem with not being able to trigger the ventilator is not in all likelihood a sensitivity issue, but rather it is the autoPEEP itself that is preventing the patient from being able to trigger the ventilator. This is because the patient's inspiratory effort has to now be sufficient enough to overcome the effect of the autoPEEP. Let's say the sensitivity is set at the standard setting for a patient controlled pressure trigger (-2 cmH$_2$O). And let's also say that the expiratory hold indicated that there is 8 cmH$_2$O of autoPEEP. In order to trigger the ventilator, this patient now has to generate a 10 cmH$_2$O effort because they also have to overcome the extra 8 cmH$_2$O being imposed by the autoPEEP. Although patients like this are still in need of having their T$_E$ increased, there is the more immediate issue of them not being able to trigger a breath because of the increased pressure being imposed by the autoPEEP. The burden of triggering a breath lies ultimately with the respiratory muscles, and although it may seem contradictory at first, it is actually applied (extrinsic) PEEP that is able to counteract the effects of the autoPEEP and thus reduce the burden that is being imposed. In situations like this, if you set the applied (extrinsic) PEEP at about 70 – 80% of the autoPEEP, it will help improve the effectiveness of the respiratory muscles such that the patient should then be able to adequately trigger the ventilator. You may also consider maximizing bronchodilator (albuterol) treatments and possibly even lavage and suction for mucus plugs.

There are several ventilator graphics that will enable you to detect autoPEEP. Shown below is the waveform you would see on the flow graphic.

AutoPEEP Detection via the Flow Waveform

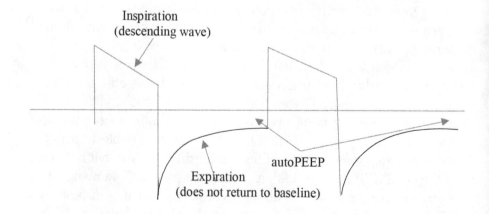

L. Weaning & Liberation from Mechanical Ventilation

Weaning is essentially a slow titration of transferring the WOB back to the patient. 80 – 85% of patients that are intubated and on mechanical ventilation are usually extubated and taken off the ventilator within 2 days. These patients typically do not need weaning. But what about the other 15 – 20% of the patients? They need to be weaned.

General Ideas

- Surgical patients tend to wean faster than medicine patients. Medicine patients are usually on the ventilator longer because they usually have other co-existing medical problems that contribute to making it more difficult for them to wean.

- An aggressive clinical approach to discontinuation of mechanical ventilation can often lead to pre-mature extubation which often leads to needing to re-intubate. This is why you need to make sure that there are no issues with things such as muscle fatigue, compromises with gas exchange, or any potential problems with the patient being able to protect their airway. Patients that end up requiring re-intubation have 8 times the likelihood of developing ventilator associated pneumonia (VAP).

- Therefore: Be less aggressive - The upside to being less aggressive is that the need to re-intubate occurs much less frequently. There are downsides to being less aggressive as well – your patient ends up spending more time on the ventilator which then statistically increases their risk for VAP as well as VILI (ventilator induced lung injury). The risk for airway trauma also increases due to them being intubated longer. Mechanical ventilation and intubation should therefore be removed as soon as possible to avoid:

1) VAP
2) VILI
3) Airway trauma from the ETT
4) Unnecessary sedation

But the key here is BALANCE

- Wean as quickly as possible
- Wean as slowly as necessary

Thinking about discontinuing mechanical ventilation is entertained when the reasons causing the need for mechanical ventilation are either resolved or very nearly resolved.

- This is the starting point for the consideration of weaning.

    A) Why were they on the ventilator in the first place
       - what was the underlying reason?

    B) Is "A" resolved or significantly improved?

Criteria for Weaning

The material in this section is consistent with accepted methodologies for weaning. If you follow the way I have organized this section and pay attention to the succinct notes that I have written, you should have a good overall understanding of how to wean a patient off a mechanical ventilator.

There are 3 overall areas of consideration when it comes to liberating a patient from the ventilator. Everything that is going to be addressed in this section falls under these 3 overall areas. These 3 overall areas are as follows:

<u>3 areas to consider when weaning a patient from the ventilator</u>

1) Has the underlying issue that got them on the ventilator in the first place been resolved or at least significantly improved?

2) Does the patient have favorable assessments of certain measurable criteria? The vast majority of this section is going to be discussing all the different assessments and tests that you will be doing to figure out if they are a candidate for weaning.

3) How did they handle the SBT (spontaneous breathing trial)?

<u>Now let us get into the specifics:</u>

A. If the patient has been on the ventilator for more than 24 hours – consider all the potential reasons that could be causing them to need the ventilator. This is consistent with making sure that the issues that got them on the ventilator in the first place are either resolved or significantly improved.

B. Here is where we are going to start to look at various different assessments to determine if the patient is ready to discontinue mechanical ventilation.

<u>Areas to be assessed (I – IV)</u>

I) Is there evidence that the underlying cause(s) of respiratory failure that necessitated mechanical ventilation have been resolved or significantly improved? To answer that question, you are going to evaluate the following:

a) <u>General Respiratory Considerations</u>

- Check breathing pattern - does patient exhibit rapid, shallow breathing?
- Is V_E stable?
- Are the respiratory muscles weak?
- Is V_D/V_T increased?
- Is there any hyperinflation going on?

- Is there any remarkable hypercapnia - is the pH ≥ 7.25?
- Is shunting present?
- Are there any issues with R_{AW} or C_L?
- Is there any obstructive sleep apnea?

b) <u>General Cardiovascular Considerations</u>

- Are there any arrhythmias?
- Do they have adequate cardiac reserves?
  - which is to say – is their heart able to work adequately enough meet any increased demands?
- They need to be able to handle the increased venous return when mechanical ventilation is discontinued.

c) <u>General Metabolic Considerations (nutrition)</u>

Consequences of overfeeding
- Be mindful that overfeeding a patient leads to increased CO_2 production and V_E.
- For COPD patients – feed them less carbohydrates and include more fat in the diet formula.

Consequences of underfeeding
- Malnutrition
- Decreased muscle mass
- Decreased surfactant

d) <u>General Neurological Considerations</u>

- Are there any remarkable findings from the neuro exam?
- Is the patient on any sedatives or narcotics that would impair neurological functioning? – (if so, they may need a sedation vacation)
- Is there any central sleep apnea?

e) <u>General Psychiatric Considerations</u>

- Any ICU psychosis going on?
- Has there been any sleep deprivation?
- Any issues with twilight awareness, or not being aware of what time it is?
- Is the patient fearful or exhibiting anxiety?

II) Is there Hemodynamic Stability?

- Make sure there is no remarkable hypotension.
- The patient should not be on any vasopressors – the only exception is low dose dopamine (1 - 5µg/kg/min).

III) Is the patient able to make an inspiratory effort on their own?

NOW:

The information derived from assessments I – III above is taken into consideration as part of the process of determining if the patient has recovered sufficiently from whatever it was that got them put on mechanical ventilation in the first place. This information is important because it contributes to the overall clinical picture of the patient.

The next area of assessments – called the physiological criteria for weaning - is what you are going to see being used extensively in real life clinical practice. Although the information derived from assessment areas I – III is very important in forming a comprehensive clinical picture of the patient, the information derived from the following physiological assessments is very specific, and they are rather strictly adhered to because of their proven reliability in being able to determine if a patient will be able to successfully wean. The various physiological criteria (indicators) that are about to be discussed are what I like to think of collectively as the "gold standard" of weaning criteria because experience has taught us that when the majority of these indicators have favorable findings, the chances for successful weaning are greatly enhanced.

IV) PHYSIOLOGICAL CRITERIA FOR WEANING

<u>7 indicators that determine if the patient has adequate **muscle strength** for weaning</u>

V_E < 10 - 15 LPM

V_T > 4 – 6 ml/kg IBW

F < 35 breaths/min.

VC > 15ml/kg IBW

RSBI (f/V_T) < 105 breaths/min./L
- *The rapid shallow breathing index (RSBI) is the single best indicator for weaning success.*
- RSBI is determined by the ratio (f/V_T) and is assessed 1 minute after the patient has been disconnected from the ventilator and O_2.
- *V_T is measured in liters – not ml.*
- f is the patient's spontaneous rate.
- Normal range for RSBI is 60 – 105 breaths/min/L
  - patients who are not able to tolerate independent spontaneous breathing tend to breath at higher frequencies and lower tidal volumes, and this is why the RSBI is a good indicator.
- The RSBI is done with a handheld spirometer that is attached to the ETT while the patient breathes room air spontaneously for one minute without any ventilator assistance.

MIP < -20 to -30 cmH₂O
- When done as a weaning assessment, MIP must be measured in an occluded airway after 20 seconds.
- You may see this called NIF (negative inspiratory force) – it means the same thing as MIP.

Breathing Pattern – stable without abnormalities.

6 indicators that determine if the patient's **oxygenation status** is adequate enough for weaning

$PaO_2 \geq 60$ mmHg with $FiO_2 \leq 40\%$

$PEEP \leq 5 - 8$ cmH$_2$O with $FiO_2 \leq 40\%$

P/F ratio $> 150 - 200$ mmHg; preferably > 250 mmHg

$P(A - a)O_2 < 350$ mmHg with FiO_2 100%

PaO_2/PAO_2 (a/A ratio) > 0.47 (47%)

Qs/Qt (shunt) $< 20 - 30$ %

3 indicators that determine if the patient will be able to handle the **WOB** associated with weaning

$C_{dyn} > 25$ ml/cmH$_2$O

$V_D/V_T < 0.6$ (60%)

CROP > 13 ml/breath/min.
- The CROP index is an equation that evaluates dynamic compliance, respiratory rate (total), oxygenation status, and MIP.
- CROP assesses the relationship between the demands that are placed on the respiratory system and the ability of the respiratory muscles to handle those demands.
- The equation is as follows:

$$\text{CROP Index} = \frac{C_{dyn} \times MIP \times (PaO_2 / PAO_2)}{f}$$

NOW – IF THE FINDINGS FROM I THROUGH IV ARE

FAVORABLE, THEN YOU CAN PROCEED TO DOING THE
SPONTANEOUS BREATHING TRIAL (SBT).

C. The Spontaneous Breathing Trial (SBT)

- The 30 – 120 minute SBT is the *BEST* indicator of the
  potential for ventilator discontinuation.

- If the patient can tolerate 30 – 120 minutes of SBT, then you
  are able to recommend that they are ready to be liberated
  from the ventilator and can be assessed for extubation.

- The SBT has close to an 85% success rate. In other words,
  roughly 85% of the patients that can tolerate the SBT can be
  successfully taken off the ventilator and extubated.

The SBT is conducted one of three ways:

1) T – piece (be aware of ETT size – it has to be ≥ 7.0)

2) Low Level CPAP (5 cmH$_2$O)

3) Low Level PSV (5 – 8 cmH$_2$O)

Assessments to make during the SBT

These assessments are made during the "screening phase" of the
SBT (i.e. – the first few minutes of the SBT)

- Respiratory Pattern – make sure the patient has a stable
  breathing pattern and a stable rate.
- Adequacy of gas exchange
- Hemodynamic stability
- Patient comfort – this is subjective

<u>Specific indications that the SBT is NOT being tolerated</u>

- The patient's spontaneous V_T < 250 – 300 ml.

- The patient's spontaneous rate is ≥ 35
  (or)
  Their spontaneous rate increases ≥ 10 from what it was before the SBT.

- Remarkable changes in heart Rate
  - an increase > 20% from what it was before the SBT,
    or if it increases to more than 140 bpm.
  - sudden onset of PVC's

- Remarkable changes in blood pressure
  - an increase or decrease of 20 mmHg in the systolic pressure,
    or if systolic pressure ≥ 180 mmHg.
  - an increase or decrease of 10 mmHg in the diastolic pressure.

- Any other clinical sign or change that would indicate that the patient is not tolerating the SBT.
  - accessory muscle usage (muscle fatigue)
  - nasal flaring
  - diaphoresis
  - anxiety or discomfort
  - decreased SpO_2
  - dyspnea
  - pain
  - cyanosis or pallor

D. Failure of the SBT

If the patient fails the SBT, you go back to I – IV and go thru the various areas of assessment to find out why they failed the SBT and try to correct any problems. When re-assessing, pay particular attention to (IV) - the physiological criteria for weaning. Try to pinpoint where they are having problems so as to determine what needs to be corrected so that they have a better chance of having success with the next SBT.

THE SBT CAN ONLY BE DONE ONCE EVERY 24 HOURS.

E. Maintaining Ventilation When the Patient Failed the SBT

The goal is to provide ventilatory support that focuses on:

A) Muscle unloading (allowing the respiratory muscles to rest)

B) Maximizing patient comfort
   * the following are things that you should be doing for any patient, but specific mention is made here insofar as they may be particularly tired or stressed after failing an SBT.
   - recommending sedation if needed
   - setting the sensitivity appropriately
   - adjusting flow if needed to meet the patient's inspiratory demand
   - using applied PEEP to mitigate autoPEEP

C) Avoiding any complications.

The modes that are traditionally used to ventilate patients that are in the process of weaning are SIMV, PSV, and T – piece (obviously T-piece is not a mode and you know that, but it's included here as it is a technique that is used regardless of the mode that is being used). Since I discussed SIMV earlier in the section on modes, I am not going to cover it again here – especially since clinical evidence has clearly shown that SIMV prolongs the weaning process and as such it is not a good mode choice for weaning.

Maintaining ventilation with PSV

Refer back to the full discussion on PSV in the mode section if necessary. PSV is one of the ways that allows for the building up of muscle strength and endurance. A patient can be considered "weaned" once the level of inspiratory pressure support is down to 5 cmH$_2$O.

- The initial setting (starting point) can be the P$_{PLT}$. That way you'll be able to get the V$_T$ you want. For patients who are able to be weaned, the initial level of pressure support should be around 5 – 15 cmH$_2$O.

- Titrate the level of pressure support until the patient is breathing at a spontaneous frequency of 15 – 20 bpm.

- Be looking for the patient to have a V$_T$ of 300 – 600ml, or 4 – 8 ml/kg IBW.

Remember that in PSV the patient controls everything – the only thing that you set on the ventilator is the pressure level and the sensitivity. If your patient develops any signs of respiratory distress or hemodynamic instability – then it is time to immediately assess and determine if the level of support is adequate.

Using the T – piece

Using the T – piece simply involves increasing amounts of time that the patient is off the ventilator. Remember that the ETT has to be ≥ 7.0

The process:

First round: 5 – 10 minutes on T – piece, 50 – 55 minutes on ventilator. This can be continued until it is felt that the patient can handle more time off the ventilator.

Second Round: 30 minutes on T – piece, 30 minutes on ventilator. As long as the patient is tolerating well, this can be continued until it is felt that the patient can handle more time off the ventilator.

Third round: 1 hour on T – piece, 1 hour on ventilator. As long as the patient tolerates the time off the ventilator, the time off the ventilator can be subsequently increased until they are completely "weaned".

The more sophisticated modes of ventilation can also be choices for weaning. Volume Support (VS), MMV, and Automode are all viable choices for weaning.

F. Removal of the ETT (extubation)

After having had a successful SBT, or having been successfully weaned, extubation of the patient is based on the following:

* *Always check the chart to see if the initial intubation was difficult.*

1) Patency of the airway - determined by the **Cuff Leak Test**

Remember that at this point they have already passed the various assessments and criteria, have had a successful SBT, and are no longer in need of being mechanically ventilated. But you need to make sure they have a patent airway. In order to determine if they have a patent airway, you are going to deflate the cuff on the ETT and look at the V_T. Be sure to take note of what their V_T was before you deflate the cuff as you need to compare this to the V_T for breaths after the cuff is deflated.

A leak (a drop in V_T) $\leq$ 110ml is indicating that you are going to have problems and probably will not have a successful extubation. With a cuff leak $\leq$ 110ml, there is significant risk for post-extubation stridor. Let me explain this: When the cuff is fully inflated it acts so as to maintain the integrity of the airway. When a breath is taken, regardless of whether it is spontaneous or mechanical, a volume of air is delivered into the lungs and the fact that the cuff is inflated makes sure that the V_T stays in the lungs. When the cuff is inflated, the only way air is getting back out is through the ETT during exhalation. But when the cuff is deflated, the integrity is lost and there is no longer a means by which to make sure that the V_T stays in the lungs. When the cuff is deflated, the ventilator should be recording a much lower V_T because a good bit of it should have leaked out since the cuff was deflated and thus not able to contain it. If there is no inflammation in the upper airway, you should be losing a lot of that V_T. Say for example that the V_T was 500ml before the cuff was deflated. Then after the cuff was deflated, the recorded V_T for a breath was 200ml. The drop in V_T was 300ml – meaning that 300ml "leaked" out. This is a good cuff leak test because it indicates that there isn't any inflammation in the airway. But now look at this example: We'll use the same 500ml V_T before the cuff was deflated, but this time the V_T after deflation is 420ml. This means that only 80ml leaked out and this is not good. Having a leak of only 80ml means that the upper airway itself is probably inflamed and it is the inflammation in the airway that is preventing the air from leaking. You may have deflated the cuff, but the inflammation in the airway is bad enough such that it is severely limiting the amount of space between the lumen of the airway and the exterior of the ETT. The clinical standard is established at 110 ml. You need to see a leak of at least this much. If the leak is less than 110ml then it is not safe to extubate. When looking at the results of the cuff leak test, consider the average of 3 values over the course of 6 consecutive breaths.

2) The ability of the patient to protect their airway.
   - they need to have an intact gag reflex.

3) The patient has an adequate cough.
   - they are able to mobilize secretions without having excessive secretions.

4) The patient is alert and has the ability to follow commands.
   - sedation should be at a minimum.

Post – extubation difficulties

Immediately after the removal of the ETT

1) Auscultate for stridor – if you hear it you treat it immediately.

- Cool aerosol with supplemental O_2
- Racemic epi via SVN

- Heliox – 70/30 via a non-rebreather
  - this will help reduce the WOB until the racemic epi takes effect.

2) If there is no response with the racemic epi

- Administer IV steroids
- Re-intubate

3) If it is too late for re-intubation

- Cricothyroidotomy at the bedside

If all goes well with extubation and stridor assessment

Put the patient on an aerosol mask with an FiO_2 that is 10% higher than what it was before when they were on the ventilator. Although an aerosol mask setup (also known as an air entrainment nebulizer or a large volume jet nebulizer) can typically deliver an FiO_2 between 21 - 100%., be mindful that the O_2 input flow rate to the device is generally limited to 10 - 15 LPM. An aerosol device operates essentially on the same principle as a venti mask so you apply the same thought process in determining if the patient is getting enough total flow to meet their demand. A visual indication that there is sufficient total flow to meet the patients demand is the presence of mist during inspiration near the exhalation ports of the mask. In lieu of an aerosol mask, you could consider using a high flow nasal cannula as that seems to be the trend now.

G. Weaning Protocols

At the beginning of this section you were given information about various assessments that need to be made in order to determine if a patient is going to be a good candidate for weaning. I labeled those areas I – IV. Then followed the discussion of the SBT. When institutions make therapist-driven protocols, what they are doing essentially is taking the information from I – IV (particularly IV) and the SBT, and organizing it in the form of a flow chart or algorithm. This flow chart or algorithm is "the protocol". This way a non-physician clinician (respiratory therapist) is able to follow each step of the algorithm so as to know what to do in each step of the weaning process. These algorithms will tell you what assessments to make and what findings to look for and how to proceed according to those findings. Therapist-driven protocols for weaning will vary from institution to institution, but they are essentially all accomplishing the same thing.

M. Non – Invasive Positive Pressure Ventilation

Non-invasive positive pressure ventilation (NIPPV or simply NIV) is a way to provide ventilation to a patient without all the potential problems and issues that are associated with intubation and mechanical ventilation. It is a conservative way to try to avoid intubation and the risks related to intubation such as VAP. Although NIPPV is "mechanical" ventilation, it is non-invasive because it is delivered via a mask rather than having to intubate the patient. The idea is that in certain circumstances we can attempt to provide ventilation to a patient in a non-invasive way in an effort to minimize any complications. With NIPPV there is less need for heavy sedation, the patient retains the ability to talk and eat, and there is less need for any type of invasive monitoring. NIPPV is what you commonly know as BiPAP®. Although BiPAP is a trademark of Respironics, when referring to non-invasive ventilation in the everyday clinical setting, it is almost always referred to as BiPAP regardless of the particular brand of device that is being used.

Candidates for NIPPV

- Candidates for NIPPV are those patients who are experiencing moderate to severe respiratory distress but their diagnosis indicates that their condition could be reversed within a matter of hours to a few days.

Criteria for NIPPV

- $f > 30$
- visible signs of accessory muscle use
- $PaCO_2 > 45$ mmHg
- P/F < 200
- pH between 7.22 and 7.35

Contraindications to using NIPPV

- Cardiac or respiratory arrest (patient is not spontaneously breathing)
- Upper airway obstruction
- Non-respiratory organ failure
- Hemodynamic instability
- Facial burns or facial trauma
- Patient has high aspiration risk or cannot protect their airway - dysphagia
- Excessive secretions (unable to clear secretions)
- GI bleed
- Patient is agitated, confused, or uncooperative
- Inability to fit the mask (mask has to fit properly to minimize air leak
- Intact dentition (patient's natural teeth must be intact – dentures must be removed)
- Traumatic brain injury patients with unstable ventilatory drive

Complications of NIPPV

- Risk of aspiration
- Hypotension (with inspiratory pressures > 20 cmH$_2$O
- Mask discomfort (avoid pressure sores or skin breakdown)
- Excessive leaks
- Oral/nasal dryness (this is why you must use humidification)
- Gastric distension
- Mucus plugging

NIPPV ("BiPAP") is patient (flow) or time triggered and flow or time cycled that is pressure limited. Most NIPPV ventilators are going to have CPAP and PSV as mode options (although this can vary). Even though CPAP appears as a mode on most non-invasive ventilators, when we are talking about "BiPAP", we are talking about the PSV (pressure support) mode on the non-invasive ventilator. When the PSV mode is being used on a non-invasive ventilator, it is providing 2 levels of pressure support – an inspiratory level of support (IPAP – inspiratory positive airway pressure) and an expiratory level of support (EPAP – expiratory positive airway pressure). CPAP on the other hand provides just one level of pressure continuously. Functionally speaking, CPAP is essentially the same thing as EPAP or PEEP – it's just that it's doing it continuously. Since CPAP has no IPAP component, it is not providing ventilation. CPAP does not ventilate the patient – it's purpose is to help with oxygenation which is the same thing that PEEP does.

BiPAP®

BiPAP is usually very good at being able to increase a patient's V$_E$ and improve the quality of gas exchange. BiPAP is often considered to be the treatment of choice for acute on chronic respiratory failure when there is no concurrent cardiovascular instability. Some clinicians also prefer to use BiPAP with patients that have increased R$_{AW}$ induced autoPEEP. Further specific uses for BiPAP will be covered when the indications for NIPPV are discussed next.

BiPAP provides two levels of support as follows:

- IPAP (inspiratory positive airway pressure) – this is the inspiratory pressure support that is given when the patient is inspiring. IPAP assists with ventilation by augmenting spontaneous breaths.

  - IPAP can range from 2 to 30 cmH$_2$O
  - Initial IPAP is generally 8 – 12 cmH$_2$O

- EPAP (expiratory positive airway pressure) – this is the positive pressure that is being given while the patient is exhaling. Think of this as the same thing as PEEP because from a functional standpoint it's doing the same exact thing.

  - EPAP can range from 2 to 20 cmH$_2$O
  - Initial EPAP is generally 4 – 6 cmH$_2$O

Some notes

IPAP & EPAP are titrated for patient comfort and to ensure an adequate V$_T$ along with being in synch with the ventilator.

When you initially put the mask on the patient, keep the pressure a little lower that what it is going to actually be in order to give the patient a little time to acclimate to the mask and the pressure.

   *With a home use CPAP/BiPAP device, the pressure starts off
    lower and builds up to whatever you set it for.

When using BiPAP, if the patient's PaCO$_2$ goes up, then raise the IPAP in 1 – 2 cmH$_2$O increments to try to correct the problem. Raising the IPAP is going to increase the V$_T$ and that will ventilate them more and hopefully correct the PaCO$_2$.

If on the other hand the patient's PaO$_2$ drops, then raise the EPAP. This has the same effect as if you raised the PEEP on someone who was intubated and receiving invasive mechanical ventilation – remember that PEEP improves oxygenation – so when your patient is on BiPAP, raising the EPAP has the same effect. But also understand that the pressure difference between IPAP and EPAP is the pressure gradient that is the driving pressure for the IPAP. If you raise the EPAP in order to correct a slightly low PaO_2, then realize that you will have decreased the pressure gradient, and with less driving pressure you'll end up having a smaller V_T unless the patient exerts more effort.

If the patient is responding favorably to BiPAP – you will see the following:

- F < 30
- Decreased accessory muscle usage
- Improved gas exchange
  - P/F > 150
  - Good ABG

YOU HAVE A TWO HOUR WINDOW to figure out if BiPAP is helping your patient. The first two hours are the most significant in predicting if BiPAP is going to be successful.

IF THERE IS NO IMPROVEMENT IN 2 HOURS – PREPARE TO INTUBATE YOUR PATIENT.

Signs that your patient is failing BiPAP

- f > 30
- Accessory muscle use
- Elevated $PaCO_2$
- SpO_2 < 90%
- Decreased LOC (level of consciousness)
- Inability to clear secretions

Specific indications for NIPPV

1. Acute Respiratory Failure – Exacerbation of COPD

   - This is usually the hypercapnic respiratory failure version of acute respiratory failure.

   - BiPAP is the standard of care for these types of patients.
     - BiPAP helps decrease dyspnea.
     - With BiPAP you also usually see their frequency decrease.

   - The intubation rate used to be 50% with these patients. By using BiPAP, now only about 20% of these patients end up needing intubation.

2. Immunocompromised Patients

   - These are predominantly your HIV+ and transplant (organ & bone marrow) patients.

   - These patients are prone to sepsis, nosocomial infections, and airway hemorrhaging.

   - BiPAP is the standard of care for these patients
     - Using BiPAP decreases complications with these patients.
     - Using BiPAP provides improved outcomes.

   - By initiating BiPAP early, you decrease the intubation rate and the mortality rate. Early use of BiPAP dropped the mortality rate 30% (from 80% down to 50%).

3. Facilitating Weaning (*only* for COPD patients)

   - This is when you have a COPD patient that has had repeated failures of the SBT. In these cases you can extubate them "early" and then immediately put them on NIPPV (BiPAP).

However:

* The patient has to have been able to breath spontaneously for at least 5 minutes.

* The original intubation of this patient needs to have been considered an easy intubation.

* The patient only needs inspiratory pressures < 20cmH$_2$O.

* Hemodynamically stable

* Have minimal secretions

* Low FiO$_2$

* Functional GI with good nutritional status

* Have a strong cough

It has been found that patients that meet the above criteria and are placed on BiPAP have the following outcomes.

- They have decreased rates of needing re-intubation.

- There is a reduction in the rate of nosocomial pneumonia.

- There is decreased mortality.

- There is a reduction in the LOS (length of stay) in the ICU and/or the hospital in general.

4. Acute Cardiogenic Pulmonary Edema

Before getting into how this relates to NIPPV, let us review the basics of pulmonary edema. There are 2 types of pulmonary edema – there is hydrostatic (cardiogenic) pulmonary edema & non-hydrostatic (non-cardiogenic) pulmonary edema.

Hydrostatic Pulmonary Edema	Non-Hydrostatic Pulmonary Edema
Cardiogenic	Non-Cardiogenic
This is a FUNCTIONAL problem.	This is a STRUCTURAL problem.

Due to increased pressure in the pulmonary capillaries
- mitral valve stenosis
- left ventricular failure
- systemic fluid overload
  - renal failure
  - excessive IV fluid
	Due to damage to the alveolar epithelium
	  - irritant gases
	  - near drowning
	  - cytokine storm from a
	    pulmonary infection

	Large amounts of fluid leak through the excessively permeable & damaged capillary walls
	  - ARDS
	  - endotoxemia
	  - fat embolism
	  - decreased plasma oncotic
	    pressure from having low
	    plasma proteins secondary
	    to severe burns, liver
	    failure, or malnutrition.

In either of these two situations, the bottom line is that more fluid leaves the arterial end of the capillary than is reabsorbed at the venous end of the capillary. The presence of pulmonary edema imposes a pulmonary restriction – meaning that it will limit and/or reduce the amount of alveolar expansion that can take place and therefore it reduces the compliance of the lung. Furthermore – this leaked fluid from the capillaries will accumulate in the air spaces (alveoli) and cause shunting and thus hypoxemia.

Patients with pulmonary edema typically present with a rapid, shallow breathing pattern. They can't take in a normal V_T due to the reduced compliance of their lungs because of the edema, so they try to make up for it by taking shallow breaths more frequently. But you know by now that rapid, shallow breathing doesn't provide a truly adequate V_A because it's mostly dead space ventilation. So you need to treat this quickly and effectively.

Now – back to how this pertains to NIPPV.

When you know that it is CARDIOGENIC pulmonary edema – your first line therapy is going to be CPAP. CPAP has been compared to standard O_2 therapy and has been found to be a much better treatment strategy.

Therefore:

- CPAP – set at 8 – 12 cmH$_2$O
- CPAP
  - expands the alveoli
  - increases FRC
  - increases compliance and thus decreases the WOB
  - improves oxygenation

Treating cardiogenic pulmonary edema with CPAP reduces the overall intubation rate associated with this condition.

If the patient starts to retain CO_2, then switch them to BiPAP so as to be able to assist them with their ventilation. Note that when you are dealing with pulmonary edema you are going to want to know the $PaCO_2$ from an ABG and not the $EtCO_2$ (end-tidal CO_2). Although $EtCO_2$ is often a very good estimate for $PaCO_2$, when you have other issues going on such as pulmonary disease or cardiovascular instability, $EtCO_2$ is not as reliable and you need to get a true $PaCO_2$ from an ABG.

5. Asthma

The evidence for using NIPPV for asthma is not as strong, but it is nonetheless still an option. You will want to start BiPAP as soon as you determine that your patient is in impending ventilatory failure.

- P/F ratios tend to increase on average around 100.
- Spontaneous frequency decreases by an average of 7 breaths/ minute.
- Peak flow & FEV_1 improved more rapidly when aerosol therapy was also given in-line with BiPAP.

6. Cystic Fibrosis

By the time most cystic fibrosis patients need ventilatory support they are already in line for a lung transplant. CF occurs when the cell membrane protein responsible for chloride transport fails to work properly. A mutation of the CFTR (cystic fibrosis transmembrane conductance regulator) gene results in a gene product (the cell membrane protein) that does not work properly. When this membrane channel protein doesn't work properly, chloride ions don't get transported the way they are supposed to and you end up with dysregulation of the transport of epithelial fluid in the lungs, pancreas, liver, and GI tract. As it pertains to the lungs, the patient ends up with markedly thickened mucus in the lungs with very frequent respiratory infections. As such, these patients require:

- Aggressive pulmonary hygiene
- O_2 therapy – first at night, then eventually for 24 hours a day.
- Eventually they become hypercapnic and then it is time for BiPAP.

7. Hypoxemic Respiratory Failure

   - In the case of ALI or ARDS

   • The information is anecdotal. Studies showed that NIPPV
     (BiPAP) initially reduced intubation rates for these patients,
     but it did not decrease mortality.

   • BiPAP significantly improved the P/F within the first hour,
     but when compared to standard therapy:
       - there was no decrease in mortality.
       - there was no decrease in length of stay in the hospital.

   • Bottom line – if there is no improvement from BiPAP within
     2 hours – then intubate.

8. The DNI (do not intubate) patient.

   Obviously when a patient is DNR you do nothing, but with
a DNI status you can still make a patient comfortable and relieve
dyspnea with NIPPV.

NIPPV and nocturnal hypoventilation

   Nocturnal hypoventilation is when the patient experiences
hypoventilation at night (generally when asleep). You see this with
obstructive sleep apnea and Pickwickian Syndrome. Pickwickian
Syndrome is hypoventilation that is secondary to severe obesity, and
although these patients experience hypoventilation during the day as
well, their propensity for nocturnal hypoventilation is why it is being
included here with obstructive sleep apnea.
   Individuals with suspected obstructive sleep apnea usually
will complain of morning headaches, dyspnea, and fatigue. A
definitive diagnosis of obstructive sleep apnea is usually on the basis
of a sleep study. Apneic episodes during a sleep study are indicated

by drops in the SpO_2. Although oximetry studies (such as home oximetry) can reveal drops in the SpO_2 and thus the presence of apneic episodes, the sleep study is much more comprehensive and will also provide the information needed to determine the level of CPAP to be used. CPAP is generally the first treatment of choice for obstructive sleep apnea because the level of pressure provided by CPAP is generally sufficient to keep the airway open and eliminate the episodes of apnea and thus maintain adequate oxygenation (SpO_2) during sleep. However, in cases where the patient also has marked CO_2 retention, the choice may be made to use BiPAP instead because the IPAP part of BiPAP will help to improve ventilation so as to bring down the $PaCO_2$, and the EPAP portion of BiPAP will aid in maintaining an appropriate SpO_2 since the EPAP portion of BiPAP is functionally doing the same thing as CPAP. Always remember to provide humidification for patients that are receiving either CPAP or BiPAP – especially for those patients with issues of oral/nasal dryness and/or nasal stuffiness.

Chapter 9

Selected Topics in Pathology

A. ARDS

ARDS (Acute Respiratory Distress Syndrome) is not a particular disease per se; rather it is a collection of signs and symptoms that when viewed collectively presents a picture of widespread inflammation in the lungs. ARDS negatively effects gas exchange in a significant way due to the damage it causes to the A/C membrane and thus causes severe hypoxemia. There is no "test" for ARDS – it is diagnosed by looking at the composite clinical picture being presented by the patient. Back in the 1960's, ARDS was known as "shock lung syndrome", and the mortality rate then was as high as 90%. The mortality rate today is significantly less at around 40%, but ARDS still claims 60,000 lives a year. MSOF (multi system organ failure) along with the patient being elderly and having pre-existing conditions are the main factors that contribute to the mortality rate being what it is today.

There are a variety of insults that can trigger the onset of ARDS. An insult is simply an event or a condition that can serve as a trigger that leads to the development of ARDS. We will begin by exploring the various insults that can trigger ARDS, then look at the clinical course taken by ARDS once it begins, and then the means by which to manage and treat ARDS so as to afford the best chance for a favorable outcome.

ARDS is quite serious and these patients are very sick. They are almost always intubated and on mechanical ventilation, and usually have other co-existing medical issues occurring simultaneously. These cases are usually complicated and challenging to manage, and will require the highest level of your A game. Obviously it will require much experience before you can handle the management of an ARDS patient, but you need to understand what is going on now as you will see this frequently when you do your rotations in critical care.

Let us begin now by looking at the initial insults that are known to trigger ARDS:

Primary or Pulmonary Insults – these are considered DIRECT insults.

1. Inhalation Injury
2. Near Drowning   *One thing that all of these have*
3. Aspiration   *in common is that they cause*
4. Pneumonia   *lung consolidation.*
5. Pulmonary Contusion

Secondary or Non-Pulmonary Insults – these are considered INDIRECT insults.

1. Sepsis / Septic Shock
2. Pancreatitis   *These all*
3. Severe Burns   *involve acute*
4. Drug OD – especially Heroin   *systemic*
5. Multiple Trauma   *inflammatory*
   – especially long bone fractures *processes.*
6. Traumatic Brain Injury
7. DIC (Disseminated Intravascular Coagulation)
8. Multiple Transfusions

NOW – all of the insults listed above (both primary and secondary), can cause non-cardiogenic pulmonary edema. They all lead to an inflammatory response. This is why ARDS is an "inflammation" condition. Non-cardiogenic pulmonary edema is a significant part of the clinical picture of ARDS.

Cardiogenic vs. non-cardiogenic pulmonary edema was discussed just a few pages back in the section on specific indications for NIPPV in the last chapter. Pulmonary edema in the context of CHF be discussed later in this chapter.

As it pertains to the present discussion – since it is non-cardiogenic pulmonary edema that is part of the clinical picture of ARDS – you need to know how to clinically differentiate between cardiogenic vs. non-cardiogenic pulmonary edema.

<u>Cardiogenic Pulmonary Edema</u>:

1. PCWP ≥ 18mmHg
2. Lung lavage is (-) for protein.

PCWP was discussed in the section on pulmonary artery pressure at the end of the hemodynamics chapter.

<u>Non-Cardiogenic Pulmonary Edema</u>:

1. PCWP ≤ 18mmHg
2. Lung lavage is (+) for protein.

It's the non-cardiogenic pulmonary edema that you're looking for. If you have a PCWP ≤ 18mmHg, ***and*** the lung lavage is positive for protein, then you know that it's non-cardiogenic pulmonary edema and therefore can be considered to be part of the clinical picture for ARDS. And remember that the finding of non-cardiogenic pulmonary edema can be caused by any of the insults listed – either primary or secondary insults.

One of the other things that you need to concern yourself with is being able to distinguish between ALI (acute lung injury) and ARDS.

With both ALI & ARDS – you'll have:

- Bilateral infiltrates on CXR
- PCWP ≤ 18mmHg

But the distinguishing difference will be:

ALI will have a P/F ratio < 300, whereas ARDS will have a P/F ratio < 200. This was mentioned previously in the text.

Note that although the mortality rate for ALI is lower than ARDS – 50 – 75% of ALI cases progress into ARDS.

The Clinical Course of ARDS

ARDS follows a pattern. It is a package of signs and symptoms that follows a pattern.

1.   Initial Injury / Insult
      • Can be any of the insults (direct or indirect) that were just discussed.

2.   Stability Period (THE LAG PHASE)
      • During this time, there are no signs or symptoms of ARDS – they are "lagging behind".

3.   Initial Onset of Symptoms
      • Dyspnea
      • Tachypnea
      • A little chest tightness
      • Increased WOB (since compliance is going down)
      • Auscultation clear – maybe a little wheezing
      • ABG normal
      • CXR normal
        - CXR's are about 24 hours behind in revealing what's actually being presented clinically.

The last 3 – breath sounds (auscultation), ABG, and CXR – although they'll be normal initially, that will all change as the syndrome progresses into the exudative phase.

4.   Progressive Decompensation (see exudative phase)

5.   MSOF
      • The chances of MSOF are greatly increased when the insult is indirect (non-pulmonary). Not all cases will progress to this point.

NOW – within the overall framework of ARDS following a pattern, there are also 3 phases to ARDS - and they are the exudative phase, the proliferative phase, and the fibroproliferative phase. If you remember back in chapter 7, an exudative phase and a proliferative phase was used to describe the pathophysiology of pulmonary oxygen toxicity. There are similarities in the implications of those terms as they are being used here to describe the phases of ARDS.

Note that a patient with ARDS does not have to progress through all three phases as resolution of the syndrome can occur at any point. The most severe form of ARDS, however, will progress to the fibroproliferative phase.

The 3 phases of ARDS

The Exudative (acute) Phase

The exudative phase lasts from 1 – 3 days, but can last up to a week. It starts around a day or two following the initial insult. The insult causes diffuse alveolar damage (DAD) and damage to the endothelium of the capillaries of the lung. There is a significant inflammatory response going on during this time that involves the release of mediator molecules such as cytokines as well as the release of neutrophils and other immune system cell types. All of these mediators increase vascular permeability which in turn leads to the non-cardiogenic PE and alveolar flooding that is characterized by the leakage of fluid and plasma proteins into the alveoli and the pulmonary interstitium. Plasma proteins and inflammatory mediators that have leaked into the alveoli also inhibit and denature alveolar surfactant, and this further worsens the problem of atelectasis. Ultimately the consequences of all these events are a significant reduction in the compliance of the lung, atelectasis, and severe refractory hypoxemia. V/Q mismatching becomes so bad that you could see anywhere from a 25 – 50% shunt. Furthermore, it is possible that the areas of the lung that do remain able to be ventilated can end up as dead space ventilation in the event that profusion to these ventilated alveoli ends up being compromised due to pulmonary vasoconstriction or occlusion of the pulmonary vasculature by the various substances involved in the inflammation.

As just mentioned in the very last section – at the initial onset of symptoms just after the insult – auscultation will reveal normal breath sounds, the CXR will be normal, and the ABG will be normal.

BUT – during the exudative phase, with its non-cardiogenic pulmonary edema, is when you will see that all change:

- Auscultation will reveal crackles.
- The ABG will reveal hypoxemia and acidosis.
- The CXR will reveal diffuse bilateral infiltrates.
  - "fluffy white opacities"
- WOB will be even more increased.
- Percussion note will be flat/dull
- Dyspnea and tachypnea may have worsened
- Tachycardia
- Cough

During this time, you may also see the manifestation of symptoms that are associated with the underlying insult (pneumonia, sepsis, etc.).

Once the manifestation of symptoms begins you're going to need to start treatment. You could initially try O_2 therapy via a 35% venti mask or a non-rebreather – but realize you're dealing with a condition that within a matter of hours to a day or two is going to be causing severe hypoxemia secondary to serve shunting from ARDS. With ARDS patients, it's usually not a matter of if you're going to need to intubate, but only a matter of when. And when you do intubate them, they will need to be on a full support control mode. The mechanical ventilation of an ARDS patient will be discussed later in this section when we discuss the treatment of ARDS.

The Proliferative Phase

The proliferative phase comes after the exudative phase and usually begins approximately 3 – 7 days following the initial insult. During the proliferative phase, the inflammation starts to resolve and the alveolar epithelium begins to regenerate and heal (to include an increase in type 2 pneumocytes). Because lymphatic function is also starting to improve during this time, alveolar proteins along with all the other unwanted material begins to drain out of the alveoli. There may also be infiltration of fibroblasts and some evidence of collagen deposition during the proliferative phase. Hyaline membranes may form, although they may have been present since the exudative phase. Increased pulmonary vascular resistance and pulmonary hypertension may occur in this stage due to remodeling of the pulmonary vasculature by fibroblasts and inflammatory cells.

The Fibroproliferative Phase

The fibroproliferative phase usually occurs 3 – 4 weeks after the onset of ARDS. This phase is characterized by the widespread formation of collagenous tissue by fibroblasts and ongoing repair of the alveolar epithelium. Scarring and thickening of the lung occurs due to the disordered deposition of collagen and this can increase the WOB because it decreases the compliance of the lung by having made it stiffer. Whether or not the pulmonary interstitium thickens enough to the point of full blown pulmonary fibrosis will vary from case to case. Pulmonary fibrosis may or may not occur. If it does occur, it could be minimal or it could be severe. Obviously with more severe pulmonary fibrosis, the patient will have reduced lung compliance and will end up having to deal with the range of issues that accompany this form of restrictive lung disease. But in many patients, however, the edema and inflammation resolve without fibrosis.

Patients can often make it through the exudative phase only to end up succumbing to the syndrome in the proliferative and/ or fibroproliferative phases. There is no way of telling. This is why it is important to get ARDS diagnosed promptly and to treat it aggressively. Outcomes are generally better when it does not progress to the point of fibrosis. If all goes well, the patient will return to normal lung compliance and normal oxygenation in about 6 – 12 months. It takes this long because although the inflammation may go down, it doesn't go away completely for a while – it takes time.

The ARDS lung is not a normal lung. It is not a homogeneous structure like it is when it is healthy. There are parts that are normal – there are parts that are recruitable – and there are parts that are non-recruitable. Non-recruitable portions of the lung are usually in the dependent areas of the lung. An ARDS lung is often 2 – 3 times heavier than a normal lung, and this is because of all the consolidation from the edema – so ARDS lungs are heavy and wet. In many cases of ARDS, there may only be 25 – 30% of functional lung tissue. This is why you may often hear ARDS referred to as "baby lung". Having only 25% of the lungs available for ventilation means that when you are setting a V_T for mechanical ventilation that you must take that into consideration. This will be discussed in much more detail in the next section on treating ARDS.

Managing and Treating ARDS

Treatment for ARDS is essentially supportive. There is no specific treatment for ARDS. The overall strategy is to maintain adequate oxygenation while treating the underlying cause and providing nutritional support.

Managing and Treating ARDS - Mechanical Ventilation:

Although you may try NIPPV at first, the simple fact is that with the vast majority of ARDS cases, the level of hypoxemia is just too severe, and the increased WOB is just too much to be compatible with life. As such you are going to need to intubate and initiate mechanical ventilation.

- There is a significant decrease in lung compliance in ARDS, therefore it's going to take more pressure to deliver a breath. But the pressure of that breath must be limited in order to protect the lung. The goal is to adequately ventilate and oxygenate the patient without causing further damage to the lung until the ARDS and underlying condition are resolved enough that the patient can be weaned off the ventilator.

- The lung protective strategy when dealing with ARDS during mechanical ventilation entails:
  * Low tidal volumes with higher PEEP
  * Low P_{PLT}
  * Permissive hypercapnia

- V_T should be maintained at 4 – 6 ml/kg IBW. You may start initially with a V_T at 8 ml/kg IBW, but you need to reduce the V_T by 1ml/kg at intervals ≤ 2 hrs. until you achieve a V_T of 4 - 6ml/kg IBW.

- Initial frequency (RR) should be set to achieve the patient's baseline V_E – but not to exceed 35 breaths per minute.

- The goal with oxygenation is to maintain a $PaO_2 \geq 60mmHg$ and/or a $SpO_2 > 88\%$.

  * Regarding PEEP and FiO$_2$: PEEP should be a minimum of 5, but you will undoubtedly need it to be higher. Low V_T with high PEEP is the strategy – the low V_T's are protecting the lung while the higher PEEP is helping with oxygenation. With ARDS, the goal of PEEP is to maintain a $PaO_2 \geq 60mmHg$ at an $FiO_2 \leq 60\%$. Just be conscious that PEEP contributes to the overall amount of pressure in the lung and you have to watch pressure very carefully so as to not cause any more lung damage. Remember also the issue of oxygen toxicity and the problems that arise from using high FiO$_2$'s for too long. You are already dealing with very sick lungs – you want to be conscientious of the further damage that could be done with sustained use of a high FiO$_2$.

  * The idea is to use the highest amount of PEEP necessary (without causing pressure or hemodynamic problems) at the lowest FiO$_2$ needed - at the lowest V_T (not less than 4ml/kg IBW) and rate that will provide an adequate V_E with minimal acidosis (permissive hypercapnia) - and a $PaO_2 \geq 60mmHg$.

- The goal with P_{PLT} is to keep it ≤ 30 cmH$_2$O. With an ARDS patient, P_{PLT} should be checked every 4 hours at a minimum – and definitely must be checked every time you adjust the V_T or PEEP.

  * If the $P_{PLT} > 30$cmH$_2$O, then you need to decrease the V_T, (but not to below 4ml/kg IBW).

* If the $P_{PLT} < 25cmH_2O$ – before you make any adjustments look and see if they are improving – remember as the health of the lung improves (better compliance), it won't take as much pressure to keep the lung inflated. Are they oxygenating well? Is their PaO_2 and/or SpO_2 adequate? Is their total rate reasonable? Are they achieving an adequate V_E? If the answer to these questions is yes – then their lungs are probably starting to improve and they may be starting to move towards the direction of eventually being able to be weaned.

* If their V_T is not yet at 6ml/kg IBW, and their $P_{PLT} < 25$ cmH_2O, raise the V_T in 1ml/kg increments until it is 6ml/kg IBW and check the P_{PLT}. If P_{PLT} stays below 30 cmH_2O after raising the V_T to 6ml/kg IBW then this further substantiates that the compliance of the lung is improving. Remember that a more compliant lung can handle a larger V_T without it requiring excessive pressures. If the P_{PLT} does however exceed 30 cmH_2O after raising the V_T to 6ml/kg IBW, then take the V_T back down to what it was and continue to monitor the patient.

- Within the framework of permissive hypercapnia, pH goals in the management of an ARDS patient should be between 7.30 – 7.45.

* If pH is between 7.15 – 7.29, increase the frequency (RR) until the pH $\geq$ 7.30, but not to exceed 35 breaths per minute.

* If pH < 7.15 – then this is when some of the rules with RR, V_T, and P_{PLT} get broken in order to deal with worsening acidosis.
  - Increase the RR to 35 and see if this improves the pH. If this doesn't solve the problem, then:
    - Raise V_T in 1ml/kg IBW increments until pH > 7.15.
    - The limit of 30 cmH_2O for P_{PLT} may be exceeded.
  - Acidosis may also be managed with HCO_3^-.

- Once the ARDS and the underlying issues are sufficiently resolved, weaning and discontinuation from mechanical ventilation may be considered. Refer back to the section on weaning in chapter 8 if necessary to review the process for liberating a patient from mechanical ventilation.

Other things to be mindful of regarding mechanical ventilation

Ventilator induced lung injury (VILI) - Compromised or injured lung units are more susceptible to injury that can be induced from the ventilator. The following ventilator induced lung injuries almost mimic ARDS, so that means that if they occur with a patient who already has ARDS, the situation is going to be greatly worsened.

Barotrauma – can cause a tension pneumothorax or subcutaneous emphysema.

Volutrauma – this is mechanical stretching of the lung from over-inflation. It causes micro tears of the alveoli, and also causes an inflammatory response.

Atelectrauma – this is the result of repetitive opening and closing of the alveoli – RACE (repetitive alveolar collapse & expansion). It is a form of shear stress and it can induce an inflammatory response called SIRS (systemic inflammatory response syndrome). Shear stress in this case refers to the tearing of the alveoli, and it not only further inhibits proper gas exchange, but it generates an inflammatory response.

Barotrauma, volutrauma, and atelectrauma with its related shear stress injury all generate an inflammatory response to varying degrees. This collectively results in bio trauma, and that, along with the poor oxygenation status of the patient to begin with due to the ARDS, leads to MSOF.

APRV and PRVC are good alternatives if it becomes necessary to try other modes of mechanical ventilation. Recruitment maneuvers may also be considered in an attempt to improve oxygenation. The recruitment maneuver is consistent with an open lung approach to ventilation. It is a sustained increase in airway pressure in the form of PEEP (40 cmH$_2$O) that is applied for 40 seconds with the goal of opening atelectatic lung units, after which *adequate* PEEP is applied to keep the lungs open. Although a recruitment maneuver is done to help improve oxygenation and hopefully help decrease inflammation in the lungs, you have to be cognizant of the reality that it carries risk for barotrauma and/or volutrauma. A recruitment maneuver, however, can help reduce the susceptibility to atelectrauma because once the alveoli are opened, they are kept open with PEEP. Keeping the alveoli open minimizes the repetitive opening and closing of the alveoli and thus reduces the level of shear stress and its associated inflammatory response – hence the risk for atelectrauma is lowered. But the benefit of lowering susceptibility to atelectrauma is after the fact – you first had to get the alveoli open to being with – and the high level of PEEP used for the recruitment maneuver has the potential to cause damage through barotrauma or volutrauma. Be very careful.

Other Aspects of Managing and Treating ARDS

Treating the underlying cause

Antibiotics can often be employed to treat several of the ARDS triggers:

- Sepsis
- Intra-abdominal sepsis (from a ruptured bowel)
  - *Sepsis induced ARDS has the highest mortality*
- Pneumonia
- UTI

Other causes cannot necessarily be treated directly – e.g. trauma, multiple transfusions, etc.

Cardiovascular management

- Fluids and vasopressors

  - Restricting fluids will help decrease pulmonary edema.
  - But fluid restriction will also decrease CO and perfusion.

  - Administering diuretics will also help decrease edema.
  - But this will also decrease CO and blood pressure.

  Therefore: vasopressors are needed to maintain cardiac output and blood pressure.

- Transfusions are indicated if Hb < 10g/dl

Steroids

- IV methylprednisolone may be useful in managing uncomplicated pulmonary fibrosis following ARDS.
- The routine use of corticosteroids in the treatment of ARDS is not recommended.

Inhaled Nitric Oxide

Inhaled Nitric Oxide is an option as a salvage therapy in ARDS patients with severe refractory hypoxemia. NO was discussed at length at the end chapter 7 - revisit that material if needed.

- Nitric Oxide is a potent vasodilator.
- It is most effective on patients with increased pulmonary vascular resistance.
- It can improve shunting.
- It can improve the P/F ratio.
- It is toxic and thus care must be exercised, and furthermore, the use of inhaled NO does not appear to reduce the mortality rate or the length of stay in the hospital.

Surfactant Administration

The use of surfactant therapy is well established in infants with IRDS (infant respiratory distress syndrome) because surfactant therapy works best when there is a pure surfactant deficiency as in the case of IRDS. ARDS is much more complex than IRDS in that it isn't just a matter of there being a pure surfactant deficiency, but rather that the surfactant has either been inhibited, or has been altered by having been denatured. Recall that in ARDS there are plasma proteins and inflammatory mediators that have leaked into the alveoli as part of the edema, and these plasma proteins and inflammatory mediators both inhibit and denature alveolar surfactant. As long as plasma proteins and inflammatory mediators are present in the alveoli, the efficacy of surfactant therapy with ARDS is questionable.

ECMO (extracorporeal membrane oxygenation)

ECMO is similar to cardiopulmonary bypass. Whereas cardiopulmonary bypass is used for short-term situations like cardiac bypass surgery, ECMO is utilized for more long-term situations. ECMO provides both cardiac and respiratory support in certain cases of hypoxemic respiratory failure where the P/F ratio < 100mmHg despite all attempts to optimize the settings of the ventilatory parameters. ECMO can potentially benefit ARDS patients by significantly improving gas exchange and decreasing airway pressures and lung inflation while the lungs heal.

Placing the patient in the prone position

In ARDS, edema and injury occurs primarily in the dependent lung regions. For a patient in the supine position this would be the dorsal region. The dependent areas of the lung are those areas that are affected the most by gravity and thus are the best perfused. If you are standing upright, the dependent areas which are better perfused are the bases, whereas the non-dependent areas that are better ventilated are the apices. Whichever position an individual is in – dependent lung regions are better perfused with less ventilation, and non-dependent regions are better ventilated with less perfusion.

Results of prone positioning:

- It changes the position of the heart such that there is less pressure on the lungs.
- It decreases abdominal pressure.
- Dorsal recruitment prevails over ventral de-recruitment.
- Overall lung inflation is more homogeneous.
- PEEP is more efficient – it optimizes recruitment while decreasing alveolar hyperinflation.
- It improves V/Q matching.
- It increases PaO_2.
- There is improved airway drainage.
- There is improved lymphatic drainage.
- Prone position better protects the lung from VILI.

Indications for prone position:

- The prone position is highly recommended when the P/F ratio < 150mmHg.
- There is significant benefit with using the prone position when the P/F < 100mmHg, however there is no survival benefit to using the prone position when the P/F > 200mmHg.
- The prone position can be used as a rescue maneuver in cases of severe hypoxemia to treat atelectasis and improve airway drainage.
- There is no agreement on how long a patient can remain in the prone position. It could be anywhere from 8 – 17 hours. Patients will often require sedation and/or paralysis in order to be successful with the prone position.

Absolute contraindications to using the prone position:

- Spinal instability

- Unmonitored elevated ICP

Relative contraindications to using the prone position:

- Hemodynamic instability
- Open abdominal wounds
- Multiple trauma with unstabilized fractures
- Pregnancy
- High dependency on airway and vascular access

B. COPD

Emphysema

Emphysema is the abnormal and permanent enlargement of the airspaces distal to the terminal bronchioles. Respiratory bronchioles in affected acini are usually narrower and convoluted. Pulmonary fibrosis is usually not seen with emphysema, however the formation of scar tissue in the connective tissue of the lungs is usually a consequence of inflammation which is an ongoing complication in patients with COPD. The abnormal enlargement of the airspaces is brought about as a result of the collapse of the alveolar wall due to the destruction of elastin fibers that are contained within the wall. The enlargement of the airspaces leads to a significant loss of surface area for gas exchange as well as a lessening of the elasticity of the lungs. The destruction of the alveolar wall also leads to disruptions in certain structural arrangements of the lungs that are necessary in maintaining unobstructed open airways. These disruptions in the structural arrangements in the lung tissue results in a lessening of the amount of radial traction being exerted on a bronchiole which leads to the narrowing of a bronchiole which essentially amounts to being an obstruction.

The destruction of the alveolar wall is due to a protease – anti-protease imbalance that results in the enzymatic destruction of the elastin (elastic fibers) that exists within the alveolar wall (the alveolar septum). Elastin is the principle protein that comprises the elastic fibers of the alveolar septum. A protease is a protein that catalyzes the breakdown of a protein. The protease in question as it pertains to emphysema is neutrophil lysosomal elastase. The chemicals in cigarette smoke stimulate the accumulation of macrophages and neutrophils in the lung. Macrophages and neutrophils are normally present as part of the defense mechanism of the lungs, however the chemicals in cigarette smoke stimulate alveolar macrophages to release neutrophil chemotactic factors that cause increased recruitment of neutrophils into the lung. These neutrophils then release elastase which in turn degrades elastin and type IV collagen that are essential for the structural integrity of the alveolar wall. The body has an enzyme known as alpha-1 antitrypsin which under normal circumstances would inhibit the activity of neutrophil elastase. The problem is that stimulated neutrophils also release oxygen free radicals that inhibit the activity of alpha-1. With alpha-1 being inhibited, it is unable to stop elastase from degrading the elastin in the alveolar wall. Ultimately the consequence of all this is that elastin is destroyed such that the alveolar wall collapses, the airspaces become enlarged and thus the surface area for gas exchange is reduced, and the lungs lose elasticity.

There are some individuals who lack alpha-1 due to a genetic problem. They don't make alpha-1, so are therefore said to have an alpha-1 antitrypsin deficiency. Despite being genetically inherited at birth, many individuals with alpha-1 deficiency who are lifelong *nonsmokers* do not develop emphysema. Obviously, an individual who is alpha-1 deficient is at greater risk for developing emphysema, but in most cases, it also requires a smoking history as well in order to bring about emphysema.

Clinical characteristics of emphysema

- Barrel – chested (increased AP diameter)
- Hoover's sign
- Dyspnea
- Pursed-lip breathing and accessory muscle use (tripoding).
- Hyper-resonant percussion note.

- Auscultation - diminished breath sounds with extended expiration.
- CXR shows hyperinflation
  - dark lung fields
  - flattened diaphragm
- ABG – usually shows compensated respiratory acidosis with hypoxemia and hypercapnia.
- CBC can indicate elevated RBC, Hb, and HCT in response to chronic hypoxemia.

Chronic Bronchitis

Chronic bronchitis is characterized by the excessive production of mucus in the bronchi along with a productive cough not caused by any other reason that is present on most days for at least three months over a period of two consecutive years. As with emphysema, the main causative agent in the development of chronic bronchitis is cigarette smoking, although other inhaled toxic substances and recurrent respiratory infections can also bring about its development.

Sustained exposure and continuous irritation from cigarette smoke leads to chronic inflammation as well as morphological changes in the cells lining the respiratory tract. Repeated exposure to the chemical toxins in cigarette smoke causes hypertrophy and hyperplasia of the submucosal mucous-secreting glands which leads to hyper-secretion of mucus in the bronchi. The patient ends up having an overabundance of larger than normal submucosal mucous-secreting glands which results in excessive secretion of mucus into the airway. Persistent inflammation also leads to an increase in the number of mucous-secreting goblet cells found among the epithelial cells of the smaller airways. Excessive secretion of mucus clogs the airway, often as mucus plugs, and the mucus itself becomes an obstruction in the airway. The chemicals in the cigarette smoke also impair the functioning of the muco-ciliary escalator which further complicates the issue of obstruction as the bronchial passages, which are now faced with even more mucus, are less able to clear themselves.

Besides obstructing the airways, excessive mucus production leads to another problem that complicates the clinical management of chronic bronchitis. Excessive mucus serves as a breeding ground for bacterial growth, which in turn becomes one of the main reasons why COPD patients often experience recurrent respiratory infections. Acute episodes of infection are accompanied by inflammation and further mucus production which makes for a vicious cycle that becomes increasingly difficult to manage as the COPD continues to progress.

Clinical characteristics of chronic bronchitis

- Cyanotic appearance.
- Productive cough with copious secretions.
- Purulent sputum often tests positive for pathogens.
- Auscultation – crackles and/or wheezes.
- CXR shows increased bronchovascular markings
  - possible cardiomegaly
  - fibrosis possible with history of chronic inflammation
  * Be mindful that patients often have mixed findings on CXR. This is because you will rarely encounter a patient that is exclusively emphysema only or exclusively chronic bronchitis only. These patients almost always present as a mixture of both conditions.
- ABG – usually shows compensated respiratory acidosis with hypoxemia and hypercapnia.
- CBC can indicate elevated RBC, Hb, and HCT in response to chronic hypoxemia.
- Patients with chronic bronchitis will usually have a normal D_{LCO}.

Bronchiectasis

Bronchiectasis is characterized by the irreversible dilation and distortion of the bronchi and bronchioles. These airways are abnormally dilated with variable amounts of mucus and inflammation. Normal structural components of the bronchial wall are destroyed and oftentimes replaced by fibrous connective tissue. The exact cause of bronchiectasis is not clearly understood, but it appears to be a consequence of the manifestation of a cycle between infections, often pneumonia, and inflammation. It is known however, that Cystic Fibrosis and Kartagener's Syndrome can lead to the development of bronchiectasis. Cystic Fibrosis you are already familiar with, and Kartagener's is an autosomal recessive condition that is characterized by primary ciliary dyskinesia.

Recurrent respiratory infections lead to chronic inflammatory changes that weaken the bronchial walls such that they become dilated and distorted. Mucus and pus accumulate in these dilated areas which then contributes to the perpetuation of infection. These recurring infections continue to cause even further damage to the lungs which makes clinical management of these patients increasingly difficult. Bronchiectasis is accompanied by a chronic, loose, productive cough that contains significant amounts of foul-smelling sputum.

Clinical characteristics of bronchiectasis

- Cyanotic appearance with digital clubbing.
- Dyspnea with accessory muscle usage.
- Barrel – chested (increased AP diameter)
- Hyper-resonant percussion note.
- Auscultation – wheezes and/or diminished sounds.
- CXR – presence of parallel line opacities (tram tracks), ring opacities or cystic spaces, and the signet ring sign are all characteristic radiographic findings for bronchiectasis. Increased size and loss of definition of the pulmonary vessels and crowding of pulmonary vascular markings is common.
- ABG – usually shows compensated respiratory acidosis with hypoxemia and hypercapnia.
- CBC can indicate elevated RBC, Hb, and HCT in response to chronic hypoxemia.

Treatment of COPD

- Low flow O_2 for hypoxemia.
  - Nasal cannula flow rate of $1 - 2$ LPM.
  - Venti mask at 24% or 28%.

- Assistance with ventilation is often necessary in order to help relieve the work of breathing. Assistance with ventilation may also be necessary in the presence of hypercapnia that is beyond the level of what would be considered normal for a particular patient. Remember that these patients often have compensated acidosis that is "normal" for them. They may have chronically elevated CO_2, but their pH is normal because they are compensating for it with elevated bicarbonate. If, however, their CO_2 rises beyond what is normal for them such that their pH starts to drop, they will need ventilatory assistance.

  - Start with NIPPV (BiPAP) – BiPAP is the first treatment of choice when ventilatory assistance is needed with COPD.
  - Set IPAP at $8 - 12$
  - Set EPAP at $4 - 6$

  - Intubation with mechanical ventilation if needed.

- Bronchodilators to open the airway
  - SABA's (e.g. Albuterol)
  - LABA's (e.g. Salmeterol)
  - Anticholinergic's (e.g. Ipratropium Bromide)

- Mucolytic Agents to help break up mucus
  - N-Acetylcysteine

- Steroids to reduce inflammation
  - Prednisone

- Antibiotics to fight infection

- Bronchial hygiene and secretion clearance

- Lung expansion therapy – bronchiectasis in particular

- Lobectomy – bronchiectasis in particular

Asthma

Asthma affects 300 million people worldwide. In the United States, asthma affects 9.3% of the children (18.7 million) and 8% of adults (6.8 million). Of the children with asthma, half of them are diagnosed before they are 10 years old. In the inner city, > 1 in 4 people will have an occurrence with asthma. Asthma accounts for almost 3500 deaths a year. I am telling you all of this to reinforce the fact that asthma is one of the conditions that you will see constantly as a respiratory therapist.

Asthma is chronic, inflammatory, obstructive airway disease that occurs in the conducting airways (bronchi and bronchioles) that results in increased contractibility of the smooth muscle that surrounds the bronchi or bronchioles.

4 main components of asthma

- Bronchoconstriction
  - asthma causes serious bronchoconstriction.
- It is a chronic condition.
- It is an inflammatory condition.
- It is a reversible condition.
  - It is not curable, but it is usually reversible. *This is what separates asthma from the other forms of COPD.*

Episodes (asthmatic attacks) occur when a patient is exposed to a trigger. Triggers could be anything from infections, cold air, exercise, chemicals, stress, environmental factors, etc. When an attack occurs, there is constriction of the smooth muscle that surrounds the bronchi/bronchioles that leads to significant narrowing of the airway that is indicated by the classic asthma symptom of wheezing.

3 Types of asthma

- Atopic – IgE mediated. It is a response to an allergen.
- Idiosyncratic – A response to a common cold (non IgE) – there is a stimulus (trigger), but it is not an antigen.
- Non-classified – emotional response, cold air, etc.

At the cellular level, the asthmatic attack (response) is a consequence of the production of mediators from the degranulation of Mast Cells.

Stimulus/Antigen → Mast cell degranulation → Histamine
Bradykinin
Leukotrienes
Prostaglandins

Many patients can have stable asthma without any attacks for weeks or months, and then for no apparent reason will have an acute asthma exacerbation that can be as severe as status asthmaticus. Exacerbations of asthma are usually from a trigger (some were just mentioned), but the problem is that the particular trigger that can trigger an episode is not always known. It could be anything – pet hair, mold, dust, perfume, chemicals, etc. The episode could be brought on by an infection or stress. In any case, it is any number of these things that ultimately alters the immune system such that the airway inflammatory response is increased so as to induce an attack.

Specific pathology of an asthma attack

- Significant narrowing of the airways.
  - Decreased airway diameter due to contraction of the airway smooth muscle (bronchoconstriction).
- Increased mucus from the inflammatory process.
  - Increased secretions
- Alveolar distention
- Vascular congestion
- Bronchial wall edema

Manifestations of the pathology

- Increased airway resistance.
- Decreased FEV1
- Hyperinflation of the lungs with air trapping and autoPEEP.
- Increased WOB
- Changes in the elastic recoil of the lung.
- Abnormal distribution of ventilation and perfusion.
  - V/Q mismatching

Clinical findings in asthma

- Auscultation – Diffuse wheezing with diminished breath sounds. Oftentimes you won't even have to auscultate – you'll just be able to hear it.
- Tachypnea with accessory muscle use.
- Pursed-lip breathing
- Chest tightness
- Hyper-resonant percussion note
- Cyanosis
- Diaphoresis
- Tachycardia
- Pulsus Paradoxus in severe cases
- Cough – increased and productive with eosinophils in sputum.
- CXR
  - hyper-inflation (increased AP diameter)
  - hyperlucent lungs with reduced vascular markings
  - flattened diaphragm
- ABG
  - Initially will reveal alveolar hyperventilation and hypoxemia. May develop into hypercarbia in status asthmaticus.

- Peak Flow

  - Mild > 50% of predicted
  - Moderate > 25 – 50% of predicted
  - Severe < 25% of predicted

Treatment of asthma

In the emergency room

- O_2 to achieve an SpO_2 > 90%
- Bronchodilator Therapy
  - SABA
  - Anti-cholinergics
  - Consider continuous therapy if necessary
- Steroids (PO or IV)
- Close monitoring (including PEFR)
- Intubation and mechanical ventilation if necessary
- Adjunct therapy
  - Heliox
  - Sub-Q epinephrine
  - $MgSO_4$ – magnesium sulfate inhibits smooth muscle contraction and decreases histamine release from mast cells.

Long term maintenance

- Bronchodilators
  - SABA
  - LABA
  - Anti-cholinergics
- Steroids (inhaled)
- Mast cell stabilizers
- Asthma action plan based on PEFR monitoring
- Bronchopulmonary hygiene
- Environmental control (attempt to avoid triggers)

C. Neuromuscular Disease

Myasthenia Gravis

Myasthenia Gravis is a disease of the neuromuscular junction. It is characterized by muscle weakness and descending paralysis that is caused when the immune system inappropriately forms antibodies that block and/or destroy acetylcholine receptors on the post synaptic side of the neuromuscular junction. Through the action of these antibodies blocking/destroying acetylcholine receptors, nerve impulses are prevented from being able to trigger muscle contractions. The disease is an autoimmune synaptopathy and its etiology is unknown. Myasthenia Gravis is twice as common in women as it is in men; the onset of the disease is between 15 – 35 years of age for women whereas for men the onset is usually at age 40+. There is a neonatal form of M.G. where the baby is born with the condition, however it usually resolves on its own within 2 – 3 months of life.

Characteristics, clinical course, and diagnosis of M.G.

- The onset is gradual.
  - it will involve episodes of exacerbation – then resolving
  - it can vary in severity

- Fatigue can occur with specific muscle groups, or it may be generalized.
  - muscle weakness generally improves following rest.

- M.G. very often affects the muscles of the face and/or diaphragm.

The patient will exhibit "normal" health for weeks or even months at a time. Then the patient will begin to develop fatigue in the evening and symptoms will progress as follows:

Earlier symptoms:

  Ptosis – drooping of 1 or both eyelids

  Diplopia – double vision

  Dysarthria – motor speech impairment

  Dysphagia – difficulty swallowing

  Droopy head

Later symptoms:

- More pronounced weakness in limbs
- Unsteady gait
- Difficulty getting out of a chair
- Paresthesia (tingling) in fingers and toes
- Possible intercostal and/or diaphragm involvement

A definitive diagnosis of M.G. can take one to two years to make.

- With M.G., imaging studies will be normal.
- ACh receptor antibody levels will be elevated in 80% of Myasthenia Gravis patients.

A test known as the Edrophonium (or Tensilon) test is performed in order to differentiate if the symptoms being presented are truly that of regular M.G., or whether they are from a different form of M.G. known as Lambert – Eaton M.G. In Lambert – Eaton M.G., rather than directly attacking the ACh receptors, the antibodies disrupt the transmission of the nerve impulse by attacking pre-synaptic calcium channels.

Edrophonium is what is known as an acetylcholinesterase inhibitor. Before we go on, let us review some of the basic physiology of the synapse that occurs between two nerves or between a nerve and a muscle. In order for a nerve impulse to get from one nerve to the next, or from a nerve to a muscle, the signal has to be transmitted through the synapse. The synapse is the "space" between two nerves or between a nerve and a muscle. Getting a nerve impulse transmitted across the synapse requires the use of a neurotransmitter – there are several, but in this case we are talking about the neurotransmitter acetylcholine (ACh). Once the signal is transmitted across the synapse via ACh, the ACh has to be broken down, and the liberated choline that results from the hydrolysis of ACh is then returned to the pre-synaptic neuron that it originated from so that it can be used again by the pre-synaptic neuron to synthesize new ACh. The breakdown of ACh is facilitated by an enzyme located on the post-synaptic membrane (the muscle cell membrane) known as acetylcholinesterase (AChE).

Now – as it pertains to the edrophonium or Tensilon test. Tensilon is an AChE inhibitor – this means that in the presence of Tensilon, AChE won't work. In other words, in the presence of Tensilon, AChE will not be able to break down ACh. The implications of this from a diagnostic standpoint regarding M.G. are as follows:

- In the case of true M.G., we know that the primary problem is the issue where a malfunctioning immune system has made antibodies that are either blocking or destroying ACh receptors on the post-synaptic side of the neuromuscular junction. The ACh receptors are located in the cell membrane of the muscle cells.

- We know that muscle weakness is the predominant symptom with these patients, and that the muscle weakness is being caused by a lack of adequate stimulation of the muscle by the nerve because the receptor on the muscle end of the synapse is not able to properly bind ACh because it is being blocked or destroyed by antibodies.

- Therefore, the idea is this: Let's maximize the potential of all the available ACh that is in the synapse by preventing its breakdown. This is where Tensilon comes into play. By inhibiting AChE, Tensilon prevents the breakdown of ACh. This keeps the synapse full of functional ACh – because even though the ACh receptors on the muscle are either blocked or destroyed – they're not *all* blocked or destroyed. So, for however many receptors that *are* functional – by maintaining as high a concentration as possible of ACh in the synapse by inhibiting AChE with Tensilon, we greatly enhance the potential for transmission to be successful.

- And if the case is truly that of standard M.G. – then within 30 – 90 seconds of administration of Tensilon, the muscle weakness will resolve and it will remain resolved for 1 – 5 minutes. Tensilon is a short acting drug and is usually given as a 10mg injection. This transitory improvement in muscle strength will fade and the patient will return to baseline within 5 minutes. Some patients will get "rebound weakness" where they experience even more muscle weakness than their usual baseline weakness once the Tensilon wears off. This usually only lasts for a few hours though.

- If the Tensilon test doesn't result in any improvement with muscle strength, then the M.G. is the Lambert – Eaton type of M.G. With Lambert – Eaton M.G., the biochemistry is different – the antibodies are attacking the calcium channels that are responsible for ACh release from the pre-synaptic neuron – they're not attacking the post-synaptic ACh receptor. The net result is the same in that it interferes with transmission of the impulse and you end up with muscle weakness, but the mechanism is different and it is not effected by Tensilon. Therefore, if the Tensilon test results in no improvement with muscle strength – then it is Lambert – Eaton M.G.

- Sometimes the Tensilon test may result in making the muscle weakness even worse. When this happens, it is indicative that a cholinergic crisis is going on and this is a totally different condition than M.G. In a cholinergic crisis, there has been significant overstimulation of the neuromuscular junction due to an excess of ACh – usually because of the inactivity of AChE. As a result of the overstimulation by ACh, the muscles stop responding to ACh and become weak and the clinical picture looks similar to M.G. – but it isn't M.G. If you give a patient with a cholinergic crisis Tensilon – that's just going to make the muscle weakness even worse because the Tensilon is going to further inhibit AChE which is already inactive. If your patient experiences a worsening of their muscle weakness with the Tensilon test – give them atropine to reverse the situation.

Other aspects of the diagnostic process will be the physical examination done by the physician to assess neurological status. If M.G. is suspected there are blood tests that can detect the presence of the antibody to the ACh receptor. An EMG (electromyography) nerve conduction study can also be done to rule out M.G., however this test can be painful.

A patient can sometimes experience what is called a myasthenic crisis where they have an acute onset of symptoms and everything is amplified – meaning that the muscle weakness is extreme and/or they can't move their jaw or their eyelids. They may also experience respiratory distress that may include periods of apnea. Assessment of their respiratory status is necessary to determine if they will require ventilatory assistance.

Treatment of Myasthenia Gravis

M.G. is treated with Neostigmine or Pyridostigmine. These are both AChE inhibitors. Pharmacologically they act like Tensilon does by inhibiting AChE – it's just that whereas Tensilon only acts for a few minutes, Neostigmine and Pyridostigmine have much longer action. That's why Tensilon is only used to test for M.G. rather than treating it - because it is too short acting.

Dosing has to be appropriate as too much will cause overstimulation. Potential side effects are also nausea, vomiting, muscle cramps, and tachycardia.

Although not the preferred method of treatment, corticosteroids have been found to be helpful with these patients. The side effects of prednisone (the steroid usually used with M.G.) include immune compromise, infections, GI bleeds, & osteoporosis.

And obviously – mechanical ventilation if needed as per the criteria for initiating mechanical ventilation. Non-Invasive ventilation (NIPPV) is often useful in the early stages of M.G.

Guillain - Barré Syndrome

Guillain–Barré Syndrome is characterized by muscle weakness that is fairly rapid in its onset. It begins in either the hands or the legs and moves upward, hence the use of the descriptive "ascending paralysis". The exact etiology of Guillain–Barré Syndrome is still not understood. It is suspected that a previous infection, particularly either gastroenteritis or a respiratory tract infection, could be a possible trigger. Regardless of the initiating factor, the issue is that of an autoimmune disorder where the immune system begins to attack peripheral nerves. Guillain–Barré Syndrome can attack a neuron in one of two ways. In the demyelinating form, GBS damages the myelin sheath that surrounds the axon of a neuron. Proper myelination of a neuron is essential for proper transmission of a neural signal. In the axonal form, GBS directly attacks the axonal cell membrane. With either of these forms, the resulting polyneuropathy renders the nerve unable to properly transmit a signal and hence the presentation of symptoms characteristic of GBS. GBS is fairly rare, affecting only 1 - 2 per 100,000 adults and 0.8 per 1,000,000 children.

Characteristics, clinical course, and diagnosis of GBS

- It begins with numbness, tingling, and/or pain in hands and/ or feet that is equally bilateral, and becomes progressively worse over time.

- Then rapidly evolving muscle weakness – it begins in the hands or feet, and ascends up the arm or leg.

- The ascension can be to the point of the respiratory muscles, laryngeal muscles, and the face. Therefore, there is the possibility of dysarthria & dysphagia, and/or the need for mechanical ventilation due to respiratory muscle weakness.

- Weakness can be severe enough that the patient can't walk.

- Diminished or absent reflexes.

The symptoms of GBS develop over the course of 8 – 24 hours. The disease usually peaks at about the point of 10 days, and most cases are resolved within 4 weeks.

Be careful with using sedation with GBS patients as some patients develop profound hypotension with sedation. Ideally these patients should be on a monitor as they can become bradycardic at any time and are also susceptible to experiencing shifts in their blood pressure swinging from hypertension to hypotension. Insofar as these patients are immobilized, make sure appropriate prophylaxis is taken to prevent a pulmonary embolus from a DVT. Know that in the vast majority of cases, GBS is self-limiting and it will end.

The diagnosis of GBS is based on the evaluation of the signs and symptoms in conjunction with the following:

- Evidence of rapidly developing muscle weakness/paralysis that is consistent with the clinical presentation of GBS.

- Diminished and/or absent reflexes.

- Absence of fever - although it may have been a febrile viral illness that triggered GBS, *GBS itself does not present with fever* - this is one of the key features that enables you to differentiate GBS from other illnesses.

- Analysis of CSF (cerebrospinal fluid) demonstrates albuminocytologic dissociation. Albuminocytologic dissociation is when there is increased protein in the CSF without an increase in cell count. This is a finding in 90% of GBS cases.

- Nerve conduction studies.

Treatment of Guillain–Barré Syndrome

- Upwards of 30–50% of GBS cases will progress to respiratory failure, therefore intubation and mechanical ventilation are to be initiated as per the criteria for initiating mechanical ventilation. The average length of stay on the ventilator with GBS is roughly 40 days. As such, within a week these patients will receive a tracheotomy with the placement of a tracheostomy tube. During mechanical ventilation, take all precautions to prevent VAP and VILI.

- Appropriate prophylaxis to prevent a pulmonary embolus from a DVT.

- Bedside passive range of motion exercises to prevent muscular atrophy.

- Plasmapheresis – (plasmapheresis is also sometimes used in treating Myasthenia Gravis)

  * Plasmapheresis involves removing whole blood from the patient and separating the plasma from the cells. In the process of separating plasma from the cells - the cells are separated from antibodies, immune complexes, cytokines,

and other inflammatory mediators that are contained within the plasma. Once separated from these other substances in the plasma that are involved in the GBS disease process, the cells are infused back into the body along with albumin or prepared fresh frozen plasma. Sometimes the original plasma that was removed from the patient is treated and then it is returned to the patient.

* Plasmapheresis usually involves 5 exchanges of 3 liters a day for 8 – 10 days. If plasmapheresis is initiated within the first seven days of the onset of GBS, the patient usually ends up spending significantly less time on the ventilator.

- Immunoglobulin Therapy

    * Through the administration of intravenous immunoglobulin therapy (IVIg), the patient receives good antibodies that are able to help boost their immune system.

    * IVIg also disrupts and/or neutralizes the harmful antibodies that are part of GBS.

    * IVIg lessens the inflammation and the autoimmune attacks on the nervous system.

Comparison of Myasthenia Gravis and Guillain–Barré Syndrome

	M.G.	G.B.
Past Hx.	Gradual onset of weakness that improves with rest.	Febrile illness -viral
Appearance	Ptosis, diplopia, dysphagia	Acute weakness in limbs, diminished/absent reflexes
Auscultation	Shallow – diminished, crackles - maybe rhonchi	Shallow – diminished, crackles – maybe rhonchi
Diagnostics	- Tensilon test - Serology for ACh receptor antibodies - Electromyography	- Lumbar puncture reveals elevated protein in CSF - Patient is afebrile - Nerve conduction studies - May have elevated IgM
	- Decreased V_T, VC, & MIP - ABG – acute vent. failure with hypoxemia and $PaCO_2 > 45mmHg$ - PFT – decreased FVC	- Decreased V_T, VC, & MIP - ABG – acute vent. failure with hypoxemia and $PaCO_2 > 45mmHg$ - PFT – decreased FVC
Tx.	Intubation & mechanical ventilation. Carefully watch MIP, VC, & V_T	Intubation & mechanical ventilation. Carefully watch MIP, VC, & V_T
	O_2 for hypoxemia	O_2 for hypoxemia
	Hyperinflation therapy	Hyperinflation therapy
	Pulmonary hygiene	Pulmonary hygiene
	Steroids	Plasmapheresis
	Thymectomy	IV Immunoglobulins
	Plasmapheresis	
	Neostigmine	

Muscular Dystrophy

   Although there are over 30 types of Muscular Dystrophy (MD), the common theme among all of them is the gradual deterioration and weakening of skeletal muscle over time. The predominant form of MD in children is called Duchenne Muscular Dystrophy, and it accounts for about half of all the cases of MD. Duchenne MD occurs at the rate of 1out of every 3,500 – 5,000 males at birth (Duchenne's only affects males). Other forms of MD such as Limb-girdle, Facioscapulohumeral, Congenital, Myotonic, Oculopharyngeal, & Distal affect both males and females. Some forms begin in childhood whereas others don't strike until adulthood. Becker MD is very similar to Duchenne MD except that the progression is much slower and the symptoms are much less severe. The onset of Becker is much later in life and patients with Becker MD live much longer – into their 60's and 70's.

   MD is an inherited disorder with no known cure. The disease occurs within the muscle tissue directly as a result of mutations in the genes that are responsible for making certain muscle proteins. There is no neurological involvement. The genetic mutations result in either a particular muscle protein not being produced, or the assembly of malfunctioning muscle proteins such that muscle contraction then leads to disruptions of the outer membrane of the muscle cells. Destroyed muscle fibers start to be replaced with fat and fibrous tissue, and this in turn furthers the weakening and deterioration of the muscle.

Characteristics, clinical course, and diagnosis of Muscular Dystrophy

   The onset of Duchenne MD can be as early as infancy, but it is usually between 3 – 6 years of age. Signs and symptoms are:

- Muscle weakness – mainly the calves, thighs, shoulders, and pelvis initially, then progression to the arms and neck and respiratory muscles (mainly the diaphragm).

- Difficulty with walking or running – may also manifest itself with walking on the toes to compensate for the muscle deterioration in the muscles of the knee.

- Increasing difficulty with motor skills.

- Lumbar hyperlordosis

- Scoliosis

Patient's with Duchenne's usually lose their ability to walk by age 10 – 12. The prognosis is not good and most of these patients will not live to see their 30's or 40's. The underlying genetic issue that is affecting the skeletal muscle will also affect heart muscle as well, therefore these patients will also develop dilated cardiomyopathy and arrhythmias. The universal outcome of MD is respiratory failure which means that they will need mechanical ventilation to remain alive.

Diagnosis is made on the basis of signs and symptoms and the clinical presentation of the patient, however there are specific tests that can be looked at to confirm the diagnosis of MD.

- Elevated Creatine Kinase – the disruptions in the muscle cell membrane enable CK to leak out of the muscle cell and thus it will be elevated in a blood test.

- DNA tests/Western Blot – to look for mutations in Dystrophin. Dystrophin is the main protein in question that is either not getting made, or not getting made correctly due to a genetic mutation. It is the either the lack of Dystrophin – which is the case with Duchenne's, or malfunctioning Dystrophin – which is the case with Becker's, that is at the heart of the MD problem.

- A muscle biopsy can also be done to stain for Dystrophin.

Treatment of Muscular Dystrophy

There is no cure for MD. Treatment is aimed at slowing the progression of the disease and attempting to provide for a better quality of life in the meantime.

- Glucocorticoids – steroids can be helpful in slowing down the muscle degeneration, but they can't stop it completely. Steroids also always come with the price of side effects such as weight gain.

- Physical Therapy and Conditioning – PT and conditioning can help enhance the quality of life for a while, but it will not reverse the condition.

- Orthopedic appliances may be used to provide support until the point is reached where a wheelchair becomes necessary.

- Treatment of cardiac issues.

- Treatment of respiratory failure – with the progression of MD will come the eventual need for intubation and mechanical ventilation. These patients will in all likelihood receive a trach because they may very well be to the point of being ventilator dependent for the rest of their lives. You will have to take this on a case by case basis depending upon the particular nuances of each case. If it's a situation where their respiratory failure is such it is thought that they may be able to recover enough to return to breathing on their own such that they will only need ventilatory support for less than 3 weeks, then intubation may be appropriate. But if the point has been reached where they no longer have the muscle strength to breathe on their own because of the MD, then they'll need to receive a tracheal airway.

D. Lung Cancer

Lung cancer is one of the leading causes of death, and 85% of lung cancer is directly attributed to cigarette smoking. Unfortunately, only 15% of these cases are found in the early stages.

Most lung cancer tumors originate in the mucosa of the tracheobronchial tree. Tumors (a neoplasm that has formed into a mass), can either be benign or malignant – which at the simplest level is to say that they are either non-invasive or invasive. Benign tumors are isolated to a specific area and do not spread, whereas malignant tumors not only spread throughout the tissue in which they originate, but they can spread through the blood and/or lymphatics and invade other tissue as well.

Bronchogenic carcinoma is a malignant neoplasm of the bronchus, bronchi, or bronchioles. It is often discovered accidentally during the course of an examination regarding another issue.

The signs and symptoms of lung CA are as follows:

- Chronic cough
- Chest pain that is aggravated by deep breathing
- Hoarseness
- Weight loss/loss of appetite
- Hemoptysis
- Recurring infections (bronchitis, pneumonia)
- Fever (low grade) of unknown origin
- New onset of wheezing
- Dyspnea

As you can see, the s/s of lung cancer are similar to many other conditions – therefore it is necessary to obtain further testing in order to definitively determine a diagnosis of lung CA.

Diagnosing lung cancer

When a patient presents with the signs and symptoms just indicated, the following are necessary:

1.   A complete history needs to be obtained, and a thorough examination needs to be done.

2.   Initial Imaging Tests – Chest X-ray

       - If anything abnormal is going to be seen on a CXR, it has to be at least 1 cm in diameter. Anything smaller than 1 cm will not be detected on a CXR.

       * 1 cm diameter tumor ≈ 1 billion cells.
       * If a tumor ≤ 3 cm, it is called a nodule.
       * If a tumor > 3 cm, it is called a mass.

3.   Subsequent Imaging

       CT and/or MRI

       - A CT scan or MRI gives much more information than a CXR.
       - A CT scan or MRI can detect lymph node involvement and metastases.

4.   Sputum Cytology

5.   Bronchoscopy – usually to obtain a biopsy

6.   Needle Biopsy

       - Done under fluoroscopy: Using fluoroscopic technique enables direct observation and visualization of the tumor while the sample tissue is obtained via the fine needle. This is the most reliable way to obtain a biopsy sample.

Performing a needle biopsy carries the risk of causing a pneumothorax. A CXR must be done right after the procedure to make sure there is no pneumothorax. The patient is to then lie flat for 4 hours and then a second CXR is to be done before the patient is released from recovery.

7.   PET scan (Positron Emission Tomography)

- Cancer cells are much more metabolically active than normal cells. With a PET scan, the patient is injected with radioactive glucose and then scanned. Because of their increased metabolic activity, cancerous cells will take more of the radioactive glucose than normal cells, and thus they will light up like a Christmas tree on the scan.

8.   Blood tests

Determining the cancer cell type

1.   Non-small cell (NSCLC)
2.   Small cell (SCLC)

NSCLC

1.   Squamous Cell Carcinoma

- Usually starts in the proximal airways.
- Usually stays in the thorax.
- Usually DOES NOT metastasize.
- This is the form of lung CA with the BEST prognosis.
- Doubling time of cancer cells = 100 days.

2.   Adenocarcinoma

- This is the most common type – 40% of lung CA cases.
- Usually starts in mucous glands – hence the presentation of increased mucus and coughing.

- It initially manifests as a single tumor, but it DOES metastasize.
- Pleural effusions are common on CXR along with the tumor. It is called a malignant effusion.
- Doubling time = 200 days.

3.   Large Cell Carcinoma

- Usually starts in the central airways.
- This form is usually determined by the characteristics it doesn't have.
- There is early metastatic spreading.
- Doubling time = 100 days.

NSCLC Staging (I – IV)

I.   * Tumor localized. Two types – T1a & T1b
        * T1a $\leq$ 2 cm
        * 2 cm < T1b $\leq$ 3 cm
        * NO lymphatic involvement.
        * NO metastases.

II.   * Tumors are bigger.
        * 3 cm < T2a $\leq$ 5 cm
        * 5 cm < T2b $\leq$ 7 cm
        * There is lymphatic involvement in the chest.

III.   * T3 > 7 cm
        * There is lymphatic involvement all the way to the center of the chest.

IV.   * Full Metastases

SCLC

1.   Oat Cell Carcinoma

- This form is almost exclusive to smokers.
- It starts in the proximal airways.
- There is early metastatic spreading.
- Doubling time = 30 days.
- This form has the WORST prognosis – Oat Cell doesn't go into remission and the 5-year survival rate is only 1%.

SCLC Staging

1.   Limited: Confined to one lung and lymph nodes on the same side of the chest.

2.   Extensive: Metastases – even other lung involvement is considered metastases.

Lung cancer treatment strategies

Treatment is based upon the staging of the cancer.

1.   Surgery: For localized tumors – resection of the tumor and surrounding tissue.

- Wedge resection
- Segmentectomy
- Lobectomy
- Pneumonectomy

2.   Chemotherapy

The goal of chemotherapy is to either kill cancer cells or to prevent them from dividing. Chemotherapy can be either a primary treatment or an adjunct therapy to other forms of treatment.

Chemotherapy cocktails consisting of 2 drugs are more effective. Most Chemo drugs are platinum based drugs (e.g. Cisplatin, Carboplatin).

- Dose intensity is the amount of drug delivered per unit of time. It is dose intensity that determines the response to therapy.

- Goal is to give as close to the max. dose as possible, and to give it as frequently as possible.

- Treatments in chemotherapy are called cycles.
  - e.g. 1 Tx/week x 10 weeks, then 1 month off
  - e.g. 1 Tx/every 2 weeks x 16 weeks
  - regardless of the way the cycle is set up, the goal is max. cell kill of cancerous cells.

- Patients undergoing chemotherapy need to have their CBC (complete blood count) checked regularly.
  - Neulasta can be given to help stimulate WBC growth if needed.
  - Erythropoietin can be given for RBC growth if needed.

- After the first cycle of chemotherapy:
  - There are always some cancer cells left behind.
  - There are always some cancer cells that are drug resistant.

  Therefore, another cycle has to be done.
  - But since some of the cancer cells will have mutated and become more resistant to chemo, it may be necessary to change the drugs in the cocktail.

3.   Radiation

Radiation therapy is used when you are able to target an individual tumor. It kills cancer cells and prevents them from dividing. The usual course of radiation treatment is 5 times a week for 4 – 8 weeks. The two days off per week are to enable the cancer cells to re-oxygenate since a hypoxic cancer cell is 2 – 3 times more resistant to radiation.

- Side effects of radiation (specifically the thorax)

    - Esophagitis: swallowing can be so painful that a patient may not even be able to eat.

Other cancer treatments in development

- Immunotherapy

    - Immunotherapy attempts to "train" the immune system to recognize cancer cells.
    - Immunotherapy also attempts to create antibodies against cancer cells in the laboratory.

- Gene therapy

    - Gene therapy is very complex, but fundamentally the process involves the insertion of DNA to help the immune system recognize cancer cells.

- Anti-angiogenesis

    - Anti-angiogenesis involves techniques aimed at cutting off the blood supply to tumors.

Respiratory therapy for lung cancer patients is consistent with what you have already learned. Whether it is oxygen therapy, mechanical ventilation, non-invasive mechanical ventilation, and/ or other respiratory therapy modalities - these respiratory specific treatments and modalities are utilized as needed per the criteria for their use.

E. Pulmonary Embolism

A pulmonary embolism is what is described as a dead space condition. An embolus is a substance that essentially blocks the flow of blood through a blood vessel. In the case of a pulmonary embolism (PE), it is a blockage that is occurring somewhere along the path of the pulmonary arterial circulation that ends up compromising blood flow to the pulmonary capillaries that are distal to the embolus. When this happens, you either have greatly reduced perfusion, or no perfusion at all through those pulmonary capillaries. This greatly disrupts V/Q because you have adequate ventilation to the alveoli, but there is inadequate perfusion – hence why it is called a dead space condition (Q is greatly diminished compared to V). Remember that dead space ventilation is when you have adequate ventilation without perfusion.

There are several types of emboli that are capable of causing the blockage that leads to the inadequacy of perfusion. The following are some of the varieties of emboli that can cause a blockage:

- Blood clots
- Cholesterol plaque
- Fat globules (fat emboli)
- Gas bubbles (gas/air emboli)
- Foreign bodies

Prolonged bed rest, immobility, trauma, recent surgery, and fractures are examples of some of the things that can lead to the formation of an embolus. When you have a patient that is essentially bed-ridden and immobile, it is always important to ensure that steps are being taken for DVT (deep vein thrombosis) prophylaxis in order to prevent a PE. If a patient develops a blood clot in one of the deep veins (particularly in the leg), that clot can dislodge and travel and then find its way into the pulmonary circulation where it can then block blood flow to the pulmonary capillaries. Early ambulation of the post-surgical patient as well as active and passive exercises (to the level of patient tolerance) are also good ways to help prevent the formation of an embolus.

Symptoms of a PE

- Tachypnea
- Crackles or wheezing on auscultation
- Pleural rub
- Diaphoresis
- Cyanosis
- Tachycardia, chest pain, decreased blood pressure
- Hemoptysis or blood tinged sputum

Diagnosing a PE

- CXR – The CXR may be normal, or there may be wedge infiltrates.
- Presence of respiratory alkalosis with hypoxemia – in response to a PE, the body will start to hyperventilate in an attempt to remove CO_2.
- Increased pulmonary artery pressure
- Spiral CT scan
- V/Q scan – to see if there is abnormal perfusion
- Pulmonary angiogram
- Blood test for D-dimer. D-dimer is a small protein fragment present in the blood after a blood clot is broken down.
- Use capnography and check the end-tidal CO_2 (EtCO2).
  - since a PE causes an increase in dead space ventilation, you will see a decrease in EtCO2 in the presence of a pulmonary embolism.

Treatment of a pulmonary embolism

- Oxygen therapy – FiO2 of 100% initially. Titrate to maintain $PaO_2 \geq 80mmHg$.
- Low dose Heparin or Coumadin
- Digoxin for circulation
- Streptokinase or tPA (tissue plasminogen activator) to break down blood clots.
- Embolectomy

F. Congestive Heart Failure/Pulmonary Edema

Pulmonary edema was previously discussed in the NIPPV section of the mechanical ventilation chapter as acute cardiogenic pulmonary edema is one of the indications for NIPPV. In this section we are going to review and expand upon that information.

There are 2 types of pulmonary edema – there is hydrostatic (cardiogenic) pulmonary edema & non-hydrostatic (non-cardiogenic) pulmonary edema.

Hydrostatic Pulmonary Edema	Non-Hydrostatic Pulmonary Edema
Cardiogenic	Non-Cardiogenic
This is a FUNCTIONAL problem.	This is a STRUCTURAL problem.

Due to increased pressure in the pulmonary capillaries.
- mitral valve stenosis
- left ventricular failure
- systemic fluid overload
- renal failure
- excessive IV fluid
	Due to damage to the alveolar epithelium.
	  - irritant gases
	  - near drowning
	  - cytokine storm from a
	    pulmonary infection

	Large amounts of fluid leak through the excessively permeable & damaged capillary walls.
	- ARDS
	- endotoxemia
	- fat embolism
	- decreased plasma oncotic
	  pressure from having low
	  plasma proteins secondary
	  to severe burns, liver
	  failure, or malnutrition.

CHF (congestive heart failure) can either be right sided heart failure or left sided heart failure, or a combination of both. Right sided failure (right ventricular failure) is going to cause blood to

back up in the systemic circulation and give rise to peripheral edema
- usually seen in the dependent areas (legs/ankles). Left sided
failure (left ventricular failure) however causes blood to back up in
the pulmonary circulation, and this causes the pressure inside the
pulmonary capillaries to increase which then results in cardiogenic
pulmonary edema.

With either cardiogenic or non-cardiogenic pulmonary
edema, the bottom line is that more fluid leaves the arterial end of
the capillary than is reabsorbed at the venous end of the capillary.
The presence of pulmonary edema imposes a pulmonary restriction
– meaning that it will limit and/or reduce the amount of alveolar
expansion that can take place, and therefore it reduces the compliance
of the lung. Furthermore – this leaked fluid from the capillaries will
accumulate in the air spaces (alveoli) and cause shunting and thus
hypoxemia.

Patients with pulmonary edema typically present with a
rapid, shallow breathing pattern. They can't take in a normal V_T due
to the reduced compliance of their lungs because of the edema, so
they try to make up for it by taking shallow breaths more frequently.
A rapid, shallow breathing pattern, however, doesn't provide a truly
adequate V_A because it's mostly dead space ventilation.

Patients with pulmonary edema secondary to CHF typically present
with the following:

- Pink / frothy secretions
- Tachypnea
- Orthopnea
- Cyanosis
- Diaphoresis
- Increased tactile/vocal fremitus
- Crackles

Other clinical findings consistent with pulmonary edema

- CXR – fluffy opacities with butterfly pattern
- Hypoxemia with respiratory alkalosis
- Increased PCWP

- BNP (Brain Natriuretic Peptide) > 100 pg/ml. BNP will be elevated in CHF. BNP gets its name from the fact that it was originally identified in pig brain. In humans however, BNP is secreted by the ventricles of the heart when it has to work harder than usual over an extended period of time.

- Hyponatremia - with CHF

Treatment

- Immediately put the patient in Fowlers and give 100% O_2.

- Then get them on CPAP right away.
  - set CPAP at 8 – 12 cmH$_2$O

  - CPAP helps to keep the alveoli open.
  - It increases FRC.
  - It increases compliance and thus decreases the WOB.
  - It improves oxygenation.

- Treating cardiogenic pulmonary edema with CPAP reduces the overall intubation rate associated with this condition.

- If the patient starts to retain CO_2, then switch them to BiPAP so as to be able to assist them with their ventilation. Note that when you are dealing with pulmonary edema you are going to want to know the $PaCO_2$ from an ABG and not the $EtCO_2$ (end-tidal CO_2). Although $EtCO_2$ is often a very good estimate for $PaCO_2$, when you have other issues going on such as pulmonary disease or cardiovascular instability, $EtCO_2$ is not as reliable and you need to get a true $PaCO_2$ from an ABG.

- Furosemide (Lasix)
- Digitalis / Dopamine / Positive Inotropes
- Afterload reduction agents (ACE inhibitors)
- Nitroprusside
- Electrolyte replacement

G. Pneumothorax/Hemothorax

PNEUMOTHORAX
Air in Pleural Space

- Tracheal shift AWAY from
  affected side. Increased volume
  on effected side.
- Increased respiratory rate.
- Hyper-resonant percussion note.

Small Pneumo
- Increased HR & BP
Large Pneumo
- Decreased HR & BP, and
  Pulsus Paradoxus.

CXR
- hyperlucency without
  vascular markings.
- depressed diaphragm.

ABG
Small Pneumo
- Acute hyperventilation
  with hypoxemia
Large Pneumo
- Acute ventilatory failure
  with hypoxemia.

Tx:

Small Pneumo: < 20% lung collapse.
- Bedrest with limited activity. Small
  pneumo usually heals by itself within
  30 days.
Large Pneumo: > 20% lung collapse.

HEMOTHORAX
Blood in Pleural Space

- Tracheal shift AWAY from
  affected side.
- Severe chest pain.
- Increased respiratory rate
- Flat percussion note.
- Increased HR & BP
- Hemoptysis

CXR
- Increased radiodensity

ABG
- Hyperventilation and
  hypoxemia

CBC
- Decreased RBC, Hb,
  and HCT.

Tx

- Thoracentesis or chest tube
  to drain blood.
- O_2 for hypoxemia
- Incentive spirometry after
  chest tube is removed.
- Mechanical ventilation
  with PEEP if needed for
  ventilatory failure.

- Evacuate with chest tube. If patient is hemodynamically unstable, do a
  needle decompression instead. O_2 therapy for hypoxemia. Incentive
  spirometry after chest tube is removed. Mechanical ventilation with
  PEEP if needed for ventilatory failure.

Chapter 10

Respiratory Pharmacology

This chapter consists of a fairly comprehensive drug list to include drug class, generic names, mechanism of action, side effects, delivery routes, and recommended dosages of the drugs that you will encounter most often as a respiratory therapist. It is presented with the understanding that you have either already taken, or are presently enrolled in a pharmacology course that is part of your curriculum. This caveat is made insofar as you are expected to already have a working knowledge of the vocabulary that pertains to drug classifications and the descriptions of their mechanisms of action. The information in this chapter is also presented with the understanding that it is always your responsibility to double check the most current information that is available before administering medication to your patients – particularly with regards to dosing and contraindications. Every attempt has been made to ensure the accuracy of the information in this chapter, but you must always check the most current information that is available to verify dosage information, methods and duration of administration, and contraindications. The most current source of information comes from the drug manufacturers themselves, and that will usually be contained in the package insert that accompanies the medication. Current, reliable, and comprehensive drug information can also be found at the following websites: *www.drugs.com* or *www.rxlist.com*.

Patient safety is the highest priority. Drug errors are a big area of concern when it comes to patient safety, and the more knowledgeable you are, the better you are able to protect your patients. All health care personnel can make mistakes. Despite the best of intentions - physicians, nurses, and respiratory therapists can and do make mistakes. Doing your due diligence and always maintaining an attitude of vigilance towards the care of your patients however will keep errors to a minimum.

PHARMACOLOGY DRUG LIST

DRUG NAME	MECHANISM OF ACTION	SIDE EFFECTS	ROUTE GIVEN	ADULT DOSING *unless otherwise noted*
ULTRA SHORT ACTING ADRENERGIC BRONCHODILATORS				
1 Epinephrine Adrenalin Chloride EpiPen *onset: 3 - 5 min.* *peak: 5 - 20 min.* *duration: 1 - 3 hr.*	Alpha, beta 1, & beta 2 agonist; vasoconstriction, bronchodilation, CNS stimulation, cardiac stimulant	hypertension, tachycardia, ventricular arrhythmias, paradoxical bronchospasm	SC, IM,	Anaphylaxis/Bronchospasm SC/IM: 0.3 - 0.5mg (0.3 - 0.5ml) of 1:1000 epi. 1:1000 epinephrine is supplied as a 1ml soln. of 1mg/ml. Repeat q 5 – 10 min. PRN. Not to exceed 0.5 mg/dose.
2 Racemic Epinephrine MicroNefrin Nephron *onset: 3 - 5 min.* *peak: 5 - 20 min.* *duration: 0.5 - 2 hr.*	Alpha & beta agonist; α - vasoconstriction β - bronchodilation	tachycardia, nausea, anxiety, headache	SVN	2.25% solution - 0.25 – 0.5ml, qid.
SHORT ACTING ADRENERGIC BRONCHODILATORS				
3 Metaproterenol Alupent *onset: 1 - 5 min.* *peak: 60 min.* *duration: 2 - 6 hr.*	Selective β-2 agonist; bronchodilation	tachycardia, dizziness, nausea, headache	SVN, PO	SVN: 10 to 15mg (0.2 to 0.3ml of 5% solution) q 4 – 6 hours. PO: 20mg, tid - qid.
4 Albuterol Sulfate Proventil Ventolin *onset: 15 min.* *peak: 30 - 60 min.* *duration: 5 - 8 hr.*	Selective β-2 agonist; bronchodilation	tachycardia, anxiety, dry mouth, fine tremor, headache	SVN, MDI, PO	SVN: 0.5% soln.; 0.5ml (2.5mg) q 4 - 6 hrs. *(2.5 to 5mg once - followed by 2.5mg q 20 min. for acute bronchospasm)* MDI: 90μg /puff, 2 puffs, tid - qid. PO: (tablets) 2 - 8mg, bid - qid. (syrup) 2mg/5ml, 1 - 2 tsp., tid - qid. [1 tsp. = 5ml]

5 Pirbuterol Acetate Maxair Autohaler *onset: 5 min.* *peak: 30 min.* *duration: 5 hr.*	Selective β-2 agonist; bronchodilation	shakiness in arms, hands, legs, or feet; fast, pounding, or irregular heartbeat or pulse	MDI	200µg/puff, 2 puffs q 4 - 6 hrs.
6 Levalbuterol Xopenex *onset: 15 min.* *peak: 30 - 60 min.* *duration: 5 - 8 hr.*	Selective β-2 agonist; bronchodilation	tachycardia, chest pain or tightness, dizziness	SVN, MDI	SVN: 0.31mg, 0.63mg, or 1.25mg per 3ml - tid. As concentrate – 1.25mg/0.5ml - tid. MDI: 45µg/puff, 2 puffs q 4 - 6 hrs.

LONG ACTING ADRENERGIC BRONCHODILATORS

7 Salmeterol Xinafoate Serevent Diskus *onset: 20 min.* *peak: 2 - 5 hr.* *duration: 12 hr.*	Selective β-2 agonist; bronchodilation	dizziness, sinus infection, migraine headache	DPI	50µg/inhalation - 1 inhalation bid. (every 12 hrs.)
8 Formoterol Fumerate Performist Foradil *onset: 15 min.* *peak: 30 - 60 min.* *duration: 12 hr.*	Selective β-2 agonist; bronchodilation	angina, hyper or hypotension, tachycardia, arrhythmias	SVN, DPI	SVN: 20µg/2ml unit dose - bid. DPI: 12µg/inhalation - bid.
9 Arformoterol Tartrate Brovana *onset: 15 min.* *peak: 30 - 60 min.* *duration: 12 hr.*	Selective β-2 agonist; bronchodilation	peripheral edema, dyspnea, diarrhea	SVN	15µg/2ml unit dose - bid.

INHALED ANTICHOLINERGIC BRONCHODILATORS

10 Ipratropium Bromide Atrovent *onset: 15 min.* *peak: 1 - 2 hr.* *duration: 4 - 6 hr.*	Anticholinergic – i.e.: an anti-parasympathomimetic acting as a muscarinic antagonist; bronchodilation	dry mouth, sedation, tachycardia, headache	SVN, HFA-MDI	SVN: 0.02% soln. (0.2mg/ml) 500µg/unit dose vial (2.5ml), tid – qid. HFA-MDI: 17µg/puff, 2 puffs qid.
11 Ipratropium Bromide & Albuterol Combivent Duoneb *Onset: 15 min.* *peak: 1 - 2 hr.* *duration: 4 - 6 hr.*	Muscarinic antagonist & selective β-2 agonist; bronchodilation	bronchitis, headache, chest pain, cough	SVN, MDI	SVN: Ipratropium 0.5mg & albuterol 2.5mg /3ml unit dose vial, tid - qid. MDI: Ipratropium 18µg/puff & albuterol 90µg/puff, 2 puffs qid.
12 Tiotropium Bromide Spiriva *onset: 30 min.* *peak: 3 hr.* *duration: 24 hr.*	Muscarinic antagonist; bronchodilation	chest pain, nausea, SOB, tachycardia	DPI	18µg/inhalation, once daily.

MUCOLYTIC AGENTS

13 N-Acetylcysteine Mucomyst	Mucolytic - acts by breaking disulfide links in the mucoproteins of mucus.	nausea, bronchospasm, dizziness	SVN	10 or 20% soln. 3 – 5ml, tid – qid.

CORTICOSTEROIDS AND COMBINATION MEDICATIONS

14 Beclomethasone Dipropionate QVAR	Glucocorticoid steroid; potent anti-inflammatory mainly through inhibition of prostaglandins and leukotrienes.	cough, oral candida, headache, visual changes	MDI	40 or 80µg/puff - 40 - 80µg bid. or 40 - 160µg bid.
15 Flunisolide Hemihydrate AeroSpan	Glucocorticoid steroid; potent anti-inflammatory mainly through inhibition of prostaglandins and leukotrienes.	dysphonia, sore throat, headache	MDI	80µg/puff, 2 puffs bid.

16 Fluticasone Propionate
Flovent HFA MDI
Flovent Diskus DPI

Glucocorticoid steroid; potent anti-inflammatory mainly through inhibition of prostaglandins and leukotrienes.

throat irritation, headache, sinusitis, fever

MDI, DPI

MDI: 44, 110, or 220µg/puff - 88µg bid, 88 - 220µg bid, or 880µg bid.

DPI: 50, 100, or 250µg/inhalation - 100µg bid, 100-250µg bid, or 1000µg bid.

17 Budesonide
Pulmicort Flexhaler DPI
Pulmicort Respules SVN

Glucocorticoid steroid; potent anti-inflammatory mainly through inhibition of prostaglandins and leukotrienes.

nasopharyngitis, headache, fever, insomnia

DPI, SVN

DPI: 90µg/inhalation & 180µg/inhalation - 180 - 360µg bid (if taking inhaled corticosteroids previously. 360 - 720µg bid (if taking oral corticosteroids previously.

SVN: (pediatric) 0.5mg/ml - 0.5mg total dose given qd or bid in divided doses.

18 Fluticasone Propionate & Salmeterol
Advair Diskus
Advair HFA

Glucocorticoid steroid; potent anti-inflammatory mainly through inhibition of prostaglandins and leukotrienes. Selective β-2 agonist; bronchodilation

pharyngitis, hoarseness/dysphonia, bronchitis, cough, headache

DPI, MDI

DPI: 100µg fluticasone/50µg salmeterol, 250µg fluticasone/50µg salmeterol, 500µg fluticasone/50µg salmeterol 1 inhalation bid. Max rec. dose - 500µg fluticasone/50µg salmeterol bid.

MDI: 45, 115, or 230µg fluticasone/21 µg salmeterol - 2 puffs bid.

NONSTEROIDAL ASTHMA MEDICATIONS

19 Cromolyn Sodium
NasalCrom
Gastrocrom

Mast cell stabilizer; acts by preventing the release of substances that cause inflammation. Inhibits sensitized mast cell degranulation, release of mediators from mast cells, and both immediate and non-immediate bronchoconstrictive reactions to inhaled antigens.

throat irritation/dryness, bad taste, cough, nausea

SVN, PO, Spray

SVN: 20mg/ampule or 20mg/2ml - 20mg qid.

PO: (Gastrocrom) 100mg/5ml ampule - 2 ampules qid, 30 minutes a.c. and at bedtime.

Spray: 40mg/ml (4%) - 1 spray in each nostril every 4 - 6 hrs.

20 Montelukast
Singulair

Leukotriene receptor antagonist; binds to cysteinyl 1 leukotriene (CYSLTR1) receptors found in the airway (including airway smooth muscle cells and airway macrophages), and on other proinflammatory cells (including eosinophils and certain myeloid stem cells). Inhibits physiologic actions of leukotriene D4 at the CYSLTR type 1 receptor.

headache, pharyngitis, influenza, fever, sinusitis, diarrhea

PO

10mg tablets - 1 tablet daily.

INHALED ANTI-INFECTIVE MEDICATIONS

21 Pentamidine
Nebupent

Antimicrobial agent; mechanism not fully understood. It is suspected to interfere with DNA, RNA, phospholipid and protein synthesis.

hypotension, cough, arrhythmias, chest pain, bronchospasm

Respirgard II nebulizer

300mg once every 4 weeks via Respirgard II nebulizer. Administer at 5 - 7 LPM from 50 PSI air or O_2 source until chamber is empty, $\approx$ 30 - 45 min.

22 Ribavirin
Virazole

Pediatric specific medication

Anti-viral action via nucleoside inhibition; mechanism unknown; suspected to act as a guanosine analog.

worsening of respiratory status, bronchospasm, pulmonary edema, hypoventilation, cyanosis, dyspnea

SPAG Nebulizer

20mg/ml continuous aerosol administration 12 - 18 hrs./day for 3 - 7 days.

Ribavirin is only to be used under strict physician supervision, and only by staff that are trained in the use of a SPAG nebulizer.

BENZODIAZEPINES

23 Diazepam
Valium

Benzodiazepines exert anxiolytic, sedative, muscle-relaxant, anticonvulsant, and amnestic effects. It is thought that Benzo's exert these effects mechanistically by potentiating GABA - i.e.: facilitating the action of GABA which is the most ubiquitous inhibitory CNS neurotransmitter.

drowsiness, fatigue, muscle weakness, ataxia

PO

2 - 10mg, bid – tid.

| 24 **Midazolam** Versed | Same as Diazepam | decreased tidal volume &/or respiratory rate, BP/HR variations, desaturation | IM, IV | IM: 0.07 - 0.08mg/kg up to 1 hr. before surgery.

IV: <u>Initial</u>: 1 - 2.5mg over a period of $\geq$ 2 min.; use less if patient is pre-medicated with narcotics or CNS depressants. <u>Titrate</u>: wait $\geq$ 2 min. and increase by small increments if needed; wait $\geq$ 2 min. after each increment. |
| 25 **Lorazepam** Ativan | Same as Diazepam | respiratory depression/failure, hypotension, somnolence, hypoventilation | IM, IV | IM: pre-anesthetic sedation - 0.05mg/kg given at least 2 hrs. prior to surgery.

IV: 2mg or 0.044mg/kg (whichever is smaller) 15 - 20 min. prior to procedure.

Max dose: 4mg IM/IV. |

ANTIBIOTICS

| 26 **Erythromycin** PCE Tablets | Macrolide antibiotic; inhibits protein synthesis by binding 50S ribosomal subunits of susceptible organisms. | nausea/vomiting, abdominal pain, diarrhea | PO | Administer in the fasting state (at least ½ hr., and preferably 2 hrs. before food).

<u>Usual dose</u>: 333mg q 8 hrs. or 500mg q 12 hrs. May increase up to 4g/day according to severity of infection. |
| 27 **Gentamicin** Isotonic Gentamicin Sulfate | Aminoglycoside antibiotic; inhibits normal protein synthesis in susceptible microorganisms. | nephrotoxicity, neurotoxicity, ototoxicity | IV, IM | <u>Serious Infections</u>: 3mg/kg/day given in 3 equal doses q 8 hrs. <u>Life-Threatening Infections</u>: Up to 5mg/kg/day given in 3 or 4 equal doses; reduce to 3mg/kg/day as soon as clinically indicated. <u>Usual Duration</u>: 7 - 10 days; may need longer course in difficult and complicated infections. |

28 Tobramycin
Nebcin

Aminoglycoside antibiotic; inhibits normal protein synthesis in susceptible microorganisms.

nephrotoxicity, neurotoxicity, ototoxicity

IV, IM

Serious Infections: 3mg/kg/day given in 3 equal doses q 8 hrs.
Life-Threatening Infections: Up to 5mg/kg/day given in 3 or 4 equal doses; reduce to 3mg/kg/day as soon as clinically indicated.

29 Ciprofloxacin
Cipro

Fluoroquinolone antibiotic; inhibits the enzymes Topoisomerase II (DNA Gyrase) and Topoisomerase IV which are required for bacterial DNA replication, transcription, repair, and recombination.

tendinitis, tendon rupture, nausea/vomiting, diarrhea

IV, PO

Infuse IV over 60 minutes.
UTI's: Mild/Moderate:
200mg q 12 hrs. for 7 - 14 days.
Severe/Complicated:
400mg q 12 hrs. for 7 - 14 days.
LRTI's/SSSI's: Mild/Moderate:
400mg q 12 hrs. for 7 - 14 days.
Severe/Complicated:
400mg q 8 hrs. for 7 - 14 days.
Nosocomial Pneumonia:
400mg q 8 hrs. for 10 - 14 days.
Bone and Joint Infections: Mild/Moderate:
400mg q 12 hrs. for ≥ 4 - 6 weeks.
Severe/Complicated:
400mg q 8 hrs. for ≥ 4 - 6 weeks.
Complicated Intra-Abdominal Infections:
(used in conjunction with Metronidazole)
400mg q 12 hrs. for 7 – 14 days.
Acute Sinusitis: Mild/Moderate:
400mg q 12 hrs. for 10 days.

PO: Uncomplicated UTI:
500mg q 24 hrs. for 3 days.
Complicated UTI or Acute
Uncomplicated Pyelonephritis:
1000mg q 24 hrs. for 7 - 14 days.

30 Azithromycin
Zithromax

Macrolide antibiotic; inhibits protein synthesis by binding 50S ribosomal subunits of susceptible organisms.

nausea/vomiting, abdominal pain, diarrhea

IV, PO

Infuse IV over ≥ 60 minutes.
Community Acquired Pneumonia:
500mg qd for at least 2 days - then 500mg PO (two 250mg tabs) qd to complete a 7 – 10 day course.

Just PO: Acute Bacterial Exacerbations of COPD (Mild-Moderate):
500mg qd for 3 days or 500mg single dose on day 1 followed by 250mg qd for days 2 – 5.
Acute Bacterial Sinusitis:
500mg qd for 3 days.

31 Vancomycin
Vancocin

Tricyclic glycopeptide antibiotic; inhibits cell wall biosynthesis. Also alters bacterial cell membrane permeability and RNA synthesis.

nausea, vomiting, abdominal pain, diarrhea, hypokalemia

IV. PO

IV: <u>bacterial infections</u>: 15 - 20 mg/kg q 8 - 12 hrs. 2 - 3 g/day with a loading dose of 25 – 30 mg/kg can be considered for seriously ill patients.

PO: <u>Clostridium Difficile</u>: 125mg qid for 10 days. <u>Enterocolitis</u>: 500mg - 2g/day in 3 or 4 divided doses for 7 - 10 days.

32 Isoniazid
Isoniazid

Isonicotinic acid hydrazide; inhibits mycolic acid synthesis and acts against actively growing tuberculosis bacilli.

hepatitis, epigastric distress, pyridoxine deficiency, elevated serum transaminases

IM, PO

For active TB: 5mg/kg (up to 300mg) qd given IM or PO - or 15mg/kg (up to 900mg) 2 - 3 times a week. Treatment is usually for 6 months.

33 Ceftriaxone
Rocephin

Cephalosporin (3rd generation) bactericidal agent that acts through inhibition of bacterial cell wall synthesis.

injection site reactions, eosinophilia, thrombocytosis

IV, IM

1 - 2g given IV/IM once daily or in equally divided doses bid depending on the type and severity of infection. <u>Staphylococcus Aureus Infections</u>: 1 - 2g/day. Max: 4g/day. <u>Uncomplicated Gonococcal Infections</u>: 250mg IM single dose. <u>Surgical Prophylaxis</u>: 1g IV single dose 1/2 - 2 hrs. before surgery. <u>General course of therapy</u>: Continue therapy for ≥ 2 days after signs and symptoms of infection have disappeared. Usual duration is 4 - 14 days; complicated infections may require longer therapy. <u>Streptococcus pyogenes Infections</u>: Continue therapy for ≥ 10 days.

When there is hepatic dysfunction and/ or significant renal disease the maximum dose is 2 g/day.

34 Levofloxacin
Levaquin

Fluoroquinolone antibiotic; inhibits the enzymes Topoisomerase II (DNA Gyrase) and Topoisomerase IV which are required for bacterial DNA replication, transcription, repair, and recombination.

tendinitis, tendon rupture, nausea/vomiting, diarrhea

PO, IV

PO: 750mg qd for 5 days or 500mg qd for 7 - 14 days.

IV: Infuse 500mg q 24 hrs. for 7 – 14 days or 750mg q 24 hrs. for 5 days.

CARDIAC & VASOACTIVE DRUGS

35 Sodium Nitroprusside Nitropress	Vasodilator; relaxes vascular smooth muscle and dilates peripheral arteries, veins, and coronary arteries.	excessive hypotension, cyanide toxicity, methemoglobinemia	IV	Initial: 0.3mcg/kg/min. Titrate: May increase every few min. until the desired effect is achieved, or the max infusion rate has been reached. Max: 10mcg/kg/min. Treatment of Acute CHF: Titration of the infusion rate must be guided by the results of invasive hemodynamic monitoring with simultaneous monitoring of urine output.
36 Nitroglycerin Nitroglycerin	Nitrate vasodilator; relaxes vascular smooth muscle and consequently dilates peripheral arteries and veins.	headache, chest tightness, tingling in hands/feet	IV	Initial: 5mcg/min. Titrate: Increase by 5mcg/min. at intervals of 3 - 5 min. If no response at 20mcg/min., may use increments of 10 and even 20mcg/min. Once some hemodynamic response is observed, dosage increments should be smaller and less frequent.
37 Dopamine Hydrochloride Intropin	Inotropic agent; catecholamine; acts directly by exerting an agonist action on β-adrenoreceptors and indirectly by causing release of norepinephrine from storage sites in sympathetic nerve endings.	tachycardia, palpitations, ventricular arrhythmia, dyspnea,	IV	Initial: 2 - 10mcg/kg/min. (≥ 5mcg/kg/min. in more seriously ill patients). Titrate: Increase gradually using 5 - 10mcg/kg/min increments up to 20 - 50mcg/kg/min. PRN. If rates in excess of 50mcg/kg/min. are required, check urine output frequently. Consider dose reduction if urine flow begins to decrease in the absence of hypotension. Additional increments may be employed in an effort to produce an appropriate arterial pressure and central perfusion in patients who do not respond to these doses with adequate arterial pressure or urine flow. Dosage should be adjusted based on patient's response.

38 **Digoxin** Lanoxin Digitek	Cardiac glycoside; inhibits Na^+/K^+ ATPase, which is responsible for maintaining the intracellular milieu throughout the body by moving Na+ ions out of cells and K+ ions into cells.	cardiac arrhythmias, nausea/vomiting, abdominal pain, intestinal ischemia	IV, PO	Dosing can be initiated either with a LD followed by maintenance dosing if rapid titration is desired, or initiated with maintenance dosing without a loading dose (LD). <u>(IV): LD</u>: 8 - 12mcg/kg. <u>Maint</u>: (Normal Renal Function): 2.4 - 3.6mcg/kg/dose qd. <u>(PO) Initial</u>: LD: 10 - 15mcg/kg. <u>Maint</u>: (Normal Renal Function) 3.4 - 5.1mcg/kg/day qd. <u>Titrate</u>: May be increased every 2 weeks according to clinical response, serum drug levels, and toxicity. * Give 1/2 the total LD, then 1/4 the LD every 6 – 8 hrs. twice, with careful assessment of clinical response and toxicity before each dose.
39 **Norepinephrine** Lovaphed	Alpha & beta adrenergic agonist; α-adrenergic action - peripheral vasoconstriction. β-adrenergic action - inotropic stimulator of the heart and dilator of the coronary arteries.	ischemic injury, bradycardia, arrhythmias, anxiety, headache, respiratory difficulty	IV	<u>Average Dosage: Initial</u>: 8 - 12mcg/min. (2 - 3mL) as IV infusion until low normal BP (80 - 100mmHg systolic) is established and maintained by adjusting rate of flow. <u>Maint</u>: 2 - 4mcg/min (0.5 - 1mL). <u>High Dosage</u>: Individualize dose as high as 68mg base/day). <u>Elderly</u>: Start a lower end of dosing range.
40 **Nitric Oxide** INOmax *Pediatric Specific Medication* Treatment of term and near-term (>34 weeks) neonates with hypoxic respiratory failure associated with pulmonary HTN in conjunction with ventilatory support and other appropriate agents.	Pulmonary vasodilator; relaxes vascular smooth muscle by binding to the heme moiety of cytosolic guanylate cyclase and activating guanylate cyclase thus increasing intracellular levels of cyclic guanosine 3', 5'- monophosphate, which leads to vasodilation. Selectively dilates the pulmonary vasculature when inhaled. Appears to increase partial pressure of arterial oxygen (PaO_2) by dilating pulmonary vessels in better ventilated areas of the lung, redistributing pulmonary blood flow away from lung regions with low ventilation/perfusion (V/Q) ratios toward regions with normal ratios.	hypotension, may increase risk of methemo-globinemia with nitric oxide donor compounds e.g. sodium, nitroprusside, nitroglycerin, or prilocaine	Gas Inhalation	Term/Near-Term (>34 Weeks) Neonates: Usual: 20ppm. Maintain treatment for up to 14 days or until underlying oxygen desaturation has resolved and the neonate is ready to be weaned from therapy.

41 Dobutamine
Dobutrex

Synthetic catecholamine; a sympathomimetic that acts by direct stimulation of β1 adrenoreceptors of the heart.

hypertension, angina, arrhythmias, tachycardia

IV

The infusion rate needed to increase cardiac output usually ranges from 2.5 to 15 mcg/kg/min. The initial dosage may be titrated upward by 2.5 mcg/kg/min. as tolerated to maintain systemic blood pressure and urine output. Administration rates greater than 40mcg/kg/min. may be necessary in serious situations.

OTHER STEROIDS

42 Prednisone
Rayos
Sterapred

Glucocorticoid - steroidal anti-inflammatory; Specifically acts to inhibit phospholipase A2 in cell membranes. This action effectively shuts down the eicosanoid pathway.

anaphylactoid reactions, hypertension, osteoporosis, muscle weakness, impaired wound healing

IV, PO

Initial: 5 - 60mg/day, depending on disease being treated. Maintain/adjust initial dose until satisfactory response is noted. If no satisfactory clinical response after a reasonable period, d/c and transfer to other appropriate therapy.
Maint. Decrease dose by small amounts to lowest effective dose. Withdraw gradually.

43 Triamcinolone Acetonide
Allernaze

Corticosteroid; shown to have a wide range of effects on multiple cell types (e.g. mast cells, eosinophils, neutrophils, macrophages, lymphocytes), and mediators (e.g. histamines, eicosanoids, leukotrienes, cytokines) involved in inflammation.

headache, back pain, pharyngitis, asthma

Spray

Initial: 2 sprays/nostril qd. If a faster onset of relief is desired, you may consider starting with 4 sprays per nostril qd, or 2 sprays per nostril bid.
Titrate to minimum effective dose.
Max: 4 sprays/nostril qd or 2 sprays/nostril bid.

ANALGESICS

44 Morphine Sulfate Duramorph	Opioid analgesic; analgesia involves at least 3 anatomical areas of the CNS: the periaqueductal-periventricular gray matter, the ventromedial medulla, and the spinal cord. Interacts predominantly with μ-receptors distributed in the brain, spinal cord, and trigeminal nerve.	respiratory depression/arrest, convulsions, dysphoric reactions, toxic psychoses	IV	For continuous IV infusion, morphine sulfate must be diluted to a concentration of 0.1 – 1mg/ml in 5% dextrose and administered via a controlled infusion device. Rate of infusion is individualized as per patient response.
45 Fentanyl Fentanyl Citrate	Narcotic analgesic; produces analgesic and sedative effects. Alters respiratory rate and alveolar ventilation, which may last longer than analgesic effects.	respiratory depression, apnea, rigidity, bradycardia	IM, IV	Individualize dose. <u>Premedication prior to surgery</u> 50 – 100mcg IM 30 – 60 min. prior to surgery. <u>Adjunct to general anesthesia</u> Minor surgery: 2mcg/kg Major surgery: 20 – 50mcg/kg <u>Adjunct to regional anesthesia</u> 50 – 100mcg IM or slow IV over 3 – 5 min. <u>Post-operative</u> 50 – 100mcg IM, repeat q 1 – 2 hrs. PRN.
46 Meperidine hydrochloride Demerol	Narcotic analgesic; produces actions similar to morphine. Principal actions involve the CNS and organs that contain smooth muscle. Produces analgesic and sedative effects.	lightheadedness, dizziness, sedation, nausea/vomiting sweating, respiratory &/or circulatory depression	IM, IV	<u>Pain:</u> Usual: 50 - 150mg IM q 3 – 4 hrs. PRN. <u>Preop:</u> Usual: 50 – 100mg IM 30 – 90 min. before anesthesia. <u>Anesthesia Support:</u> Use slow IV inj. of fractional doses or continuous IV infusion of a more diluted soln. (1ml/mg). Titrate PRN.

ANESTHESIA RELATED DRUGS

47 Sufentanil
Sufenta

Opioid analgesic; analgesia involves at least 3 anatomical areas of the CNS: the periaqueductal-periventricular gray matter, the ventromedial medulla, and the spinal cord. Interacts predominantly with μ-receptors distributed in the brain, spinal cord, and trigeminal nerve.

respiratory depression, skeletal muscle rigidity, bradycardia, HTN, hypotension

IV

Individualize dose. Premedication: Based on patient's needs. Analgesic: Total dose: 1 - 8mcg/kg. Maint: Incremental from 10 - 50mcg. Infusion: Based on induction dose not to exceed 1mcg/kg/hr. Anesthetic: Total Dose: 8 - 30mcg/kg. Maint: Incremental 0.5 - 10mcg/kg. Infusion: Based on induction dose not to exceed 30mcg/kg.

48 Dexmedetomidine Hydrochloride
Precedex

Alpha 2 agonist - Selective α2 adrenergic agonist; possesses sedative properties.

hypotension, HTN, bradycardia, dry mouth, tachycardia, N/V, atrial fibrillation, fever, anemia, hypovolemia, hypoxia, atelectasis, agitation, respiratory depression/failure

IV

Individualize dose. Administer by continuous infusion (using a controlled infusion device) not to exceed 24 hrs. Intensive care Unit Sedation: LD: 1mcg/kg IV infusion over 10 min. May not be required for patients being converted from alternate sedative therapy. Maint: 0.2 - 0.7mcg/kg/hr. Adjust infusion rate to achieve desired level of sedation.

49 Propofol
Diprivan

Sedative-hypnotic agent; Suspected to produce effects by the positive modulation of the inhibitory function of the neurotransmitter gamma-aminobutyric acid (GABA) through the ligand-gated $GABA_A$ receptors.

bradycardia, arrhythmia, hypotension, HTN, decreased cardiac output, respiratory acidosis during weaning

IV

General Anesthesia: < 55 yrs: Induction: 40mg IV q10 seconds until onset (2 - 2.5mg/kg). Maint: 100 - 200mcg/kg/min. IV or may be given in increments of 20 - 50mg IV intermittent bolus PRN. Elderly/Debilitated- Induction: 20mg IV q10 seconds until onset (1 - 1.5mg/kg). Maint: 50 - 100mcg/kg/min. IV. ICU Sedation: Initial: 5mcg/kg/min IV for at least 5 min., then increased by increments of 5 – 10mcg/kg/min. IV over 5 - 10 min. until desired clinical effect. Maint: 5 – 50mcg/kg/min. IV or higher may be required. Max: 4mg/kg/hr.

PARALYTICS & MUSCULAR BLOCKING AGENTS

50 Succinylcholine Chloride
Anectine
Quelicin

Depolarizing skeletal muscle relaxant; combines with cholinergic receptors of the motor end plate to produce depolarization and subsequent inhibition of neuromuscular transmission.

respiratory depression, apnea, cardiac arrest, malignant hyperthermia, arrhythmia, bradycardia, tachycardia, HTN, hypotension, hyperkalemia

IV, IM

Individualize dose. Short Surgical Procedure: 0.6mg/kg IV. Optimum dose: 0.3 - 1.1mg/kg IV. Blockade develops in 1 min., may persist up to 2 min. Long Surgical Procedure: Depends upon the duration of the surgical procedure and need for muscle relaxation. 2.5 - 4.3mg/min. IV or 0.3 - 1.1mg/kg initial IV, then 0.04 - 0.07mg/kg IV at appropriate intervals. IM (if vein not accessible): Up to 3 - 4mg/kg IM, but not greater than 150mg/total dose. Observe effect in 2 - 3 min.

51 Pancuronium Bromide
Pancuronium

Nondepolarizing neuromuscular blocking agent; acts by competing for cholinergic receptors at the motor-end plate.

skeletal muscle weakness, paralysis, salivation, rash, severe allergic reactions

IV

Individualize dose. Initial: 0.04 - 0.1mg/kg IV. May use later incremental doses starting at 0.01mg/kg. Skeletal Muscle Relaxation For Endotracheal Intubation: 0.06 - 0.1mg/kg bolus.

OTHER MISCELLANEOUS DRUGS

52 Pentobarbital
(barbiturate - insomnia/anti-seizure)
Nembutal

Barbiturate; CNS depressant. Depresses sensory cortex, decreases motor activity, alters cerebellar function, and produces drowsiness, sedation, and hypnosis.

somnolence, agitation, hypoventilation, bradycardia, N/V, headache

IM, IV

Individualize dose. Consider age, weight, and condition. IM: Usual: 150 - 200mg (max 5mL/inj.) as a single deep inj. IV: Inject slowly (max 50mg/min.). Monitor closely.

53 Haloperidol
(anti-psychotic)
Haldol

Butyrophenone; mechanism not fully established. Haloperidol is a typical butyrophenone type antipsychotic that exhibits high affinity dopamine D2 receptor antagonism and slow receptor dissociation kinetics. The drug binds preferentially to D2 and Alpha 1 receptors at low dose (ED50 = 0.13 and 0.42 mg/kg, respectively), and 5-HT2 receptors at a higher dose (ED50 = 2.6 mg/kg). Given that antagonism of D2 receptors is more beneficial on the positive symptoms of schizophrenia and 5-HT2 receptors on the negative symptoms, this characteristic underlies haloperidol's greater effect on delusions, hallucinations and other manifestations of psychosis.

Extrapyramidal symptoms - TD, dystonia; EKG changes, ventricular arrhythmias, tachycardia, hypotension, HTN

PO, IM

Individualize dose. (PO) Initial: Moderate Symptoms/Elderly/Debilitated: 0.5 - 2mg bid or tid. Severe Symptoms/Chronic/Resistant: 3 - 5mg bid or tid. Doses up to 100mg/day may be needed to achieve optimal response. Doses >100mg/day have been used for severe resistant patients, but safety with prolonged use has not been demonstrated. (IM) 2 - 5mg IM for prompt control of acute agitation with moderately severe or very severe symptoms. May give subsequent doses as often as every hour, although 4 to 8 hr. intervals may be satisfactory, depending on response.

54 Neostigmine Bromide
(used to treat Myasthenia Gravis)
Prostigmin

Cholinesterase inhibitor - Anticholinesterase agent; Inhibits the hydrolysis of acetylcholine by competing with acetylcholine for attachment to acetylcholinesterase. At sites of cholinergic transmission it enhances cholinergic action by facilitating the transmission of impulses across the neuromuscular junction.

Salivation, bowel cramps, diarrhea, anaphylaxis, dizziness, convulsions, cardiac arrhythmias, respiratory depression

PO

Individualize dose. Range: 15 - 375mg/day. May exceed 375mg/day, but possibility of cholinergic crisis must be recognized. Average: 150mg (10 tabs.) over 24 hrs. Give larger portions of total daily dose when more prone to fatigue (e.g. afternoon, mealtimes, etc.).

55 Furosemide
(diuretic)
Lasix

Loop diuretic; primarily inhibits the reabsorption of Na^+ and Cl^- in the Loop of Henle.

pancreatitis, jaundice, anorexia. diarrhea, N/V, photosensitivity, fever, dizziness aplastic anemia, eosinophilia

PO, IV

Individualize dose. (PO) Edema: Initial: 20 - 80mg as a single dose. Titrate: May repeat the same dose if needed, or increase dose by 20mg or 40mg; give dose no sooner than 6 - 8 hrs. after the previous dose until desired effect has been obtained.
(Inj.) Edema: Initial: 20 - 40mg

as a single dose IV. Give IV dose slowly (1 - 2 min). Titrate: May repeat the same dose if needed, or increase by 20mg not sooner than 2 hrs. after the previous dose. Give individually determined single dose qd or bid. Acute Pulmonary Edema: Initial: 40mg IV slowly (over 1 - 2 min.). Titrate: May increase to 80mg IV slowly (over 1 - 2 min.) if satisfactory response does not occur within 1 hr.

56 Warfarin Sodium *(anticoagulant)* Coumadin	Vitamin K-dependent coagulation factor inhibitor; thought to interfere with clotting factor synthesis by inhibition of the C1 subunit reductase enzyme complex of the vitamin K epoxide, thereby reducing the regeneration of vitamin K1 epoxide.	hemorrhage, necrosis of the skin and other tissues, systemic atheroemboli, cholesterol microemboli, hypersensitivity, tracheal/tracheobronchial calcifications IV, PO	Individualize dose and duration of therapy. Adjust dose based on INR and condition being treated. Coumadin IV dose is the same as PO dose. Initial: 2 - 5mg qd. Maint: 2 - 10mg qd.
57 Naloxone *(reverses the effects of narcotic drugs)* Narcan	Opioid antagonist; prevents or reverses effects of opioids - including respiratory depression, sedation, and hypotension by competing for the mu, kappa, and sigma opiate receptor sites in the CNS. Greatest affinity is for the mu receptor	HTN, IV, IM, SQ hypotension, ventricular tachycardia and fibrillation, dyspnea, pulmonary edema, cardiac arrest	Opioid Overdose: Initial: 0.4 - 2mg IV. If desired response not obtained, may repeat at 2 - 3 min. intervals up to 10mg. Administer IM/SQ if IV route not available. Post-Operative Opioid - Induced Depression: Initial: 0.1 - 0.2mg IV at 2 - 3 min. intervals to the desired degree of reversal. May repeat doses within 1 - 2 hr. intervals depending on the amount, type, and time interval since last administration of opioid. Supplemental IM doses produce longer lasting effect.
58.Budesonide/ Formoterol Fumerate Symbicort	Budesonide: Corticosteroid; shown to have inhibitory activities on multiple cell types and mediators involved in allergic and nonallergic mediated inflammation. Formoterol: LABA; attributable to stimulation of intracellular adenyl cyclase that catalyzes the conversion of ATP to cAMP. Increased cAMP levels cause relaxation of bronchial smooth muscle and inhibits the release of mediators of immediate hypersensitivity from cells - especially mast cells.	nasopharyngitis, MDI headache, upper respiratory tract infection, pharyngolaryngeal pain, sinusitis, influenza, bronchitis	Asthma: 2 puffs bid (am and pm, approximately q 12hr.). Initial: Based on severity. 80/4.5 mcg/puff, 2 puffs bid. If not responding after 1 – 2 weeks of therapy with 80/4.5 mcg, then replace with 160/4.5 mcg/puff, 2 puffs bid for better asthma control. COPD: 160/4.5 mcg/puff, 2 puffs bid.

Bibliography

Alberts, Bruce, et. al. *Molecular Biology of the Cell.* 4th ed. New York: Garland Science, 2002.

Beachey, Will. *Respiratory Care Anatomy and Physiology.* 2nd ed. St. Louis: Mosby Elsevier, 2007.

Boron, Walter F., and Emile L. Boulpaep. *Medical Physiology.* Philadelphia: Elsevier Saunders, 2005.

Cairo, J.M., *Pilbeam's Mechanical Ventilation.* 5th ed. St. Louis: Elsevier Mosby, 2012.

Green Jr., Robert J. *Emphysema and Chronic Obstructive Pulmonary Disease.* San Diego: Aventine Press, 2005.

Kacmarek, Robert M., James K. Stoller, and Albert J. Heuer. *Egan's Fundamentals of Respiratory Care.* 10th ed. St. Louis: Elsevier, 2013.

Owens, William. *The Ventilator Book.* First Draught Press, 2012.

PDR Staff, *Physician's Desk Reference.* 71st ed. Montvale: PDR Network, 2016.

Stryer, Lubert. *Biochemistry.* 4th ed. New York: W.H. Freeman and Company, 1995.

West, John B. *Pulmonary Pathophysiology: The Essentials.* 6th ed. Philadelphia: Lippincott, Williams, and Wilkins, 2003.

Index